Controversies in Oral and Maxillofacial Surgery

Editors

LUIS G. VEGA
DANIEL J. MEARA

ORAL AND MAXILLOFACIAL SURGERY CLINICS OF NORTH AMERICA

www.oralmaxsurgery.theclinics.com

Consulting Editor
RICHARD H. HAUG

November 2017 • Volume 29 • Number 4

ELSEVIER

1600 John F. Kennedy Boulevard • Suite 1800 • Philadelphia, Pennsylvania, 19103-2899

http://www.oralmaxsurgery.theclinics.com

ORAL AND MAXILLOFACIAL SURGERY CLINICS OF NORTH AMERICA Volume 29, Number 4
November 2017 ISSN 1042-3699, ISBN-13: 978-0-323-54895-3

Editor: John Vassallo; j.vassallo@elsevier.com
Developmental Editor: Colleen Dietzler

Oral and Maxillofacial Surgery Clinics of North America (ISSN 1042-3699) is published quarterly by Elsevier Inc., 360 Park Avenue South, New York, NY 10010-1710. Months of issue are February, May, August, and November. Business and Editorial Offices: 1600 John F. Kennedy Blvd., Suite 1800, Philadelphia, PA 19103-2899. Periodicals postage paid at New York, NY and additional mailing offices. Subscription prices are $385.00 per year for US individuals, $653.00 per year for US institutions, $100.00 per year for US students and residents, $455.00 per year for Canadian individuals, $783.00 per year for Canadian institutions, $520.00 per year for international individuals, $783.00 per year for international institutions and $235.00 per year for Canadian and foreign students/residents. To receive student/resident rate, orders must be accompanied by name or affiliated institution, date of term, and the *signature* of program/residency coordinator on institution letterhead. Orders will be billed at individual rate until proof of status is received. Foreign air speed delivery is included in all *Clinics* subscription prices. All prices are subject to change without notice. **POSTMASTER:** Send address changes to *Oral and Maxillofacial Surgery Clinics of North America,* Elsevier Periodicals **Customer Service, 11830 Westline Industrial Drive, St. Louis, MO 63146. Tel: 1-800-654-2452 (U.S. and Canada); 314-447-8871 (outside U.S. and Canada). Fax: 314-447-8029. E-mail: journals customerservice-usa@elsevier.com (for print support); journalsonlinesupport-usa@elsevier.com (for online support).**

Reprints. For copies of 100 or more, of articles in this publication, please contact the Commercial Reprints Department, Elsevier Inc., 360 Park Avenue South, New York, NY 10010-1710. Tel.: 212-633-3874; Fax: 212-633-3820; Email: reprints@elsevier.com.

Oral and Maxillofacial Surgery Clinics of North America is covered in *MEDLINE/PubMed* (*Index Medicus*), *Science Citation Index Expanded* (*SciSearch®*), *Journal Citation Reports/Science Edition*, and *Current Contents®/Clinical Medicine*.

Contributors

CONSULTING EDITOR

RICHARD H. HAUG, DDS
Professor and Chief, Oral Maxillofacial Surgery,
Carolinas Medical Center, Charlotte, North
Carolina

EDITORS

LUIS G. VEGA, DDS
Associate Professor, Oral and Maxillofacial
Residency Program Director, Department of
Oral and Maxillofacial Surgery, Vanderbilt
University Medical Center, Nashville,
Tennessee

DANIEL J. MEARA, DMD, MS, MD, FACS
Chair, Department of Oral and Maxillofacial
Surgery & Hospital Dentistry, Christiana Care
Health System, Wilmington, Delaware

AUTHORS

TARA L. AGHALOO, DDS, MD, PhD
Professor, Section of Oral and Maxillofacial
Surgery, Assistant Dean for Clinical Research,
UCLA School of Dentistry, Los Angeles,
California

SCOTT B. BOYD, DDS, PhD
Professor, Oral and Maxillofacial Surgery,
Retired, Vanderbilt University School of
Medicine, Nashville, Tennessee

BRANDO DELGADO, BS
Dental Student, UCLA School of Dentistry,
Los Angeles, California

CAROLYN C. DICUS BROOKES, DMD, MD
Assistant Professor, Interim Division Chief,
Division of Oral and Maxillofacial Surgery,
Froedtert & the Medical College of Wisconsin,
Milwaukee, Wisconsin

ROBERT DIECIDUE, DMD, MD, MBA, MPH
Professor, Department of Oral and
Maxillofacial Surgery, Sidney Kimmel Medical
College, Thomas Jefferson University,
Philadelphia, Pennsylvania

ADAM P. FAGIN, DMD, MD
Resident, Oral and Maxillofacial Surgery,
Department of Oral and Maxillofacial Surgery,
Oregon Health & Science University, Portland,
Oregon

LIONEL GOLD, DDS
Professor, Department of Oral and
Maxillofacial Surgery, Sidney Kimmel Medical
College, Thomas Jefferson University,
Philadelphia, Pennsylvania

MICHAEL S. JASKOLKA, DDS, MD, FACS
Director, New Hanover Regional Medical
Center Children's Surgery, New Hanover
Regional Medical Center Cleft and Craniofacial
Program, Adjunct Assistant Professor,
Department of Surgery, School of Medicine,
Department of Oral and Maxillofacial Surgery,
UNC School of Dentistry, Chapel Hill, North
Carolina

LEWIS C. JONES, DMD, MD
Assistant Professor, Oral and Maxillofacial
Surgery, Department of Surgical and Hospital
Dentistry, University of Louisville, Louisville,
Kentucky

BRETT J. KING, DDS
Assistant Professor, Division of Plastic and Reconstructive Surgery, Departments of Oral and Maxillofacial Surgery and General Surgery, LSU Health New Orleans, New Orleans, Louisiana

ANTONIA KOLOKYTHAS, DDS, MS, FACS
Associate Professor, Chair, Program Director, Department of Oral and Maxillofacial Surgery, University of Rochester Strong Memorial Hospital, Eastman Institute for Oral Health, Rochester, New York

DEEPAK G. KRISHNAN, DDS, FACS
Associate Professor of Surgery, Residency Program Director, Division of Oral Maxillofacial Surgery, Department of Surgery, University of Cincinnati, Cincinnati, Ohio

ADAM LEVINE, MD
Professor, Departments of Anesthesiology, Perioperative and Pain Medicine, Pharmacological Sciences, and Otolaryngology, Vice Chair of Education, Residency Program Director, Mount Sinai Health System, Icahn School of Medicine at Mount Sinai, New York, New York

AARON LIDDELL, DMD, MD, FACS
Diplomate, Fellow, American Board of Medical Specialties, Colorado Oral and Maxillofacial Surgery, Denver, Colorado

MARTIN MARDIROSIAN, DDS, MD
Chief Resident, Section of Oral and Maxillofacial Surgery, UCLA School of Dentistry, Los Angeles, California

DANIEL J. MEARA, DMD, MS, MD, FACS
Chair, Department of Oral and Maxillofacial Surgery & Hospital Dentistry, Christiana Care Health System, Wilmington, Delaware

ZACHARY S. PEACOCK, DMD, MD, FACS
Assistant Professor, Department of Oral and Maxillofacial Surgery, Massachusetts General Hospital, Harvard School of Dental Medicine, Boston, Massachusetts

DANIEL E. PEREZ, DDS
Associate Professor, Oral and Maxillofacial Surgery, The University of Texas Health Science Center at San Antonio, San Antonio, Texas

DANIEL PETRISOR, DMD, MD, FACS
Assistant Professor, Oral and Maxillofacial Surgery, Director, Head and Neck Oncologic and Microvascular Reconstructive Surgery, Department of Oral and Maxillofacial Surgery, Oregon Health & Science University, Portland, Oregon

ARMANDO RETANA, DDS, MD
Associate Oral and Maxillofacial Surgeon, Associate Cosmetic Surgeon, Capital Center for Oral and Maxillofacial Surgery, Washington, DC

DANIEL TAUB, DDS, MD
Associate Professor, Department of Oral and Maxillofacial Surgery, Sidney Kimmel Medical College, Thomas Jefferson University, Philadelphia, Pennsylvania

JOHN S. VORRASI, DDS
Assistant Professor, Department of Oral and Maxillofacial Surgery, University of Rochester Strong Memorial Hospital, Eastman Institute for Oral Health, Rochester, New York

ANDREW YAMPOLSKY, DDS, MD
Instructor, Department of Oral and Maxillofacial Surgery, Sidney Kimmel Medical College, Thomas Jefferson University, Philadelphia, Pennsylvania

JACOB G. YETZER, DDS, MD
Private Practice, Head and Neck Surgery, Nebraska Oral and Facial Surgery, Lincoln, Nebraska; Assistant Professor, Department of Surgery, Creighton University School of Medicine, Omaha, Nebraska

Contents

> Dentoalveolar surgeries are among the more common procedures performed by oral maxillofacial surgeons. It is only natural that there are several controversies associated with many aspects of this type of surgery. Although good scientific evidence is the basis of most oral maxillofacial procedures, some of what is accepted as common wisdom may not meet strict guidelines of evidence-based practice. This article explores some controversies that are relevant to the current practice of dentoalveolar surgery.

> Craniomaxillofacial trauma management has continued to improve and evolve as a result of advances in technology and scientific inquiry. Controversies exist where there is little evidence-based literature to guide treatment in frontal sinus management, rigid versus absorbable fixation, open versus closed treatment of mandibular condyle fractures, extraction of teeth in the line of fracture, optimal timing for repair of mandible fractures, antibiotic use for facial wounds and fractures, and reconstructive materials in orbital fracture reconstruction. This article reviews current literature to resolve some of the controversies, and to improve patient care by reducing variability and uncertainty in the optimal management of patients with facial trauma.

> Traditional reconstruction of the head and neck has significantly evolved over the past 20 to 30 years with advances in microvascular surgery, biologic materials such as bone morphogenic protein, and dental implant predictability. Earlier and more definitive reconstruction can now be achieved with combining therapies, allowing patients immediate restoration of function and improved cosmetics. Antiresorptive medications, such as denosumab and bisphosphonates, have complicated bony reconstruction treatments with altered biology and less-predictable results. Virtual surgical planning is a major advancement for reconstruction pretreatment planning and designing of intraoperative tools to expedite the operation and achieve more predictable results.

> The effectiveness and reliability of microvascular reconstruction for large defects in the head and neck is no longer disputed; however, many controversies still persist in the ideal perioperative management of patients undergoing free tissue transfer. The optimal method of postoperative monitoring, the use of vasoconstrictors in the perioperative period, and the use of anticoagulants in the postoperative period remain topics of debate. This article offers recommendations on each of these controversies based on a review of the current literature.

Controversy has accompanied orthognathic surgery since its adaptation for the correction of dentofacial deformities. With the development of less invasive and less morbid osteotomy designs, questions regarding overall osteotomy stability have abounded. The transition from prolonged intermaxillary fixation and wire osteosynthesis to rigid internal fixation has spurred questions regarding the most effective fixation technique, and challenged previously accepted hierarchies of stability. These questions represent only the surface of a sea of debate and discussion, as measures have been taken to optimize patient outcome, minimize patient morbidity, and maximize operating room productivity.

Facial cosmetic surgery techniques are constantly updated to meet the expectations of patients who demand less invasive procedures and less recovery time. Current trends in lower eyelid surgery call for periorbital fat repositioning instead of excision of fat. Controversies still exist in chin augmentations regarding osseous genioplasty versus alloplastic chin implant. The benefits, disadvantages, and considerations of these procedures are discussed.

 Video content accompanies this article at http://www.oralmaxsurgery.theclinics.com.

Metopic craniosynostosis is being reported with an increasing incidence and is now the second most common type of isolated suture craniosynostosis. Numerous areas of controversy exist in the workup and management, including defining the diagnosis in the less severe phenotype, the association with neurodevelopmental delay, the impact of surgical treatment, and the applicability of various techniques and their timing on outcomes.

The management and treatment of odontogenic infection, and its frequent extension into the head and neck, remains an important section of oral and maxillofacial surgical practice. This area of maxillofacial expertise is widely recognized by the medical community and an essential component to the hospital referral system. Although the general principles of infection management have not changed, there have been modifications in the timing of treatment sequences and treatment techniques. These modifications are influenced by the development of diagnostic methods and advances in bacterial genetics and antibiotic usage. This article reviews treatment considerations and controversies surrounding this subject.

Several benign pathologic entities that are commonly encountered by the oral and maxillofacial surgeon remain controversial. From etiology to treatment, no consensus exists in the literature regarding the best treatment of benign lesions, such as the keratocystic odontogenic tumor, giant cell lesion, or ameloblastoma. Given the need for often-morbid treatment to prevent recurrence of these lesions, multiple less-invasive treatments exist in the literature for each entity with little agreement. As the molecular and genomic pathogenesis of these lesions are better understood, directed treatments will hopefully lessen the contention in management.

Imaging studies are essential components of tumor diagnosis, staging, assessing tumor response to neoadjuvant and adjuvant therapies, and postoperative surveillance on completion of definitive treatment. Treatment of early-stage clinically node-negative oral cavity squamous cell carcinoma is controversial. Approximately 3% of all head and neck tumors arise within the parotid gland and most often within the superficial lobe, lateral to the facial nerve; approximately 80% are benign and most are pleomorphic adenoma. In patients with dry eyes failing multiple other treatment modalities and facing ongoing pain and loss of vision, microvascular transplant of the submandibular gland is a viable option.

Obstructive sleep apnea (OSA) is a common chronic disease characterized by repetitive pharyngeal collapse during sleep. OSA is associated with cardiovascular disease and increased mortality, among other issues. Continuous positive airway pressure (CPAP) is considered first-line therapy for OSA, but is not always tolerated. Both nonsurgical and surgical alternative management strategies are available for the CPAP-intolerant patient. This article explores controversies surrounding airway evaluation, definition of successful treatment, and surgical management of the CPAP-intolerant patient with moderate to severe OSA. Controversies specific to maxillomandibular advancement also are discussed.

The future of office-based anesthesia for oral and maxillofacial surgery is at risk. Oral and maxillofacial surgeons have been on the forefront of providing safe and effective outpatient anesthesia for decades. Recent changes in Medicare policies have had, and will continue to have, a significant effect on the training of oral and maxillofacial surgery residents regarding anesthesia. The outcome of these changes can have a major effect on the specialty of oral and maxillofacial surgery and a cornerstone of the profession.

Dental implants are a mainstream treatment protocol to replace missing teeth. Patient and clinician demands have led to shorter length and narrower diameter implants, immediately placed implants into infected sites, and the use of implants in children. This article reviews some of the controversial topics in implant dentistry, and presents the evidence that supports and challenges these newer techniques. Because long-term studies are often not available, especially for implants in infected sites, mini implants, and implants in the growing patient, the field continues to evolve.

ORAL AND MAXILLOFACIAL SURGERY CLINICS OF NORTH AMERICA

ISSUE OF RELATED INTEREST

Atlas of the Oral & Maxillofacial Surgery Clinics, March 2017 (Vol. 25, No. 1)
Advances in the Management of Mandibular Condylar Fractures
Martin B. Steed, *Editor*
Available at: www.oralmaxsurgeryatlas.theclinics.com

THE CLINICS ARE NOW AVAILABLE ONLINE!
Access your subscription at:
www.theclinics.com

Preface

Controversies in Oral and Maxillofacial Surgery

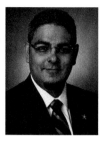
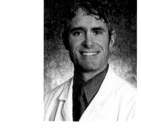

Luis G. Vega, DDS   Daniel J. Meara, DMD, MS, MD, FACS
Editors

The most damaging phrase in the language is:
We've always done it this way.
—*Grace Hopper*

It is our great pleasure to present the most current issue of the *Oral and Maxillofacial Surgery Clinics of North America* dedicated to "Controversies in Oral and Maxillofacial Surgery."

Since the inception of our specialty, controversy has been both a fortunate and an unfortunate part of our daily professional life. The influence of controversy reaches our surgical decision making and shapes our training and scope of practice. Controversy has been defined as a prolonged state of public debate involving conflicting views or opinions. In medicine, time, research, and technology attempt to address and extinguish controversy. Inevitably, however, new controversies arise from the ashes in a seemingly never-ending chain. Controversies in oral and maxillofacial surgery are abundant as some old arguments and opinions have withstood the test of time. On the other hand, new controversies are created regularly from peer-review journals, scientific meetings, and individuals who challenge the status quo.

In this issue, we attempt to address the predominant controversies in oral and maxillofacial surgery pertaining to a variety of topics as presented by a young generation of enthusiastic surgeons who have gracefully accepted our challenge to present the greatest controversies they face in their clinical practice each day. Each of these surgeons was granted the freedom to explore what they thought were the most critical controversies they currently face. We are forever thankful for their time and efforts, and we hope that the readers enjoy their work as much as we have. We would like to extend our thanks to the Elsevier editorial team for their patience and support throughout this project. We would also like to thank our families for their unconditional love and support. Last, much gratitude and thanks are due to our past, present, and future residents, who are always pushing us forward. This issue of the *Oral and Maxillofacial Surgery Clinics of North America* is for you.

Luis G. Vega, DDS
Department of Oral and Maxillofacial Surgery
Vanderbilt University Medical Center
1211 21st Avenue South. Suite 332
Nashville, TN 37212, USA

Daniel J. Meara, DMD, MS, MD, FACS
Department of Oral and Maxillofacial Surgery &
Hospital Dentistry
Christiana Care Health System
501 West 14th Street, Suite 2W40
Wilmington, DE 19801, USA

E-mail addresses:
luis.vega@vanderbilt.edu (L.G. Vega)
DMeara@ChristianaCare.org (D.J. Meara)

Oral Maxillofacial Surg Clin N Am 29 (2017) ix
http://dx.doi.org/10.1016/j.coms.2017.09.001
1042-3699/17/© 2017 Published by Elsevier Inc.

Controversies in Dentoalveolar and Preprosthetic Surgery

Deepak G. Krishnan, DDS, FACS

KEYWORDS

- Controversies in dentoalveolar surgery • Third molars and periodontal disease
- Drug holiday in ONJ • Dental clearance for sepsis • Bone grafting the extraction socket

KEY POINTS

- Identify scientific evidence and current consensus in evidence-based practice of dentoalveolar surgery.
- Explore the scientific evidence behind the fact that asymptomatic third molars can be responsible for progression of future periodontal disease.
- Clarify the rationale behind drug holidays in ONJ.
- Investigate the claim that dental disease can cause systemic disease.
- Inspect the current evidence and rationale for bone grafting extraction sockets.

INTRODUCTION

Given that dentoalveolar surgeries are the most common procedures undertaken by oral maxillofacial surgeons, there are several controversies associated with many of its related aspects. Although good scientific evidence is the basis of most things oral maxillofacial surgeons do, some of what is accepted as common wisdom may not meet strict guidelines of evidence-based practice. This article explores some controversies that are relevant to the current practice of dentoalveolar surgery.

THE THIRD MOLAR DEBATE: THE ASYMPTOMATIC THIRD MOLAR CAN CAUSE PERIODONTAL DISEASE IN THE FUTURE

It is only apt that we begin this article with the debate that seems to most consume the specialty: the third molar (M3) and the indications for removing the asymptomatic tooth.

A recent update on the prevalence of periodontitis in the US adult population using combined data from the 2009 to 2010 and 2011 to 2012 cycles of the National Health and Nutrition Examination Survey estimates that in 2009 to 2012, a total of 46% of US adults representing 64.7 million people had periodontitis with 8.9% having severe periodontitis.[1] Most epidemiologic studies investigating periodontal disease tend to define periodontitis by combinations of clinical attachment loss and periodontal probing depth (PD) from six sites per tooth on all teeth, except M3. Therein lays the challenge when one attempts to investigate the relationship of partially impacted M3 on periodontal disease.

Seeking Clarity: Is There a Relationship Between Partially Impacted Third Molars and Progression of Periodontal Disease?

Steed recently presented an elegant synopsis of the current evidence on the indications for removal of M3.[2] He summarized that "evidence based clinical data from prospective investigations show that an asymptomatic third molar does not necessarily reflect an absence of disease."

Division of Oral Maxillofacial Surgery, Department of Surgery, University of Cincinnati, Cincinnati, OH 45219, USA
E-mail address: deepak.krishnan@uc.edu

Oral Maxillofacial Surg Clin N Am 29 (2017) 383–390
http://dx.doi.org/10.1016/j.coms.2017.06.001
1042-3699/17/© 2017 Elsevier Inc. All rights reserved.

Strong scientific evidence suggests that significant periodontal pathology exists in the area of M3 and second molar (M2), especially when M3 was visible in the oral cavity.[3] Partially impacted M3 is associated with higher rates of periodontal disease, especially at M2 sites, even in asymptomatic patients. In fact, M3 may be the site of initial presentation of periodontal disease in many patients.

Research on periodontal pathogens in erupting or partially impacted M3 of otherwise periodontally healthy patients suggests that these sites harbor species of bacteria that cause severe pericoronal infections. Species, such as *Porphyromonas gingivalis*, was positive even in 20% of the symptom-free cases. Studies that have looked at changes in periodontal status of mandibular M2 after surgical extraction of adjacent M3 suggest that removal of partially erupted M3 can improve periodontal health in younger patients.[4] Retained partially impacted M3s are associated with more severe periodontal disease in older patients.

Periodontal Disease Associated with the Partially Impacted Third Molar

Regardless of whether patients exhibit symptoms, there is significant evidence that partially impacted M3 is associated with increased PD around these teeth and distal to the M2. This increased PD is associated with attachment loss in nearly all patients, even young healthy adults with good periodontal health. However, there are several studies that suggest that if the PD is greater than 5 mm, there are elevated levels of inflammatory mediators present in the subgingival samples from these sites.

Studies of microbial colonization of partially erupted follicles show that these are populated by periodontal pathogens even in healthy subjects without evidence of periodontal disease. Numerous studies have implicated the same bacterial species found around a partially impacted tooth in local colonization leading to pericoronitis, upper respiratory tract infections, and possibly systemic invasion.

There is credible evidence that shows that the red and green bacterial complexes seen around M3s visible in the oral cavity may be responsible for initiation of periodontal disease in young healthy adults. These bacterial species have been detected at M2/M3 sites in otherwise periodontally healthy patients in larger quantities if the tooth is partially exposed in the mouth or if the PD is deeper. The presence of these complexes heralds a higher risk of progression of periodontal disease at these sites. Furthermore, M3 periodontal pathology is a significant risk factor during pregnancy for progression of generalized periodontal disease. In studies that have investigated periodontal pathology in older patients, the presence of partially erupted M3 was associated with more severe periodontal disease.

The elimination of a partially impacted M3 eliminates a focus for periodontal pathogens at these sites. An improvement of periodontal health distal to M2 in particular and the posterior quadrant in general has been suggested by researchers who have looked at this following removal of M3 in young periodontally healthy patients. They have found a positive effect on generalized periodontal health and demonstrated gain in distal M2 alveolar bone following extraction of M3.

A Consensus?

Although the term "partial impaction" or "partial visibility" in the oral cavity may be applied to any M3, maxillary or mandibular, a thorough review of the literature that pertains to scientific studies on the subject reveals that most investigations focused on the mandibular M3 and extrapolated that data to the maxillary M3. However, clinicians are aware and accept that the far reaches of the oral cavity, whether in the maxilla or the mandible, remain limited in access to cleansing and tend to attract more plaque and debris deposition.

Dodson[5] developed a practical guide for clinicians to establish the presence or absence of disease in light of presence or absence of symptoms. The system exposes that the absence of symptoms does not necessarily mean the absence of disease.

Partial impaction or partial visibility is associated with increased PD around M3. White and coworkers[6] found that this increased PD and associated loss of attachment in nearly all patients. In a related study,[7] they found that a cross-sectional analysis of data from healthy young adults with periodontal pathology was detected more frequently on asymptomatic M3s compared with first/second molar teeth; caries experience was detected more frequently on first/second molars compared with M3s. Their extensive work spanning a wide spectrum of clinical scenarios led to findings that the prevalence of periodontal pathology with erupting M3s or a visible M3 was almost three times greater compared with M3s below the occlusal plane.[8] Furthermore, there was significantly elevated levels of inflammatory mediators present if the PD around these M3s was greater than 5 mm. While looking for microbial complexes in the subgingival plaque samples in the M3 areas, Blakey and coworkers found that if M3s were at or above the occlusal plane and vertical or distal in position, targeted microorganisms were as likely to be detected at levels of equal to or greater than 10^4 compared with M3s below the occlusal plane and mesioangular or horizontal in position. This was true whether a PD equal to or greater than 5 mm was found in the M3 region or not.[9] Even in the groups of essentially healthy young people without periodontitis studied, the clinical findings of increased periodontal PDs and loss of periodontal attachment compounded by detection of presence of periodontal pathogens suggest that clinical and microbial changes in periodontitis may begin at the M3 sites.

Data from White's studies looking at inflammatory mediators at the sites of asymptomatic M3s suggest that patients who have PD equal to or greater than 5 mm in the M3 region, have increased levels of biochemical mediators of inflammation compared with patients with PD less than 5 mm.[10] Additionally, by looking at clinical measures (PD) and biochemical markers (interleukin-1β) of periodontal disease, they conclude with the concept that early periodontitis in young adults is initiated in the M3 region and these sites are associated with increases in key inflammatory mediators even in the absence of clinical symptoms. They suggest that sampling of M3 sites for inflammatory markers may be a useful tool in predicting advancement of periodontitis.

Assay analyses of gingival crevicular fluid inflammatory mediators as indicators of the degree of oral inflammation have proven that chronic oral inflammation begins at the sites of M3s with increased PDs and leads to progression of periodontal disease. In addition, it has been shown that at least one visible M3 makes periodontal outcomes significantly worse during pregnancy.

Colonization of partially erupted follicles around M3s occurs by periodontal pathogens even in healthy subjects without evidence of periodontal disease.[11] Teeth follicles, especially in the partially impacted, partially visible or erupting M3s, have been reported to harbor pathogens that contribute to local and upper respiratory tract infections.[12] Rajasuo's work[11] isolating periodontal pathogens in the partially impacted M3s of periodontally healthy subjects showed that the species of bacteria isolated in 94% of acute pericoronitis was *Prevotella intermedia*. They also found a significant collection of other periodontopathogens residing lavishly in the M3 sites especially when the tooth was partially erupted in the mouth.

Partially impacted M3s may influence gingival health status because they influence the patient's ability to maintain proper hygiene at those sites. Laskin and colleagues concluded that removal of partially impacted M3s provided some benefit in terms of improved gingival health while evaluating plaque and gingival indices around M2, 6 weeks after M3.[13] They also reported that plaque and gingival indices were worse in the presence of an impacted M3 especially when there was no osseous wall present between an M2 and an M3.

A partially visible M3 was associated with 1.5 times the odds of PD of greater than 5 mm on the adjacent M2, while controlling for other factors associated with the presence of M3s and periodontal disease in a study assessing the association of periodontal pathology and a visible M3 in middle aged and older Americans.[14] The investigators of that study conclude that more severe periodontal conditions associated with visible M3s in these middle-aged and older adults indicates that M3s may continue to have a negative impact on periodontal health well into later life and called for more longitudinal studies to support their finding.

Montero and Mazzaglia investigated the effect of removing an impacted M3 on the periodontal status of M2.[4] Their investigation of 48 patients who underwent surgical removal of shallow or deeply impacted M3s 1 year later showed improved plaque and gingival indices in the regions and an actual gain in distal M2 alveolar bone. They found that their flap design does not influence PD or attachment level. However, the osteotomy design/extent affected attachment and the deeper the level of impaction, the higher the baseline probing and greater the change. A single operator standardized their study. The finding that removal of M3s significantly improved the periodontal status of the distal surfaces of the M2s was also found in studies reported by others.[15,16]

For more than half a millennium, clinicians have known about the negative impact of the partially impacted M3.[17] Astute clinicians have always placed common sense above all while making clinical decisions about removal of the asymptomatic partially impacted M3s. Over the period of several years, an overwhelming amount of scientific evidence has accrued that convincingly suggests that biomarkers of inflammation are concentrated at the site of M3s even when there is no clinical evidence of disease. This combined with emerging evidence from longitudinal studies prompts the recommendation that the partially impacted M3 has a negative influence on the overall periodontal health of patients and they are indicated for removal.

DRUG HOLIDAY IN MEDICATION-RELATED OSTEONECROSIS OF THE JAWS: DOES CESSATION OF THE ANTIRESORPTIVE MEDICATION OF A PERIOD OF TIME DECREASE THE RISK OF MEDICATION-RELATED OSTEONECROSIS OF THE JAWS?

Medication-related osteonecrosis of the jaws (MRONJ) is a poorly understood condition that presents as necrotic exposed bone in the jaws of patients who have been exposed to certain medications that can affect bone turnover. Although it is known that such factors as minimal trauma during surgery and local and systemic variations can influence precipitation of occurrence of MRONJ following dentoalveolar procedures, there is some controversy as to whether cessation of the medication can actually be a logical step in the prevention of the condition.

The American Association of Oral and Maxillofacial Surgeons 2014 position paper on bisphosphonate-related osteonecrosis of the jaw mentions that the original position paper from 2009 recommended discontinuing oral bisphosphonates for 3 months before and 3 months after invasive dental surgery, systemic conditions permitting.[18] The updated guidelines emphasizes that there is "no evidence that interrupting bisphosphonate therapy alters the risk of ONJ..." The American Dental Association council for scientific affairs also looked at current evidence and revised their previous recommendation of a drug holiday. In 2011 the Food and Drug Administration produced a summary document on the long-term safety of bisphosphonate therapy for osteoporosis, and categorically stated that there are no data available to guide decisions regarding the initiation or duration of a drug holiday.[19]

The premise of the recommendation of drug cessation for a period of time may sound logical, but there is little actual evidence to support the idea when one examines bone physiology and the pharmacokinetics of antiresorptive medications. There is, however, the theoretic consideration that Damm and Jones proposed of a creative interdisciplinary patient care model that has the potential to reduce prevalence of MRONJ.[20] The authors present the idea that deposition of bisphosphonates is not uniform in the osteoclasts and osteocytes, and that a "full understanding of bone remodeling and the pharmacokinetics of nBP (aminobisphosphonates) allow for the modification of the antiresorptive therapy and the timing of the surgical procedure in a manner that minimizes the prevalence of osteonecrosis while at the same time continuing to protect the patient's skeleton from osteoporotic fracture." They describe how 50% of the antiresorptives in the serum undergo renal excretion and the major depot of the remaining drugs is the osteoclasts. These cells only have a lifespan of 2 weeks. Hence, they extrapolate that because most free serum drug would be low 2 months following the last administration, and the cellular depot would have been exhausted, a 2-month drug-free period should be adequate before an invasive surgical intervention. To the average practitioner this is an appealing theory, but in fact, there is a low level of evidence to support it.

Current Evidence

Most recently, the Japanese Study Group of Cooperative Dentistry with Medicine performed a multicenter retrospective study examining risk factors associated with MRONJ following tooth extractions in patients on oral bisphosphonate therapy, looking in particular at drug holidays and the intervention of attempting primary wound closure.[21] They found no evidence supporting the efficacy of a pre-extraction short-term drug holiday from oral bisphosphonates in reducing the risk of MRONJ.

The duration of administration of the antiresorptive has been identified as a risk factor in the development of the condition. There is no current evidence-based guideline that recommends drug holidays for patients who have been on these medications long term, whether oral or parenteral. In those patients who have been on an oral bisphosphonate for less than 4 years, drug holidays have been supported as a strategy to reduce the risk of development of MRONJ following a surgery. The 2-month holiday remains the current recommendation. Complete osseous healing is to be established before restarting the medication.

In patients who are on oral bisphosphonate therapy for high risk of osteoporosis, a period of drug holiday may be risky and may not necessarily provide any benefit. Thus in view of the lack of current evidence supporting the idea of a drug holiday, it is only prudent to suggest that clinicians consider individualizing the choice, duration, and length of a drug holiday for each patient. There is evidence to suggest that bone mineral density does significantly decrease proportional to the duration of the drug holiday. There are emerging data on using bone turnover markers to help guide resumption of treatment in real-life clinical setting.

There is not a body of evidence available yet regarding drug holidays in patients who have been on intravenous bisphosphonates. Intravenous drug doses tend to be higher and tend to accumulate in bone providing some residual antifracture reduction for several years following cessation of active treatment. Endocrinology literature makes mention of recommendation of mandatory 5- to 10-year drug holidays following intravenous bisphosphonate treatment.[22] This is based on fracture risk assessment and the pharmacokinetics of the bisphosphonate used.

There is also not adequate evidence available in regard to drug holidays in patients with established MRONJ (clinical stages 1, 2, or 3) to guide the clinician. The recommendation is to personalize a drug holiday in communication with the physician prescribing the medication and to make a risk versus benefit decision for the patient.

THE DENTAL CLEARANCE: DO ORAL INFECTIONS INCREASE SYSTEMIC MORBIDITY AND MORTALITY?

It is not unusual for hospital-based oral and maxillofacial surgeons to be consulted on patients admitted for a variety of reasons to rule out "dental sepsis" or obtain "dental clearance." These are often patients who are admitted with elevated white blood cell counts without a clear source of infection, presurgical admissions for cardiac procedures, in particular valvular repairs or pretransplant patients awaiting your "clearance."

Robert Koch famously suggested as a part of his focal theory of inflammation that the human mouth is a focus of inflammation as early as 1890s. Frank Billings gave a series of lectures at Stanford University in the beginning of the previous century that were recorded by Stanford University, stating that steps in treating systemic diseases included elimination of "focal infections" by extractions of teeth and removal of tonsils. By the 1920s, popular medical literature was suggesting that the standard of care for management of oral and systemic maladies begin with teeth extractions.

The tide has resurfaced recently with the linkage of oral health and systemic health with reports that maintaining healthy teeth and gums may reduce the risk for pneumonia and chronic obstructive pulmonary disease and teeth loss may be linked to memory loss. Most often, these studies are those that generate associations, and do not necessarily establish a cause-effect relationship and thus belong to the bottom of the evidence pyramid and can best be presented as background information when considered as scientific evidence.

Neiderman and Richards[23] attempted a meta-analysis within evidence-based dentistry, to answer the question, "do oral infections increase systemic morbidity or mortality?" They looked at the current status of the cause-effect relationship between oral infections and systemic disease in current literature. Examination of systematic reviews with meta-analysis identified six trials addressing pregnancy, seven addressing coronary heart disease/stroke, eight addressing diabetes, and one addressing pneumonia/chronic obstructive pulmonary disease. Their article makes the following summary statements:

- A systematic review appraising randomized controlled trials examining the effect of periodontal therapy on preterm low birth weight stated: "Results of this meta-analysis do not support the hypothesis that periodontal therapy reduces preterm birth and LBW [low birth weight] indices."
- A systematic review appraising randomized controlled trials testing the effect of periodontal therapy on glycemic control stated: "There is some evidence of improvement in metabolic control in people with diabetes, after treating periodontal disease." ("There are few studies available, and individually these lacked the power to detect a significant effect.")

The problem with digging deep into literature for pure scientific evidence is that one often is faced with the following dilemma. Although straightforward and clear-appearing data represent the current highest level of evidence, it often contradicts the appealing intuitive hypothesis that oral disease has an adverse effect on systemic health. The clinician often has to balance such information based on one's own clinical experiences that identify an association between oral and systemic diseases versus a handful of powerful systematic reviews.

Astute clinicians know that absence of evidence is not evidence of absence. However, reliance on lower levels of evidence can lead to false conclusions, and the persistence of these incorrect conclusions can continue long after definitive studies are published. There is the reality of practicing in a litigious society, with legal practices focusing on malpractice, which forces the clinician to believe that treatment of oral disease is clearly beneficial in and of itself. However, current evidence does not support oral treatment for the prevention of systemic morbidity or mortality.

Specific Clinical Indications for Dental Clearance

Transplant patient with dental disease

In patients awaiting organ and marrow transplants, extensive dental examination and treatment is a prerequisite. Most patients are required to have comprehensive dental care before the transplant to alleviate the risk of infection from the oral cavity adversely affecting the posttransplant outcome. Sometimes, the dental treatment creates a delay in the patient receiving the much needed transplant. The evidence supporting this recommendation is weak and the necessity for such pretransplant treatments has been questioned. In a retrospective study in Germany, dental status was assessed in patients who received lung transplantation and evaluated for 3 years posttransplant for infectious foci.[24] Their results did not show any complications associated with dental infections in their patients. They questioned the need for these extensive dental interventions including extractions before lung transplants.

Such data are not as forthcoming in kidney or liver transplant patients and the chances of ever conducting an institutional review board–approved double-blinded prospective clinical trial are slim to none. Until we have a body of evidence to contradict the common practice, we continue to abide by the practice of pretransplant dental treatment.

Prosthetic valves and prophylaxis as it relates to dentoalveolar procedures

The risk of prosthetic valve endocarditis from dental foci has prompted the American Heart Association to present guidelines and recommendations as it pertains to these patients in the preoperative and postoperative phases of management. It is accepted that only an extremely small number of cases of infectious endocarditis (IE) might be prevented by antibiotic prophylaxis for dental procedures even if such prophylactic therapy were 100% effective. Despite that, the current guidelines suggest the following: (1) IE prophylaxis for dental procedures should be recommended only for patients with underlying cardiac conditions associated with the highest risk of adverse outcome from IE; (2) for patients with these underlying cardiac conditions, prophylaxis is recommended for all dental procedures that involve manipulation of gingival tissue or the periapical region of teeth or perforation of the oral mucosa; and (3) prophylaxis is not recommended based solely on an increased lifetime risk of acquisition of IE.

Although multiple studies have questioned the validity of the data that support these recommendations, until we have a multinational randomized controlled clinical trial, we may not be able to define the role of dental clearances before valvular repair and the role of antibiotic prophylaxis to prevent IE.[25]

Brain abscess from dental infection?

Septic cavernous sinus thrombosis (CST) and brain abscesses have been reported with an odontogenic source being implicated as the primary source of infection. The contiguous spread of infection from maxillary teeth to the cavernous sinuses through the pterygoid plexus is theoretically possible. Thus, hematogenous spread of septic emboli to the cavernous sinus or brain would also be possible. In the preantibiotic era, septic CST was almost always fatal, with mortality rates approaching 100%. Currently, the mortality rate remains in the range of 20% to 30%. Of those who survive, more than 50% have residual deficits, such as blindness, cranial nerve palsy, oculomotor weakness, and pituitary insufficiency.

To attribute septic CST to an odontogenic cause, at least three of the four have to be true: (1) confirm the diagnosis of CST by clinical presentation and imaging, (2) precisely match the isolated pathogens from intracranial/extracranial sites with identical DNA homology, (3) document a plausible pathway of hematogenous spread of infection, and (4) show anatomic evidence of contiguous spread of infection.

Brain abscesses have an incidence of about 1% to 8.5%. Brain abscess secondary to dental infection will continue to be a diagnosis of exclusion. Evidence-based studies with matching bacterial serotypes and identical DNA homology, an obvious contiguous focus, and a documented pathway replace anecdotal reports.[26]

ALVEOLAR RIDGE PRESERVATION: IS THERE A NEED TO GRAFT ALL EXTRACTION SOCKETS TO PRESERVE ALVEOLAR RIDGE HEIGHT?

It has become common practice to attempt alveolar ridge preservation and reconstruction of the extraction socket with grafting using biomaterials following dental extractions, especially in those patients who desire rehabilitation of the missing tooth with dental implants. The practice ensures preservation of marginal bone height for future implant reconstructions. In a comprehensive overview of systematic reviews, the following were identified as surgical and patient factors affecting marginal bone loss in integrated implants[27]:

1. Marginal bone loss was significantly more in patients with periodontitis than in periodontally healthy patients
2. Significantly greater in generalized aggressive periodontitis patients compared with chronic periodontitis patients
3. Significantly less in alveolar socket preservation techniques

4. Significantly more in alveolar ridge augmentation sites
5. Significantly more in men than in women
6. Significantly more in smokers than in nonsmokers
7. Smokers also have significantly more marginal bone loss in the maxilla than in the mandible

In the esthetic zone there is some clinical relevance to achieve good marginal height for proper emergence profiles, but is there a need for socket preservation and graft reconstruction of every extraction socket? Regardless of the technique or graft biomaterial used, some of the biologic processes of postextraction bone resorption and bone modeling are inevitable.

Studies have clearly shown that when alveolar ridge preservation techniques are attempted, it limits the contour changes and bone resorption following tooth extraction. These sites show better preservation of facial keratinized tissue when compared with control sites and when ready for implants, can accommodate longer and wider implants when compared with nongrafted sites.[28]

Other studies have shown that implants placed in grafted sockets showed similar clinical performance in 3-year follow-up studies compared with the nongrafted sites in a different study; however, the grafted sites allowed for placement of larger implants and required less augmentation procedures at implant placement.[29] When alveolar ridge preservation is not preferred, and immediate implants are performed following extractions, the socket walls show some dimensional changes that are most pronounced on the buccal aspects. Whether or not this has an impact on the long-term performance of the implant is not been investigated conclusively.

Although there is not much controversy among practitioners that grafting an extraction socket is beneficial, the debate about the safety and efficacy of some of the graft materials has emerged. Bone morphogenic protein has been used in its recombinant form in multiple craniofacial reconstructive procedures including alveolar ridge preservation. Additionally, some of these treatments are expensive.

As tissue engineering evolves, it is making its way into the doctor's office, providing options touted as new and improved. Whether there is sound science behind that investment for patients remains to be seen. Most studies seem to be focused on particular techniques and often have short follow-up on their results. One thing is clear in reviewing the literature: alveolar ridge augmentation procedures are often technique- and operator-experience-sensitive, and implant survival may be a function of residual bone supporting the dental implant rather than grafted bone. In time, one can expect long-term, multicenter studies that might provide further insight into augmentation procedures to support dental implant survival.

SUMMARY

Dentoalveolar surgery is practiced worldwide with variations in technique, rationale, and philosophies. Just about everything in dentoalveolar surgery is wrought with controversy. There is argument in scientific forums about the indications for removal of asymptomatic M3s and pathology-free impacted mesiodenses. There is debate over the choice of bone graft materials and tissue engineering techniques. Clinicians compare and contrast their belief in dry sockets and some question its very existence. There is an attempt to rationalize the decision to recommend a drug holiday in patients. Oral maxillofacial surgeons cannot come to terms with the choices of individual instruments in operatories. As with any other field, the science and thus practices continue to evolve and new solutions emerge helping oral maxillofacial surgeons and patients. As long as oral maxillofacial surgeons remain curious and intuitive, this emerging and dynamic specialty will keep everything controversial.

REFERENCES

1. Eke PI, Dye BA, Wei L, et al. Update on prevalence of periodontitis in adults in the United States: NHANES 2009-2012. J Periodontol 2015;17:1–18.
2. Steed MB. The indications for third-molar extractions. J Am Dent Assoc 2014;145(6):570–3.
3. Blakey GH, Gelesko S, Marciani RD, et al. Third molars and periodontal pathology in American adolescents and young adults: a prevalence study. J Oral Maxillofac Surg 2010;68(2):325–9.
4. Montero J, Mazzaglia G. Effect of removing an impacted mandibular third molar on the periodontal status of the mandibular second molar. J Oral Maxillofac Surg 2011;69(11):2691–7.
5. Dodson TB. How many patients have third molars and how many have one or more asymptomatic, disease-free third molars? J Oral Maxillofac Surg 2012; 70:S4–7.
6. Golden BA, Baldwin C, Sherwood C, et al. Monitoring for periodontal inflammatory disease in the third molar region. J Oral Maxillofac Surg 2014; 73(4):595–9.
7. Garaas RN, Fisher EL, Wilson GH, et al. Prevalence of third molars with caries experience or periodontal

pathology in young adults. J Oral Maxillofac Surg 2011;69(9):e2–3.

8. Ahmad N, Gelesko S, Shugars D, et al. Caries experience and periodontal pathology in erupting third molars. J Oral Maxillofac Surg 2008;66(5): 948–53.

9. White RP Jr, Madianos PN, Offenbacher S, et al. Microbial complexes detected in the second/third molar region in patients with asymptomatic third molars. J Oral Maxillofac Surg 2002;60(11):1234–40.

10. White RP, Offenbacher S, Phillips C, et al. Inflammatory mediators and periodontitis in patients with asymptomatic third molars. J Oral Maxillofac Surg 2002;60(11):1241–5.

11. Rajasuo A, Sihvonen OJ, Peltola M, et al. Periodontal pathogens in erupting third molars of periodontally healthy subjects. Int J Oral Maxillofac Surg 2007; 36(9):818–21.

12. Meurman JH, Rajasuo A, Murtomaa H, et al. Respiratory tract infections and concomitant pericoronitis of the wisdom teeth. BMJ 1995;310(6983):834–6.

13. Giglio JA, Gunsolley JC, Laskin DM, et al. Effect of removing impacted third molars on plaque and gingival indices. J Oral Maxillofac Surg 1994;52(6): 584–7.

14. Elter JR, Offenbacher S, White RP, et al. Third molars associated with periodontal pathology in older Americans. J Oral Maxillofac Surg 2005;63(2): 179–84.

15. Dicus-Brookes C, Partrick M, Blakey GH, et al. Removal of symptomatic third molars may improve periodontal status of remaining dentition. J Oral Maxillofac Surg 2013;71(10):1639–46.

16. Blakey GH, Parker DW, Hull DJ, et al. Impact of removal of asymptomatic third molars on periodontal pathology. J Oral Maxillofac Surg 2009;67(2): 245–50.

17. Ash M, Costich ER, Hayward R. A study of periodontal hazards of third molars. J Periodontol 1962;33:209–15.

18. Ruggiero SL, Dodson TB, Assael LA, et al. American Association of Oral and Maxillofacial Surgeons position paper on bisphosphonate-related osteonecrosis of the jaws–2009 update. J Oral Maxillofac Surg 2009;67(2).

19. Available at: https://www.fda.gov/downloads/AdvisoryCommittees/CommitteesMeetingMaterials/drugs/DrugSafetyandRiskManagementAdvisoryCommittee/ucm270958.pdf. Accessed May 20, 2017.

20. Damm DD, Jones DM. Bisphosphonate-related osteonecrosis of the jaws: a potential alternative to drug holidays. Gen Dent 2013;61:33.

21. Hasegawa T, Kawakita A, Ueda N, et al. A multicenter retrospective study of the risk factors associated with medication-related osteonecrosis of the jaw after tooth extraction in patients receiving oral bisphosphonate therapy: can primary wound closure and a drug holiday really prevent MRONJ? Osteoporos Int 2017;28(8):2465–73.

22. Watts NB, Diab DL. Long-term use of bisphosphonates in osteoporosis. J Clin Endocrinol Metab 2010;95(4):1555–65.

23. Niederman R, Richards D. What is evidence-based dentistry, and do oral infections increase systemic morbidity or mortality? Oral Maxillofac Surg Clin North Am 2011;23(4):491–6.

24. Walterspacher S, Fuhrmann C, Germann M, et al. Dental care before lung transplantation: are we being too rigorous? Clin Respir J 2013;7(2):220–5.

25. Taubert KA, Wilson W. Is endocarditis prophylaxis for dental procedures necessary? Heart Asia 2017.

26. Akashi M, Tanaka K, Kusumoto J, et al. Brain abscess potentially resulting from odontogenic focus: report of three cases and a literature review. J Maxillofac Oral Surg 2017;16(1).

27. Ting M, Tenaglia MS, Jones GH, et al. Surgical and patient factors affecting marginal bone levels around dental implants: a comprehensive overview of systematic reviews. Implant Dent 2017;26(2): 303–15.

28. Barone A, Ricci M, Tonelli P, et al. Tissue changes of extraction sockets in humans: a comparison of spontaneous healing vs. ridge preservation with secondary soft tissue healing. Clin Oral Implants Res 2013;24(11):1231–7.

29. Barone A, Orlando B, Cingano L, et al. A randomized clinical trial to evaluate and compare implants placed in augmented versus non-augmented extraction sockets: 3-year results. J Periodontol 2012;83(7):836–46.

Controversies in Maxillofacial Trauma

Daniel J. Meara, DMD, MS, MD, FACS[a],*, Lewis C. Jones, DMD, MD[b]

KEYWORDS

- Facial fractures • Titanium and absorbable fixation • Timing of surgical repair
- Open versus closed treatment • Antibiotics for facial injuries

KEY POINTS

- The decision regarding open versus closed treatment of mandibular condyle fractures is multifactorial, and patient-specific factors often determine the most appropriate management.
- The evolution of absorbable fixation materials and techniques have made it a viable option in the management of facial fractures, although it must be used with caution in adult mandible fractures.
- Extraction of teeth in the line of fracture is guided by the condition of the tooth and the associated risk of poor healing as well as its impact on bony reduction.
- Current literature suggests that mandible fracture repair outcomes are not improved with immediate versus delayed repair.
- There is little evidence to support the routine use of antibiotics in the treatment of facial wounds and fractures.

INTRODUCTION

Controversies in craniomaxillofacial trauma still exist despite advances in technology, surgical techniques, and peer-reviewed literature. The purpose of this article is to highlight current areas of controversy in facial trauma management and to review the most applicable literature in an attempt to provide some clarity, and possibly resolution, to the presented topics. At minimum, these topics should generate discussion. For many situations and treatments, definitive indications and contraindications do exist. A surgeon, however, is often required to make clinical decisions that lie within the gray zone—where there is no clear indication or contraindication. The result is that the surgeon is required to make a judgment call, and the best surgeons are those who couple the existing scientific literature with clinical experience. This way, the treatment and healing process can move forward and any subsequent complications can be addressed and anticipated. This is the authors' opinion—and like the rest of these topics, is up for debate.

OPEN VERSUS CLOSED REDUCTION FOR CONDYLAR FRACTURES

Condylar fractures do not plague all facial surgeons—just those who care about restoring patients to optimal occlusion. The debate regarding open versus closed treatment of these fractures has been discussed, and it lives on because there is no single parameter that exists to determine the necessity of an open reduction or acceptability of a closed reduction. Even with regard to closed reduction of condylar fractures, the method for closed reduction (wire vs elastic maxillomandibular fixation) and the length of time in treatment vary. Regardless of the treatment modality,

Disclosure: The authors have no disclosures.
a Department of Oral and Maxillofacial Surgery & Hospital Dentistry, Christiana Care Health System, 501 West 14th Street, Suite 2W40, Wilmington, DE 19801, USA; b Department of Surgical and Hospital Dentistry, University of Louisville, 501 South Preston Street, Louisville, KY 40241, USA
* Corresponding author.
E-mail address: dmeara@christianacare.org

complications can occur. These complications were outlined by Ellis in 1998[1] to include malocclusion, hypomobility, asymmetry, degeneration, and iatrogenic injury.

Few clear indications for open reduction exist. In 1983, Zide and Kent[2] published the definitive indications for open reduction of a condyle. These include the following 4 conditions:

1. Displacement of the condyle into the middle cranial fossa or external auditory canal
2. Lateral extracapsular dislocation
3. Contaminated open joint wound
4. Inability to obtain adequate occlusion

The first 3 conditions are binary and leave little wiggle room. The last clause, obtaining adequate occlusion, is where the real controversy exists. First, a surgeon has to decide what constitutes "adequate." For the conscientious facial surgeon, the goal is restoration of premorbid occlusion, when possible. Some trauma results in loss of teeth and alveolar bone such that restoration of premorbid occlusion is no longer possible and the challenge to obtain the best possible result ensues. When there is no loss of dentition or alveolar bone, attaining premorbid occlusion should be possible; thus, the need to open a subcondylar fracture to help obtain this occlusion must be determined.

Conservative treatment can avoid the risks associated with open reduction, which includes injury to the branches of the facial nerve, postoperative malocclusion, sialocele formation, and facial scarring. The complication of facial nerve weakness has been demonstrated at 12% to 30% with resolution by 6 months postoperatively.[3–5] Open reduction results have demonstrated sound restoration of occlusion, improved range of motion, and the ability for functional convalescence. Subcondylar fractures should be approached with considerations and principles in mind that help guide the treatment to attain restoration of premorbid occlusion and function. The following are considerations in the optimal management of subcondylar fractures:

1. Is it a unilateral subcondylar fracture or bilateral subcondylar fracture?
2. Where is the level of the fracture?
3. Is the fracture displaced?
4. What is the degree of displacement?
5. What is the condition of the remaining dentition?
6. Are there other facial fractures?
7. Is the patient skeletally mature?

Many unilateral fractures can be treated closed with proper follow-up and patient compliance.

Bilateral subcondylar fractures, on the other hand, present more frequently with loss of facial height, resultant apertognathia, and difficulty with restoration of premorbid occlusion/function with closed reduction.[1] For the bilateral fractures, open reduction has demonstrated statistically and clinically significant improved function (opening/excursion/protrusion) and occlusion in comparison with closed reduction.[6]

The level of the fracture is assessed to ensure that adequate bone exists on the superior fractured segment to allow for placement of internal fixation. A variety of methods and plates exist for subcondylar fractures, but the bone must be adequate to allow for placement of some form of fixation if the fracture is opened.[7,8]

Displacement of the fracture is a consideration, because it would be difficult to justify an open procedure for a nondisplaced fracture. Ellis[9] has demonstrated that degree of displacement (measured on Towne and panoramic views) correlated to the clinical finding of dropback on examination at the time of surgery. This requires correlation of clinical and radiographic examination (with emphasis on the clinical examination) to aid in the determination for the need for an open procedure—the surgeon should also note that even a closed reduction can result in additional displacement.[10]

The condition of remaining dentition also has implications in the treatment of subcondylar fractures. Presence of intact posterior dentition aids with maintaining the vertical dimension during the healing period of closed treatment. A lack of posterior teeth can allow for collapse in the vertical dimension and development (or persistence) of a malocclusion.

The presence of other facial fractures, especially in the bilateral subcondylar fracture patient, may require the surgeon to open at least one side to re-establish the vertical dimension of the mandible for facial reconstruction.

A skeletally immature patient has significant healing and remodeling potential.[11] Therefore, the initial treatment of these patients is closed treatment if possible.

The decision to open a subcondylar fracture is not always a simple one, but it can be guided by careful thought and consideration of these factors.

TEETH IN THE LINE OF THE FRACTURE

Another conundrum a facial trauma surgeon encounters is when to extract a tooth in the line of a mandible fracture. Some investigators/surgeons have advocated for retention of healthy teeth in the line of fracture with the use of rigid fixation (with few caveats).[12] A tooth left in the line of fracture, however, can lead to localized infection, hardware infection/failure, and osteomyelitis and contribute to postoperative pain. Unfortunately, this is a commonly encountered problem as approximately 50% to 85% of mandibular fractures present with a tooth in the line of fracture.[13,14] Alpert's[13] investigation in 1978 demonstrated that 32% of patients with a tooth in the line of fracture went on to experience some form of morbidity. Ellis[14] study in 2002 demonstrated a 19% infection rate of angle fractures whether the tooth was retained or extracted.[14] A meta-analysis of angle fractures with teeth in the line of fracture demonstrated an infection rate of 10.7% for fractures where the tooth was removed and 11.1% where the tooth was retained. In all 3 studies, the complications occurred irrespective of the management of the tooth (extraction vs retention). Thus the debate rages on. Should the tooth be extracted, and does it matter if it is extracted?

Again, there are myriad variables, including condition of the teeth, type and location of fracture, and planned method of fixation, to name a few, which complicate the decision-making process. Considerations with regard to extraction of teeth in the line of fracture (as well as the timing of any extractions to be performed) include

1. Does the tooth help with the fracture reduction?
2. Does the tooth aid in proximal control?
3. Is there any evidence of existing disease/infection associated with the tooth?
4. Will bone need to be removed to perform the extraction? And if so, is this bone crucial to the fixation?

If the tooth aids with reduction of the fracture, it makes little sense to extract the tooth prior to placement of fixation. This can be true of fractures anywhere in the mandible, but by anecdotal experience, is especially true in the angle region where control of the proximal segment can prove difficult and the presence of a third molar may aid in stabilizing the segment during application of fixation.

Teeth with existing disease should be extracted with débridement of adjacent affected tissues. If the tooth aids in reduction, the fracture can be first fixated and the extraction performed subsequently with careful attention to avoid displacement of the recently fixated fracture.

Occasionally, a tooth is present in the fracture site that requires significant bone removal for extraction. This is most often an impacted third molar at an angle fracture or an impacted anterior tooth at a parasymphysis fracture. Consideration should be made with regard to the implications of the bone removal on the placement of fixation. Lateral bone removal at the third molar site may preclude placement of a superior lateral border plate or external oblique (Champy) plate.

A viable treatment option for mandible fractures, although seldom selected by patients, is closed reduction. Closed reduction can be performed with low (3%) morbidity in angle fractures with partially impacted teeth in the line of fracture.[15] In angle fractures, however, closed reduction should be reserved for nondisplaced, favorable-type fractures.

PROPHYLACTIC ANTIBIOTICS IN FACIAL FRACTURES

A chasm exists between the current practice and the evidence supporting the prescription of postoperative prophylactic antibiotics for facial fractures. Studies have consistently shown that not only are they often prescribed but also the prescription of antibiotics does not correlate to a decrease in infection in the postoperative period.[16–20] Certainly, there are traumatic scenarios (a class IV wound/penetrating trauma) that warrant postoperative antibiotic therapy.[21] The practice of routine administration postoperative antibiotics, however, is not supported by the literature and should be curtailed in this era of evidence-based medicine.

A recent review of literature by Mundinger[19] (looking at 44 published studies) resulted in recommendations that included extrapolated data from orthopedic and oncologic literature. These recommendations included perioperative antibiotics within 60 minutes prior to incision (up to 120 minutes for vancomycin or clindamycin) for open fractures or clean-contaminated procedures and cessation of antibiotics within 24 hours of the procedure. Mundinger did note that "unique situations in the management of craniofacial fractures, such as contamination of fracture sites from the sinuses, exposure of fractures to intraoral bacteria from mucosal tears, and delay in fracture management, intuitively suggest that there may be benefit to preoperative and prolonged postoperative antibiotic administration in craniofacial fractures."[19] Considerations that aid this decision may include the following:

1. Is the host immunocompromised?
2. What is the mechanism of injury?
3. Which anatomic structures are involved, and is the surgical approach sterile?

An immunocompromised patient has an increased risk of postoperative infection. Conditions, such as diabetes mellitus, HIV, substance abuse, and use of immunosuppressants, increase the risk of postoperative infections. Although this is intuitive, it has been studied and correlations exist between these immunosuppressed states and increased rates of infection after facial trauma.[22–25] In cases of an increased risk inherent based on medical history, prolonged postoperative prophylactic antibiotics may be prudent.

The mechanism of injury may dictate the presence of contamination, such as animal bites or open wounds with retained foreign material. Débridement of these wounds can prove difficult and frustrating. The wound classifications encountered in facial trauma surgery are most often clean contaminated (class II) or contaminated (class III). A clean (class I) case is rarely encountered in facial trauma, and even closed fractures are often addressed with transoral approaches, rendering the case clean contaminated (class II). These wound classifications correlate with the risk for postoperative surgical wound infection rates and should be taken into consideration when determining the duration of antibiotic therapy.[26,27] Multiple studies have shown no decrease in infection rates with increased length of time of postoperative antibiotics beyond 24 hours.[28–32] Therefore, when prescribing for a timeframe beyond 24 hours postoperative, there should be a reason to justify the duration of antibiotics.

Finally, the overriding confounding factor in this discussion is a patient's expectations. Often, a patient and/or family expect to receive an antibiotic, and failure to prescribe can be perceived as inadequate care, especially if any healing complications occur. Thus, surgeons must understand the literature and should incorporate shared decision-making into everyday practice.

MATERIALS FOR ORBITAL FLOOR REPAIR

There is plenty of controversy surrounding orbital fractures—timing of repair, surgical approach, and material for reconstruction are the main culprits of controversy. This discussion only addresses the surgeon's choice of orbital implant. There are of options ranging from porous polyethylene, titanium, titanium coated with porous polyethylene, autogenous calvarium, and resorbable materials. Which material is preferable, and in what situation?

Although titanium does have its advantages, including visibility on postoperative imaging, malleability, ease of placement of fixation screws, and strength, it also has drawbacks. Titanium requires large incisions for placement and has unrefined/sharp margins when trimmed. Titanium has also been reported to cause an inflammatory response leading to orbital/ocular complications, including restriction.[33,34] Other surgeons have stated, however, that titanium implants do not cause restriction.[35,36] This exemplifies the controversy of orbital plate selection.

Titanium reinforced porous polyethylene has the rigidity, stability, and radio-opacity of titanium while avoiding the sharp margins that occur with trimming titanium. The disadvantage of this option is the decreased porosity for drainage.

Absorbable plates used in orbital reconstruction include plates made of a wide variety of materials. Details regarding the various properties have been nicely outlined in previous publications.[37–39] Early absorbable implants were made of high-molecular-weight polymerized poly L-lactide (PLLA), which degraded slowly and had a late inflammatory reaction.[40] Newer materials, such as poly L-lactide-co-glycolide and poly D-lactide/L-lactide (KLS Martin), claim to avoid much of the late inflammatory complications of PLLA and resorb within approximately 12 months to 30 months. These are not opaque on postoperative imaging but have the advantage of resorption.

Autogenous calvarial bone has the distinct (and major) disadvantage of donor site morbidity that is avoided with all the alloplastic materials. It is also difficult to contour but is biocompatible, rigid, and radiopaque.

Finally, current research in the field of patient-specific implants is performed on orbital floor repairs. This allows for a snap-in–type effect and restores the orbital volume. These are generally fabricated from titanium, and their main disadvantages are added cost and time for fabrication.

If the perfect material existed for orbital floor/wall repairs, then there is only 1 option. Because the perfect material does not exist, however, surgeons use a variety of methods depending on the scenario encountered. Bartoli and colleagues[41] study of 301 orbital floor fractures illustrates this, implementing 8 different materials for repair of the fractures. Thus, when selecting the material, the following can be taken into consideration:

1. What is the age of the patient? (Titanium is often avoided in immature orbit.)
2. What is the size of the defect? (Increased rigidity is required for maintenance of orbital volume with a large defect.)
3. Is fixation of the implant likely to be required? (Some of the absorbable options do not have the ability to be fixated).
4. What works best in each surgeon's hands? (A valid, albeit arbitrary, factor.)

Controversy will continue to exist unless studies comparing methods reach unequivocal results that illustrate a material's superiority. Recent publications elucidate some of the advantages and disadvantages of reconstructive materials, but additional analysis is required to eliminate this controversy.[42,43]

FRONTAL SINUS FRACTURES

The ideal intervention for frontal sinus fractures has been controversial, because it relates to the creation of a safe and more predictable sinus. The concern regarding mucocele and mucopyocele formation, as well as the development of sinusitis and frank meningitis, is what has seemingly created the controversy and variability in frontal sinus fracture management. Treatment options range from cranialization to nasofrontal duct and sinus obliteration to simple observation, but the implementation of endoscopic techniques for the treatment of the fontal sinus outflow tract has seemingly decreased the need for more aggressive intervention.[44] However, patients with frontal sinus fractures often need to be monitored for life, but in many cases, the patients do not continue with postoperative visits once they are healed and feeling well.

There is no real controversy regarding the need to perform surgery in patients with frontal sinus fracture–induced cosmetic deformities or the persistence of a cerebrospinal fluid leak. The controversy arises in the management of the sinus cavity and the nasofrontal ducts.

Sinus Obliteration Versus Sinus Observation

Historically, the predilection has been toward the more aggressive management of frontal sinus fractures due to the concern of delayed complications and the difficulty with predicting which patients are most at risk for downstream complications. Frontal sinus mucoceles and mucopyoceles have been reported more than 20 years after the repair of a frontal sinus fracture and many patients are lost to follow-up long before such complications can develop. In the general population, however, the frontal sinus is the most common paranasal sinus location for routine mucocele formation (unrelated to frontal sinus trauma). Mucocele cases observed decades after frontal sinus trauma may be unrelated to the trauma management.[45] Thus, with the development of endoscopic sinus surgery and coupled with the lack of definitive evidence-based guidance, the controversy rages on. So what does the literature suggest? The most recent evidence suggests that a more conservative approach is reasonable. Jafari and colleagues[46] noted that almost 90% of patients with frontal sinus outflow tract injury had spontaneous reventilation.

Advancements in Technology

The advances in technology have led to improved diagnostic imaging and treatment options. Specifically, Koento[47] highlights the enhanced imaging quality from CT, which assist surgeons in determining the significance of any FSTO involvement. Also, advances in endoscopic sinus surgery offer a rescue surgical option in the event that sinus aeration does not occur in the early healing period, or if complications arise in delayed fashion. Guy and Brissett[48] suggest that even when there are comminuted fractures of the frontal recess with narrowing of the outflow tract, endoscopic procedures, such as the Lothrop and Draf type III widening procedures, can correct this narrowing without the need for obliteration. Gabrielli and colleagues[49] discuss the use of stents along the naso-frontal outflow tract to maintain patency and allow for mucosalization during the initial healing period.

Less Is More

Pawar and Rhee[50] suggest that a more conservative approach leads to better patient outcomes as a result of reduced surgery-related morbidity.

Soft Tissue Versus Hard Tissue for Obliteration

In the event that a need to obliterate the frontal sinus is determined, no consensus exists for the best material. Rodriquez and colleagues,[51] however, discuss the benefits of calvarial bone dust plus demineralized bone matrix. The study highlights the unlimited availability of biomaterials and the avoidance of a donor site. Furthermore, the potential negatives of soft tissues, such as autogenous fat and/or muscle, is that these tissues can result in an inadequate seal of the outflow tract and the development of dead-space with resorption or necrosis.

The investigators of this article suggest that in the absence of evidence-based guidelines for treatment, that the more conservative approach should be given first consideration, in an attempt to reduce treatment variation and health care costs, but each individual case still requires a treatment plan that is tailored to the specific patient.

TIMING OF REPAIR FOR MANDIBLE FRACTURES

The unpredictability of facial trauma and the timely and convenient access to operating room time are challenges for surgeons, especially for common injuries, such as mandible fractures. Thus, the timing of mandible fracture repair and the associated complications are continued areas of controversy. Does the timing of a mandible fracture repair have an impact on the outcome? Furr and colleagues[16] in a retrospective review of 273 patients state that there were no statistically significant relationships to lag time to repair, patient demographics, fracture site, length of hospitalization, or the use of antibiotics. Furthermore, the article suggests that the development of infection and nonunion correlates most with a history of tobacco and alcohol use in patients undergoing open reduction and internal fixation.

Luz and colleagues[52] noted that a delay in fracture repair was more likely associated with the need for reoperation, as were substance abuse, dental condition, and open fracture repair. The mean time elapsed between the trauma and the initial treatment, however, was 19.1 days in the reoperated group and 13.5 days in the group without complications. The group without complications still had a delay of almost 2 weeks (average of 13.5 days) before mandible fracture repair, but only 20% of these patients had open treatment.

Biller and colleagues[53] evaluated complications and the time to repair of mandible fractures in a retrospective chart review that divided patients into 2 groups: those repaired in 3 days or less and those repaired after 3 days, from the time of injury. Furthermore, those who experienced complications were further subdivided into 2 groups: infectious and technical complications. The investigators concluded that patients with mandible fractures treated after 3 days do not have a higher risk of developing an infectious complication, but the risk is elevated in patients with substance abuse. Technical complications increased, however, with treatment delay, including weakness to the marginal mandibular nerve, malocclusion, and chronic pain. The study noted that those without any type of complication were repaired an average of 5 days after the injury.

Lucca and colleagues[54] performed a retrospective chart review of 92 patients comparing outcomes with early versus late treatment. Early treatment was rendered within 48 hours of the injury and late intervention occurred after more than 48 hours since the injury and no statistically significant difference was noted, regarding complications, among the 2 groups. Barker and colleagues[55] also found no relationship between complications and timing to repair, with the mean time to repair 6.7 days.

In the absence of an absolute need for urgent mandibular fracture repair (airway compromise, inability to take orally, uncontrolled pain, and significant displacement with inability to place bridle wire), the literature suggests that complications are rare if mandible fracture repair can occur within the first 5 to 7 days.

RIGID VERSUS ABSORBABLE FIXATION IN CRANIOMAXILLOFACIAL TRAUMA SURGERY

Absorbable fixation has become more commonplace in synostosis surgery and upper midface trauma repair, but its use in orthognathic surgery and mandibular fracture repair continues to be controversial. Benefits of absorbable fixation are the elimination of the need for plate removal, the absence of radiographic scatter, and the application to pediatric cases. Can absorbable fixation, however, be a reasonable alternative to titanium fixation? Park,[56] in his review of bioabsorbable osteofixation, discusses that 3 main materials include polyglycolic acid (PGA), poly-L-lactic acid (PLLA), and poly-D-lactic acid. PGA degrades in 6 weeks and PLLA can take 3.5 years; thus, polymers alter the behavior to allow for strength during the initial healing period but with a resorption time closer to 1 year. Inflammatory complications can occur as a result of the resorptive process.[56] Absorbable material composition affects handling, fixation stability, and resorption and is critical to its success in clinical care.

Absorbable materials are more readily accepted for use in orthognathic surgery and offer insight into their application to maxillofacial trauma. A *PLOS ONE* meta-analysis by Yang and colleagues[57] evaluating the complications of absorbable fixation in maxillofacial surgery included 20 studies and revealed that the absorbable group had significantly more complications than the titanium group, with the main issue foreign body reaction and mobility. No overall differences were noted for infection, temporomandibular disorders, fistulation, palpability, dehiscence, malocclusion, exposure and relapse. Furthermore, for the bimaxillary (orthognathic surgery) subgroup, the absorbable group did not have a significant increase in complications. No differences were noted for bilateral sagittal split osteotomies and Le Fort I osteotomies.

A 2015 systematic review by Al-Moraissi and Ellis[58] evaluated the differences in skeletal stability and material-related complications for titanium or biodegradable fixation in orthognathic surgery. The findings included no statistical difference for skeletal stability, wound problems, plate and screw removal, and palpability, but there was a difference for intraoperative fracture of plates and screws in the biodegradable group.[58]

Meara and colleagues[59] demonstrated the benefits of poly-DL-lactic acid mesh and ultrasonic welding as an alternative to titanium fixation, in Le Fort I osteotomies. No tapping for screw placement is needed, decreasing time needed for fixation. The most common complication was sterile abscess formation, occurring in only 1.9% of patients.

Bakelen and colleagues[60] in a randomized control trial at 4 institutions with 230 patients compared biodegradable and titanium fixation systems in all types of maxillofacial surgery, including fracture repair. The study resulted in the biodegradable system requiring more 2.2 times higher plate and screw than the titanium group. Almost all of the issues arose in the mandible, due mainly to abscess formation.

Mandible Fractures

Vazquez-Morales and colleagues[61] performed a prospective clinical trial of 50 mandibular fractures using an Inion 2.5-mm 4-hole absorbable plate adapted along the ideal line of osteosynthesis. Every patient, however, was placed into maxillomandibular fixation for approximately 3 weeks. Primary bone healing was achieved in all the cases, but 10 complications were noted: 5 soft tissue infections, 4 plate dehiscence, and 1 malocclusion. No malunion, nonunion, plate facture, or osteomyelitis was noted and no reoperation was performed, despite a long-term follow-up of 10 months. The article states that the Inion System is approved by the Food and Drug Administration for mandible fixation with an appropriate period of maxillomandibular fixation.[61]

Ahmed and colleagues[62] performed a prospective, randomized study to compare bioabsorbable plates with titanium plates for mandibular fractures; 34 patients were assigned to the absorbable plate group and 35 to the titanium group. The absorbable plates 90:10 poly L-lactide-co-D, L-lactide. The key finding was screw and plate breakage in the absorbable plate group, and fixations costs were significantly greater than in the titanium group.

Lee and colleagues[63] in a retrospective review of 91 patients compared titanium to biodegradable miniplates for fixation of mandibular fractures. Maxillomandibular fixation was used from a mean of 7.6 days. The overall complication rate was 4.41% and there were no significant differences between the 2 groups. Nonunion or malunion was not noted in either group.

Leonhardt and colleagues[64] compared titanium fixation to Inion in the treatment of mandible fractures and this study was notable because no maxillomandibular fixation was part of treatment. Bony healing occurred in all cases, but malocclusions at 1 week were twice as common in the Inion group. As a result, the investigators recommend a short period of maxillomandibular fixation. Wound healing complications were similar in both groups.

Absorbable fixation has a legitimate role in craniomaxillofacial trauma surgery, but its use as the sole fixation in mandible fracture repair cannot be recommended based on the existing literature.

SUMMARY

Craniomaxillofacial trauma management has continued to improve and evolve over time as a result of advances in technology and scientific inquiry. Controversies still exist, however, because there is insufficient evidence-based literature, in certain aspects of facial trauma management, to unequivocally guide treatment in areas, such as frontal sinus management, rigid versus absorbable fixation, open versus closed treatment of mandibular condyle fractures, extraction of teeth in the line of fracture, optimal timing for repair of mandible fractures, antibiotic use for facial wounds and fractures, and reconstructive materials in orbital fracture reconstruction.

The current evidence-based literature has not resolved the controversies discussed in this article but does provide some clarity around the most ideal management strategies and techniques in the optimal management of craniomaxillofacial trauma. Ultimately, the goal is to create evidence-based guidelines to guide the surgeon, to reduce variability, improve operative efficiency, and enhance patient outcomes. Thus, work remains to erase the remaining areas of controversy.

REFERENCES

1. Ellis E. Complications of mandibular condyle fractures. Int J Oral Maxillofac Surg 1998;27:255–7.
2. Zide MF, Kent JN. Indications for open reduction of mandibular condyle fractures. J Oral Maxillofac Surg 1983;41(2):89–98.
3. Ellis E 3rd, McFadden D, Simon P, et al. Surgical complications with open treatment of mandibular condylar process fractures. J Oral Maxillofac Surg 2000;58(9):950–8.
4. Kanno T, Sukegawa S, Tatsumi H, et al. Does a retromandibular transparotid approach for the open treatment of condylar fractures result in facial nerve injury? J Oral Maxillofac Surg 2016;74(10):2019–32.
5. Manisali M, Amin M, Aghabeigi B, et al. Retromandibular approach to the mandibular condyle: a clinical and cadaveric study. Int J Oral Maxillofac Surg 2003;32(3):253–6.

6. Singh V, Bhagol A, Dhingra R. A comparative clinical evaluation of the outcome of patients treated for bilateral fracture of the mandibular condyles. J Craniomaxillofac Surg 2012;40(5):464–6.

7. Bischoff EL, Carmichael R, Reddy LV. Plating options for fixation of condylar neck and base fractures. Atlas Oral Maxillofac Surg Clin North Am 2017;25(1):69–73.

8. Darwich MA, Albogha MH, Abdelmajeed A, et al. Assessment of the biomechanical performance of 5 plating techniques in fixation of mandibular subcondylar fracture using finite element analysis. J Oral Maxillofac Surg 2016;74(4):794.e1-8.

9. Ellis E 3rd. Method to determine when open treatment of condylar process fractures is not necessary. J Oral Maxillofac Surg 2009;67(8):1685–90.

10. Ellis E 3rd, Palmieri C, Throckmorton G. Further displacement of condylar process fractures after closed treatment. J Oral Maxillofac Surg 1999; 57(11):1307–16 [discussion: 1316–7].

11. Ghasemzadeh A, Mundinger GS, Swanson EW, et al. Treatment of Pediatric Condylar Fractures: A 20-Year Experience. Plast Reconstr Surg 2015; 136(6):1279–88.

12. Gerbino G, Tarello F, Fasolis M, et al. Rigid fixation with teeth in the line of mandibular fractures. Int J Oral Maxillofac Surg 1997;26(3):182–6.

13. Neal DC, Wagner WF, Alpert B. Morbidity associated with teeth in the line of mandibular fractures. J Oral Surg 1978;36(11):859–62.

14. Ellis E 3rd. Outcomes of patients with teeth in the line of mandibular angle fractures treated with stable internal fixation. J Oral Maxillofac Surg 2002;60(8): 863–5 [discussion: 866].

15. Marker P, Eckerdal A, Smith-Sivertsen C. Incompletely erupted third molars in the line of mandibular fractures. A retrospective analysis of 57 cases. Oral Surg Oral Med Oral Pathol 1994;78(4):426–31.

16. Furr AM, Schweinfurth JM, May WL. Factors associated with long-term complications after repair of mandibular fractures. Laryngoscope 2006;116(3): 427–30.

17. Adalarasan S, Mohan A, Pasupathy S. Prophylactic antibiotics in maxillofacial fractures: a requisite? J Craniofac Surg 2010;21(4):1009–11.

18. Morris LM, Kellman RM. Are prophylactic antibiotics useful in the management of facial fractures? Laryngoscope 2014;124(6):1282–4.

19. Mundinger GS, Borsuk DE, Okhah Z, et al. Antibiotics and facial fractures: evidence-based recommendations compared with experience-based practice. Craniomaxillofac Trauma Reconstr 2015; 8(1):64–78.

20. Domingo F, Dale E, Gao C, et al. A single-center retrospective review of postoperative infectious complications in the surgical management of mandibular fractures: Postoperative antibiotics add no benefit. J Trauma Acute Care Surg 2016;81(6): 1109–14.

21. Motamedi MH. Primary treatment of penetrating injuries to the face. J Oral Maxillofac Surg 2007; 65(6):1215–8.

22. Senel FC, Jessen GS, Melo MD, et al. Infection following treatment of mandible fractures: the role of immunosuppression and polysubstance abuse. Oral Surg Oral Med Oral Pathol Oral Radiol Endod 2007;103(1):38–42.

23. Passeri LA, Ellis E 3rd, Sinn DP. Relationship of substance abuse to complications with mandibular fractures. J Oral Maxillofac Surg 1993;51(1):22–5.

24. Odom EB, Snyder-Warwick AK. Mandible fracture complications and infection: the influence of demographics and modifiable factors. Plast Reconstr Surg 2016;138(2):282e–9e.

25. Ward NH 3rd, Wainwright DJ. Outcomes research: Mandibular fractures in the diabetic population. J Craniomaxillofac Surg 2016;44(7):763–9.

26. Culver DH, Horan TC, Gaynes RP, et al. Surgical wound infection rates by wound class, operative procedure, and patient risk index. National Nosocomial Infections Surveillance System. Am J Med 1991;91(3b):152s–7s.

27. Garibaldi RA, Cushing D, Lerer T. Risk factors for postoperative infection. Am J Med 1991;91(3b): 158s–63s.

28. Zix J, Schaller B, Iizuka T, et al. The role of postoperative prophylactic antibiotics in the treatment of facial fractures: a randomised, double-blind, placebo-controlled pilot clinical study. Part 1: orbital fractures in 62 patients. Br J Oral Maxillofac Surg 2013;51(4):332–6.

29. Schaller B, Soong PL, Zix J, et al. The role of postoperative prophylactic antibiotics in the treatment of facial fractures: a randomized, double-blind, placebo-controlled pilot clinical study. Part 2: Mandibular fractures in 59 patients. Br J Oral Maxillofac Surg 2013;51(8):803–7.

30. Soong PL, Schaller B, Zix J, et al. The role of postoperative prophylactic antibiotics in the treatment of facial fractures: a randomised, double-blind, placebo-controlled pilot clinical study. Part 3: Le Fort and zygomatic fractures in 94 patients. Br J Oral Maxillofac Surg 2014;52(4):329–33.

31. Lauder A, Jalisi S, Spiegel J, et al. Antibiotic prophylaxis in the management of complex midface and frontal sinus trauma. Laryngoscope 2010;120(10): 1940–5.

32. Miles BA, Potter JK, Ellis E 3rd. The efficacy of postoperative antibiotic regimens in the open treatment of mandibular fractures: a prospective randomized trial. J Oral Maxillofac Surg 2006;64(4):576–82.

33. Katou F, Andoh N, Motegi K, et al. Immuno-inflammatory responses in the tissue adjacent to titanium miniplates used in the treatment of

mandibular fractures. J Craniomaxillofac Surg 1996;24(3):155–62.

34. Lee HB, Nunery WR. Orbital adherence syndrome secondary to titanium implant material. Ophthal Plast Reconstr Surg 2009;25(1):33–6.

35. Ellis E 3rd, Messo E. Use of nonresorbable alloplastic implants for internal orbital reconstruction. J Oral Maxillofac Surg 2004;62(7):873–81.

36. Gear AJ, Lokeh A, Aldridge JH, et al. Safety of titanium mesh for orbital reconstruction. Ann Plast Surg 2002;48(1):1–7 [discussion; 7–9].

37. Potter JK, Malmquist M, Ellis E 3rd. Biomaterials for reconstruction of the internal orbit. Oral Maxillofacial Surg Clin N Am 2012;24(4):609–27.

38. Totir M, Ciuluvica R, Dinu I, et al. Biomaterials for orbital fractures repair. J Med Life 2015;8(1):41–3.

39. Boyette JR, Pemberton JD, Bonilla-Velez J. Management of orbital fractures: challenges and solutions. Clin Ophthalmol 2015;9:2127–37.

40. Bergsma EJ, Rozema FR, Bos RR, et al. Foreign body reactions to resorbable poly(L-lactide) bone plates and screws used for the fixation of unstable zygomatic fractures. J Oral Maxillofac Surg 1993; 51(6):666–70.

41. Bartoli D, Fadda MT, Battisti A, et al. Retrospective analysis of 301 patients with orbital floor fracture. J Craniomaxillofac Surg 2015;43(2):244–7.

42. Ellis E 3rd, Tan Y. Assessment of internal orbital reconstructions for pure blowout fractures: cranial bone grafts versus titanium mesh. J Oral Maxillofac Surg 2003;61(4):442–53.

43. Tabrizi R, Ozkan TB, Mohammadinejad C, et al. Orbital floor reconstruction. J Craniofac Surg 2010; 21(4):1142–6.

44. Patel S, Berens A, Devarajan K, et al. Evaluation of a minimally disruptive treatment protocol for frontal sinus fractures. JAMA Facial Plast Surg 2017;19:E1–7.

45. Palmer J, Schipor J. Frontal-orbital ethmoid mucoceles. In: Kountakis S, Senior B, Draf W, editors. The frontal sinus. New York: Springer; 2005. p. 75–81.

46. Jafari A, Nuyen B, Salinas C, et al. Spontaneous ventilation of the frontal sinus after fractures involving the frontal recess. Am J Otolaryngol 2015;36(6):837–42.

47. Koento T. Current advances in sinus preservation for the management of frontal sinus fractures. Curr Opin Otolaryngol Head Neck Surg 2012;20:274–9.

48. Guy W, Brissett A. Contemporary management of traumatic fractures of the frontal sinus. Otolarngol Clin N Am 2013;46:733–48.

49. Gabrielli MF, Gabrielli MA, Hochuli-Vieira E, et al. Immediate reconstruction of frontal sinus fractures: review of 26 cases. J Oral Maxillofac Surg 2004;62(5): 582–6.

50. Parwar S, Rhee J. Frontal sinus and naso-orbital-ethmoid fractures. JAMA Facial Plast Surg 2014; 16(4):284–9.

51. Rodriguez I, Uceda M, Lobato R, et al. Post-traumatic frontal sinus obliteration with calvarial bone dust and demineralized bone matrix: a long term prospective study and literature review. Int J Oral Maxillofac Surg 2013;42:71–6.

52. Luz J, Moraes R, D'Avila R, et al. Factors contributing to the surgical retreatment of mandibular fractures. Braz Oral Res 2012;27(3):258–65.

53. Biller J, Pletcher S, Goldberg A, et al. Complications and the time to repair of mandible fractures. Laryngoscope 2005;115:769–72.

54. Lucca M, Shastri K, McKenzie W, et al. Comparison of treatment outcomes associated with early versus late treatment of mandible fractures: a retrospective chart review and analysis. J Oral Maxillofac Surg 2010;68:2484–8.

55. Barker D, Oo K, Allak A, et al. Timing for repair of mandible fractures. Laryngoscope 2011;121: 1160–3.

56. Park Y. Bioabsorbable osteofixation for orthognathic surgery. Maxillofac Plast Reconstr Surg 2015;37(6): 1–9.

57. Yang L, Xu M, Jin X, et al. Complication of absorbable fixation in maxillofacial surgery: a meta-analysis. PLos One 2013;8(6):1–10.

58. Al-Moraissi E, Ellis E. Biodegradable and titanium osteosynthesis provide similar stability for orthognathic surgery. J Oral Maxillofac Surg 2015;73: 1795–808.

59. Meara DJ, Knoll M, Holmes J, et al. Fixation of LeFort I Osteotomies With Poly-DL-lactic acid mesh and ultrasonic welding—a new technique. J Oral Maxillofac Surg 2012;70:1139–44.

60. Bakelen N, Buijs G, Jansma J. Comparison of biodegradable and titanium fixation systems in maxillofacial surgery: a two-year multi-center randomized controlled trial. J Dent Res 2013;92(12):1100–5.

61. Vazquez-Morales D, Dyalram-Silverberg D, Lazow S, et al. Treatment of mandible fractures using resorbable plates with a mean of 3 weeks maxillomandibular fixation: a prospective study. Oral Surg Oral Med Oral Pathol Oral Radiol 2013;115:25–8.

62. Ahmed W, Bukhari S, Janjua O, et al. Bioresorbable versus titanium plates for mandibular fractures. J Coll Physicians Surg Pak 2013;23(7):480–3.

63. Lee H, Oh J, Kim S, et al. Comparison of titanium and biodegradable miniplates for fixation of mandibular fractures. J Oral Maxillofac Surg 2010;68:2065–9.

64. Leonhardt H, Demmrich A, Mueller A, et al. INION compared with titanium osteosynthesis: a prospective investigation of the treatment of mandibular fractures. Br J Oral Maxillofac Surg 2008;46:631–4.

Controversies in Traditional Oral and Maxillofacial Reconstruction

John S. Vorrasi, DDS*, Antonia Kolokythas, DDS, MS, FACS

KEYWORDS

- Reconstruction • Nonvascularized graft • Virtual surgical planning

KEY POINTS

- Traditional head and neck reconstruction has been revolutionized by advancements in preoperative surgical planning and expanded options for immediate reconstruction.
- Free tissue transfers to the head and neck have improved reconstructive options for earlier rehabilitation, function, speech, and swallowing.
- Advances in medicinal therapy including antiresorptive medications and head and neck radiation continually pose controversy regarding appropriate reconstruction.

INTRODUCTION

Historical treatments have given way to newer technologies as they relate to maxillofacial reconstruction, although controversies still exist regarding the most optimal treatment of certain conditions and in certain situations. Traditional reconstruction for maxillofacial surgery has largely relied on local vascularized tissues for soft tissue reconstruction and nonvascularized bone deposits for bony reconstruction. The paradigm shift has been to vascularized free tissue for larger soft tissue, bone, or composite defects in the head and neck and biologic agents such as bone morphogenic proteins (BMP), blood components such as platelet-rich plasma and fibrin, and tissue engineering. The successes of traditional reconstruction have been limited for large defects and may require multiple rounds of soft tissue rearrangements or bone grafting to obtain a satisfactory result. Currently, with more reconstruction options, patients have improved cosmetics, faster healing and dental rehabilitation, and preserved

or restored function. Dental implants have become reliable foundations for dental rehabilitation that have predictable behavior for osseointegration in the facial skeleton.

Advances in medicine, immunologic drugs, and antiangiogenic therapy, such as denosumab (Xgeva, Amgen, CA, USA), or bisphosphonates, such as zoledronic acid (Zometa, Novartis, Basel, Switzerland), have created a host of side effects and treatment considerations when planning patients for reconstruction. These side effects have become of published concern only over the last 20 years. These medications can dramatically alter the behavior of bone healing. The mechanism and interaction with reconstruction efforts is not entirely understood; however, the intravenous forms have been implicated in more destructive lesions and less predictable reconstructions or grafting. Most episodes of infection or bone destruction involve the mandible, but they rarely involve the entirety of the lower jaw, causing continuity defects.[1]

The addition of virtual surgical planning (VSP) and computer-aided design has revolutionized

The authors have nothing to disclose.
Department of Oral and Maxillofacial Surgery, University of Rochester Strong Memorial Hospital, Eastman Institute for Oral Health, 601 Elmwood Avenue, PO Box 705, Rochester, NY 14642, USA
* Corresponding author.
E-mail address: John_vorrasi@urmc.rochester.edu

Oral Maxillofacial Surg Clin N Am 29 (2017) 401–413
http://dx.doi.org/10.1016/j.coms.2017.06.003
1042-3699/17/Published by Elsevier Inc.

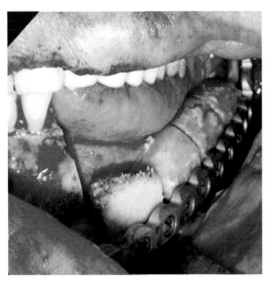

Fig. 1. Immediate reconstruction with anterior iliac crest bone graft to left mandible.

the specialty, and preoperative and intraoperative technology now allows patient-specific information to be readily available and interactive for reconstructive means and treatment planning. Traditional reconstruction, even for the experienced surgeon, required more estimation and intraoperative quick decision making than what preoperative VSP allows. Although costly, the advantages of preoperative computer engineering and planning provide insight to possible surgical obstacles and complications before the actual surgery.

MANDIBULAR RECONSTRUCTION

The incorporation of free tissue transfer into the armamentarium of reconstruction options has made reconstruction of large-span and complex defects more predictable and has allowed for earlier dental rehabilitation with dental implants. Tissue transfer has gone so far as to replace the

maxillary/mandibular complex in full-face transplants.[2,3] Controversy revolves around the extent of defects and need for vascularized bone grafts. Our specialty literature cites 9 cm as a critical length[4]; however, traditional reconstruction sources from the orthopedic literature argue that 6 cm is the maximum extent of free grafting. The significant amount of tissue vascularity and reduced load requirements of the head and neck make larger span defects amenable to free grafting; however, angiogenesis and osteogenesis may be compromised with larger spans (**Fig. 1**). Schlieve and colleagues[5] reported several benign reconstructions with successful immediate nonvascularized bone in defects greater than 6 cm (**Fig. 2**). More recent orthopedic evidence challenges the 6-cm maximum for nonvascularized bone reconstruction as unfounded and unsupported in literature.[6] Further biologic studies need to be used to examine the interface of bony union and stresses in nonvascularized versus vascularized tissue.

Controversy also exists around which grafting/reconstruction technique is used based on central, lateral, hemimandible, or combinations. Anterior mandibular defects will arguably constitute an absolute indication for reconstruction using vascularized bone.[7,8] Because of multiple osteotomies required to contour the bone, vascularized bone such as the fibula should be considered the first choice for reconstruction of anterior or large defects (**Figs. 3** and **4**). Dental implants in vascularized and nonvascularized neo-mandible are now the standard for dental rehabilitation in patients with reconstruction (**Figs. 5–8**).

MAXILLARY RECONSTRUCTION

Maxillary and midfacial defects traditionally required implants or obturators to support soft tissue. Surgical intervention involving local tissues was originally described by von Langenbeck in the 19th century.[9] Flaps from nasal septum,

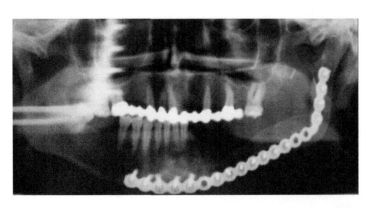

Fig. 2. Panoramic radiograph of approximately 8-cm left mandibular reconstruction with anterior iliac crest bone graft.

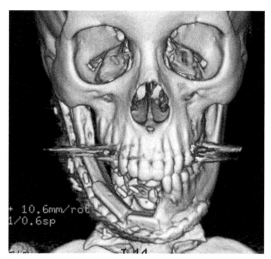

Fig. 3. Fibula reconstruction of right lateral and anterior mandible defect.

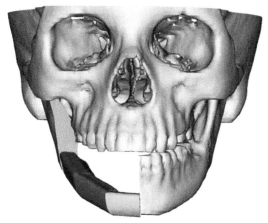

Fig. 4. VSP for fibula reconstruction of right lateral and anterior mandible.

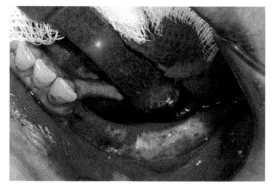

Fig. 5. Six months after anterior iliac crest graft placement.

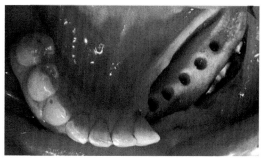

Fig. 6. Dental implant preparation of left mandibular reconstruction.

tongue, cheeks, pharynx, turbinates, scalp, and neck were commonly used for most cases.[10–12] The 1970s and 1980s brought larger myocutaneous soft tissue pedicled flaps into the lower face, midface, and intraoral reconstruction arena.[13] Brown and colleagues[14] in 2000 described both the vertical and horizontal defect after surgical procedures usually for tumor resection or pathology. The standardized description of defects may suggest components involved but does not dictate reconstructive means. Controversy traditionally revolves around use of local, regional, or distant tissue transfer to cover the defect or fabrication of a prosthesis to restore the defect. Recently, Futran and Mendez[15] reviewed historical and contemporary approaches to midface reconstruction highlighting the incorporation of multiple techniques in some cases, be it combining microvascular, local flaps, or prosthetics.[15] Theoretically, placement of an obturator could manage midface defects as an immediate reconstruction; however, hygiene, patient comfort, ease of use, and large resections involving zygoma and orbital floor result in compromised cosmetics, compromised function, and questionable patient compliance (**Figs. 9–12**).[16,17] Proximity of nasal and sinus cavities complicate nonvascularized grafting techniques and limited soft tissue envelopes.

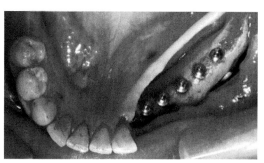

Fig. 7. Dental implants placed in left anterior iliac crest bone graft.

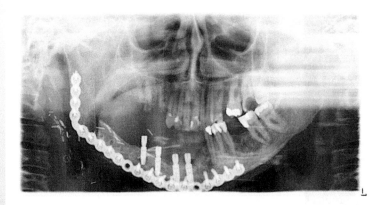

Fig. 8. Dental implant rehabilitation after right mandible resection and fibula reconstruction.

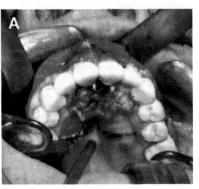
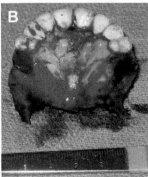

Fig. 9. (*A*) Anterior maxillectomy for squamous cell carcinoma of anterior gingiva. (*B*) Anterior maxillectomy for squamous cell carcinoma of anterior gingiva.

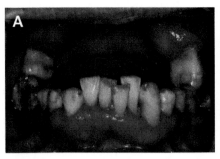
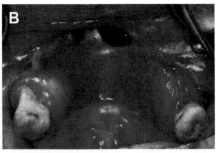

Fig. 10. (*A*) Resulting anterior maxillary defect after resection. (*B*) Resulting anterior maxillary defect after resection.

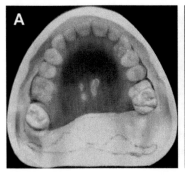
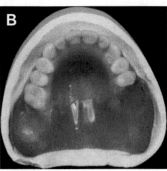

Fig. 11. (*A*) Maxillary obturator after anterior maxillectomy. (*B*) Maxillary obturator after anterior maxillectomy.

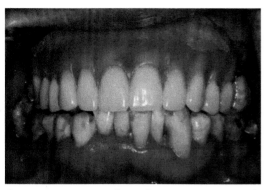

Fig. 12. Anterior maxillary obturator approximately 4 weeks after resection.

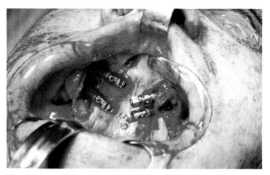

Fig. 14. Maxillary reconstruction using zygomatic implants. Cross-arch stability achieved with 4 or quad zygomatic implants.

Adequate maxillofacial prosthetic rehabilitation hopes to ensure proper form, swallowing, speech, and function, but traditionally this has been lacking. Vascularized osteocutaneous reconstructions have become the ideal composite reconstruction option to restore maxillary function using dental implants with fixed prosthetics.

VSP and reconstruction planning can be used to rehabilitate large composite defects with bone, soft tissue reconstruction, and immediate dental implant placement. Zygomatic implants have gained popularity, although they are costly for severely resorbed maxillary ridges and postsurgical maxillectomies.[18] These methods require cross-arch stability either with bar attachments or bilateral placement to minimize micromovement and implant failure[19,20] (**Fig. 13**). Chemically treated implant surfaces and more biocompatible titanium hardware are recent advancements in alloplastic materials (**Fig. 14**). These treatments allow more predictable reconstructions with long-term use.

RADIATION AND MEDICATION IMPLICATIONS ON RECONSTRUCTION

Previous radiation treatment to the head and neck further complicates wound bed vascularity, soft tissue/muscle contracture, and acceptance of

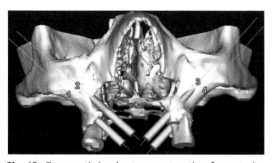

Fig. 13. Zygomatic implant reconstruction for anterior maxillary defect.

reconstruction tissue, vascularized or nonvascularized. Traditional radiation therapy is responsible for high rates of local tissue destruction and associated complications (eg, reduced salivary gland function, myositis, fibrosis, and oral mucositis). With the advent of intensity-modulated radiotherapy and image-guided radiation therapy, collateral damage to surrounding tissue is minimized; however, the resulting targeted tissue environment is hypoxic, fibrotic, and hypovascular. Traditional reconstruction in head and neck postradiation patients largely relies on local vascular beds for angiogenesis or pedicled soft tissues such as pectoralis, temporalis, or latissimus dorsi muscle. A study in 1984 by Lukash and colleagues[21] found significantly lower success in long bone reconstruction procedures of irradiated rabbits. Survival was improved with vascularized nonirradiated tissue surrounding the nonvascularized bone grafts. These conventional options have been replaced mostly with biologics and vascularized free tissue transfers as a reconstruction option for patients; however, vascularized tissue transfer in irradiated patients consistently complicates the reconstruction success with high rates of soft tissue dehiscence and nonhealing wounds.[22] In advanced osteoradionecrosis cases, vascularized tissue may be the only viable option for sufficient reconstruction.[23]

Antiangiogenetic medications (denosumab; Xgeva, Prolia, Amgen, CA, USA) and bisphosphonate medications (zoledronic acid; Zometa or pamidronate; Aredia, Novartis, Basel, Switzerland) widely used for various conditions such as multiple myeloma and metastatic cancers have further complicated reconstruction treatment planning, as the genetics and biologic behavior of bone at a cellular level is affected (**Fig. 15**). The resulting systemic effects have raised questions regarding the use of traditional nonvas cularized bone grafts in treated areas. Anecdotal evidence suggests that with proper soft tissue management and support,

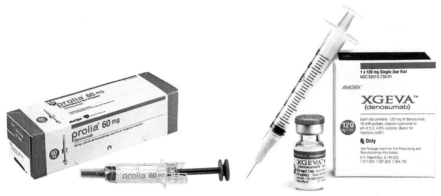

Fig. 15. Antiangiogenetic medications used to prevent metastatic disease spread are of particular interest recently with cases of maxillofacial side effects. (*Courtesy of* Amgen, Thousand Oaks, CA; with permission.)

nonvascularized bone grafting may be a viable option.[24] Long-term results with newer medications such as denosumab are not yet established to allow guidelines (**Fig. 16**). According to the most recent update by the American Association of Oral and Maxillofacial Surgeons in 2014, newer medications such as denosumab may have similar effects to bone biology as intravenous bisphosphonates.[25–27] Although the risk is low, clear understanding and communication to patients regarding risk of graft failure or loss should be detailed and well documented.

AUTOGENOUS GRAFTING VERSUS BIOLOGICS FOR MAXILLOFACIAL RECONSTRUCTION

In the late 1990s, the use of biologics such as platelet-rich plasma (PRP) and BMP gained momentum by the initial work of Marx and colleagues[28] and Moghadam and colleagues[29] The concept of enhanced grafting techniques with adjunctive biologics aimed to:

1. Reduce the time required from grafting or reconstruction to rehabilitation
2. Reduce donor site morbidity
3. Improve bone quantity and quality
4. Enhance soft tissue healing

Controversy revolved around the clinical efficacy of these products and the cost-effective nature of products that may warrant an $800 to $10,000 price tag. The plastic surgery literature has promoted PRP as a soft tissue adjunct; however, studies such as the one by Gerard and colleagues[30] were not able to improve mandibular grafts placed into dogs; however, the healing time was enhanced. These conclusions were echoed in a rabbit study by Butterfield and colleagues.[31] Meta-analysis and systemic reviews failed to show consistent efficacy with PRP use in bone grafting and dental implant healing. As an adjunctive material to autogenous grafting, BMP and PRP anecdotally seem to improve volume and healing.

Bone Morphogenic Protein

BMP was approved by the US Food and Drug Administration for orthopedic and spine cases in

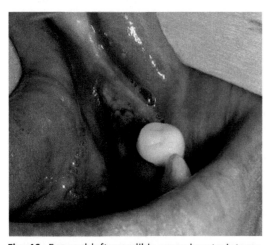

Fig. 16. Exposed left mandible secondary to intravenous bisphosphonate, zoledronic acid (Zometa).

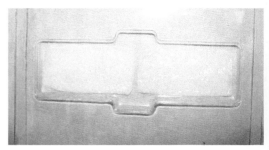

Fig. 17. BMP-2 product on collagen membranes ready for incorporation to graft.

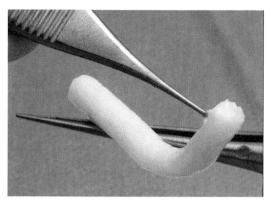

Fig. 18. Cadavaric nerve graft used for pathologic resection nerve reconnection or traumatic nerve disruptions.

2002. The use of BMP has been controversial because of lawsuits regarding bone overgrowth, possible increased cancer risk, and several other side effects. Despite these allegations, in 2007, Medtronic (Minneapolis, MN) INFUSE (rhBMP-2) was approved by the US Food and Drug Administration for dental procedures to enhance bone growth in defects (**Fig. 17**). BMP-2 is important for the development of bone and cartilage in the transforming growth factor-β family. The protein is osteoinductive and promotes osteoblast differentiation. Several studies found improved bone volume in oral bone defects and alveolar cleft defects; however, there is no evidence supporting complete replacement of traditional autogenous grafting.[32–34] Autogenous bone volume needed for mandibular reconstruction has typically

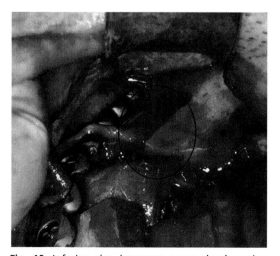

Fig. 19. Inferior alveolar nerve neurorrhaphy using collagen conduit. *Circle* indicates collagen conduit connection with native proximal inferior nerve post resection.

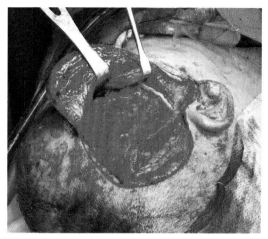

Fig. 20. Preparation of a temporalis myofascial flap for a palatal defect.

been 1 mL^3 for each centimeter of bone lost. With newer therapies such as BMP incorporation, the osteoinductive properties require less autogenous bone harvesting for defects amenable to free graft reconstruction.

Peripheral Nerves

Peripheral nerve reconstruction has advanced beyond autogenous grafting incorporating the use of allograft nerves (collagen nerve conduits) and cadaveric nerve interpositional grafts (**Figs. 18** and **19**). The goals of nerve reconstruction include inert biologic activity or resorbability, protection of nerve stumps from scar or inflammation, and guidance regenerating axons to connect along the gap.[35] Recent studies by Lohmeyer and colleagues[36] suggest that bovine collagen conduits can provide satisfactory sensory return with defects less than 12 mm. There is also evidence that the traditional 12-month period for

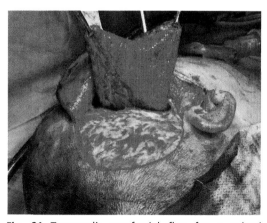

Fig. 21. Temporalis myofascial flap for a palatal defect.

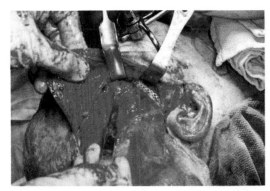

Fig. 22. Preplate and osteotomy of zygomatic arch to allow muscle flap rotation.

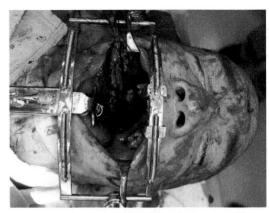

Fig. 24. Temporalis myofascial flap for a palatal defect with oral pull through.

nerve recovery may be more of a dynamic process lasting greater than a year rather than at a static endpoint for recovery.[37] Synthetic polyester materials and chitosan, a refined glycosaminoglycan, are contemporary grafting materials available for nerve reconstruction.[38]

SOFT TISSUE RECONSTRUCTION

Head and neck soft tissue reconstruction poses many complexities in restoring form, function, and esthetics. As in composite defects and bone defects, free tissue transfer has taken a major role in large soft tissue reconstructions and composite defects. Pedicled flaps for reconstruction are still used frequently with large head and neck reconstruction and in patients incapable of obtaining free tissue transfers (**Figs. 20–24**). The pectoralis major myocutaneous flap still maintains itself as the workhorse reconstruction option outside of free tissue transfer.[39–41] Additional local and regional tissue transfers such as temporalis, cervicofacial advancements, submental island, and platysma flaps all have a role in the reconstruction ladder and should be considered as options (**Figs. 25** and **26**). Free tissue transfer

has become the primary reconstruction option in many institutions for larger defects of the head and neck and will be addressed further in the article in this issue.

TECHNOLOGY ADVANCEMENTS

Traditional means of planning complex reconstruction was done intraoperatively. Preoperative dental models or facial models (facial moulage) may give insight for functional occlusion concerns or cosmetic soft tissue drapes; however, the incorporation of technology in preoperative planning has made immediate reconstruction, with composite free tissue transfers or custom implants, a real option for patients (**Figs. 27–30**).[42–44] The controversy lies around when to use this emerging technology.

This technology has been most useful in the neurosurgical and head and neck specialties. Imaging software capable of integrating 3-dimensional computed tomography units called *Hounsfield units* into stereolithic products was not available until the 1990s.[45] This technology has evolved into user-friendly, accurate, representative

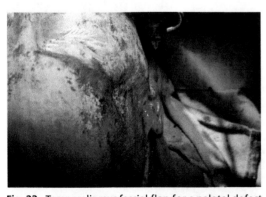

Fig. 23. Temporalis myofascial flap for a palatal defect with resulting temporal hollowing requiring implant placement.

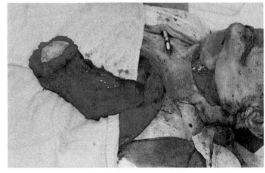

Fig. 25. Pectoralis myocutaneous flap for reconstruction of a lateral mandible and floor-of-mouth pathologic resection.

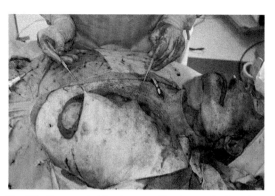

Fig. 26. Prepared skin closure after harvest of pectoralis major flap.

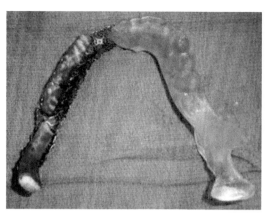

Fig. 28. Intraoperative use of stereolithic model and prebent hardware with anterior iliac crest and costochondral graft.

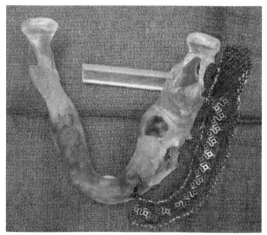

Fig. 27. Preoperative planning for benign tumor resection and immediate hardware and graft reconstruction.

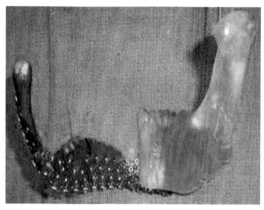

Fig. 29. A mirrored native stereolithic mandible can give accurate width and condylar height for immediate reconstruction.

Fig. 30. Panorex radiograph after left mandible reconstruction.

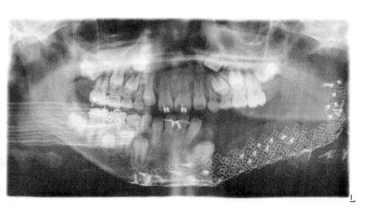

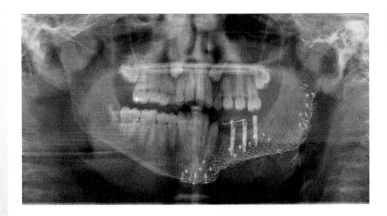

Fig. 31. Panorex radiograph after consolidation of bone graft and dental implant placement.

models and preoperative computer Web sessions that predict and guide any complicated maxillofacial reconstruction. Cost for many institutions and practitioners has been prohibitive with a high price tag attached to the models and online engineering sessions. In-house computer-aided design/computer-aided manufacturing is slowly evolving with more 3-dimensional printers, interactive low-cost software, and precision intraoperative products.[46] Workflow algorithms can now incorporate in-office cone beam computed tomography scans and digital impressions to preplan maxillofacial surgical cases. Computed tomography navigation can be used for intraoperative accuracy to assess 3-dimensional positioning in real time. Reconstructions are more accurate with VSP preoperative planning including prefabricated hardware, patient-specific models, and osteotomy guides.[47] Dental implant reconstructions have become more predictable with grafted bone, and evidence-based practices support implants in reconstructed areas (**Figs. 30–36**).

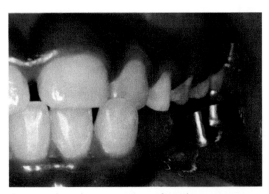

Fig. 32. Clinical presentation of implant reconstruction in final stages of dental rehabilitation.

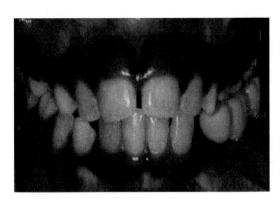

Fig. 34. Final restored left posterior occlusion.

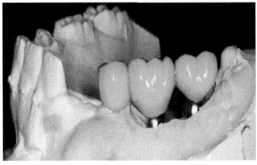

Fig. 33. Laboratory presentation of implant reconstruction in final stages of dental rehabilitation.

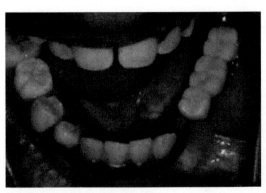

Fig. 35. Final dental restoration.

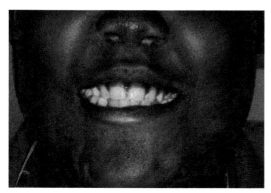

Fig. 36. Restoration restores appropriate lip support and occlusion.

DISTRACTION OSTEOGENESIS

Distraction osteogenesis was developed in the early 20th century as a method of inductive bone growth without grafting. It was not until 1973 that these principles were translated to the maxillofacial skeleton of a canine and eventually a human mandible in 1992.[48,49] This method has been further adapted to transport segments that are sections of native maxilla or mandible to help support a larger volume of periosteal stretching.[50,51] Smaller distractor devices specific for dentoalveolar reconstruction can be completely maintained within the oral cavity and successfully improve alveolar ridge height (**Fig. 37**). There is controversy as to whether distraction osteogenesis is a more effective means of skeletal expansion or reconstruction compared with traditional reconstruction or grafting. There is anecdotal evidence that progressive control of the soft tissue envelope and reduced nerve paresthesias or paralysis can be achieved more predictably with distraction; however, this has yet to be consistently proven.[52] Distraction in the oral cavity

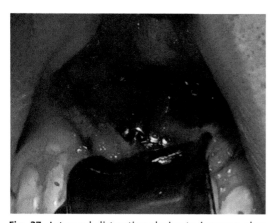

Fig. 37. Intraoral distraction device to improve alveolar height in the anterior maxilla.

may add possible options to the reconstruction armamentarium.

SUMMARY

Complex head and neck reconstruction has significantly improved over the last 2 to 3 decades, although controversies still exist. Many patients are able to obtain immediate reconstruction for conditions or defects that allows earlier rehabilitation and better quality of life. Host immunity, history of radiation or antiresorptive medication use, diagnosis of tumor/pathologic condition, prognosis, and condition of soft tissue recipient bed, play critical roles in treatment planning patients. It is important for each patient to be evaluated critically for candidacy for advanced or traditional reconstruction means. Computer-aided surgical planning or VSP and advances in free tissue transfer and microvascular reconstruction are arguably the most significant changes in head and neck reconstruction in the last 2 decades.

REFERENCES

1. Marx RE. Reconstruction of defects caused by bisphosphonate-induced osteonecrosis of the jaws. J Oral Maxillofac Surg 2009;67(5 Suppl): 107–19.
2. Siemionow M, Papay F, Alam D, et al. Near-total human face transplantation for a severely disfigured patient in the USA. Lancet 2009;374(9685):203–9.
3. Lantieri L. Face transplant: a paradigm change in facial reconstruction. J Craniofac Surg 2012;23(1): 250–3.
4. Pogrel MA, Podlesh S, Anthony JP, et al. A comparison of vascularized and nonvascularized bone grafts for reconstruction of mandibular continuity defects. J Oral Maxillofac Surg 1997;55(11): 1200–6.
5. Schlieve T, Hull W, Miloro M, et al. Is immediate reconstruction of the mandible with nonvascularized bone graft following resection of benign pathology a viable treatment option? J Oral Maxillofac Surg 2015;73(3):541–9.
6. Allsopp BJ, Hunter-Smith DJ, Rozen WM. Vascularized versus nonvascularized bone grafts: what is the evidence? Clin Orthop Relat Res 2016;474(5): 1319–27.
7. Takushima A, Harii K, Asato H, et al. Mandibular reconstruction using microvascular free flaps: a statistical analysis of 178 cases. Plast Reconstr Surg 2001;108:1555–63.
8. Cordeiro PG, Disa JJ, Hidalgo DA, et al. Reconstruction of the mandible with osseous free flaps: a 10-year experience with 150 consecutive patients. Plast Reconstr Surg 1999;104:1314–20.

9. Von Langenbeck B. Die Uranoplastik Mittelst Ablosung Des Mucoes-Periostalen Gaumenuberzuges. 1861. Arch Klin Chir 2 1861;205–87.

10. Edgerton MT, DeVito RV. Closure of palatal defects by means of hinged nasal septum flap. Plast Reconstr Surg 1963;31–33:537–40.

11. Chambers RG, Jaques DA, Mahoney WD. Tongue flaps for intraoral reconstruction. Am J Surg 1969; 118:783–6.

12. Komisar A, Lawson W. A compendenium of intraoral flaps. Head Neck Surg 1985;8:91–7.

13. Ariyan S. The pectoralis major myocutaneous flap: a versatile flap for reconstruction in the head and neck. Plast Reconstr Surg 1979;63:73–81.

14. Brown JS, Rogers SN, McNally DN, et al. A modified classification for the maxillectomy defect. Head Neck 2000;22:17–26.

15. Futran N, Mendez E. Developments in reconstruction of midface and maxilla. Lancet 2006;7:249–58.

16. Brown KE. Peripheral considerations in improving obturator retention. J Prosthet Dent 1968;20:176–81.

17. Funk GF, Arcuri MR, Frodel H. Functional dental rehabilitation of massive palatomaxillary defects: cases requiring free tissue transfer and osseointegrated implants. Head Neck 1998;20:38–48.

18. Malevez C, Daelemans P, Adriaenssens P, et al. Use of zygomatic implants to deal with resorbed posterior maxillae. Periodontol 2000 2003;33:82–9.

19. Meredith N. Assessment of implant stability as a prognostic determinant. Int J Prosthodont 1998;11: 491–501.

20. Brunski JB. Biomaterials and biomechanics in dental implant design. Int J Oral Maxillofac Implants 1988; 3:85–97.

21. Lukash FN, Zingaro EA, Salig J. The survival of free nonvascularized bone grafts in irradiated areas by wrapping in muscle flaps. Plast Reconstr Surg 1984;74(6):783–8.

22. Maurer P, Eckert A, Kriwalsky M, et al. Scope and limitations of methods of mandibular reconstruction: a long-term follow-up. Br J Oral Maxillofac Surg 2010;48(2):100–4.

23. Rice N, Polyzois I, Ekanayake K, et al. The management of osteoradionecrosis of the jaws–a review. Surgeon 2015;13(2):101–9.

24. Rahim I, Salt S, Heliotis M. Successful long-term mandibular reconstruction and rehabilitation using non-vascularised autologous bone graft and recombinant human BMP-7 with subsequent endosseous implant in a patient with bisphosphonate-related osteonecrosis of the jaw. Br J Oral Maxillofac Surg 2015;53(9):870–4.

25. Fizazi K, Carducci M, Smith M, et al. Denosumab versus zoledronic acid for treatment of bone metastases in men with castration-resistant prostate cancer: a randomised, double-blind study. Lancet 2010;377:813.

26. Stopeck A, Body JJ, Fujiwara Y, et al. Denosumab versus zolendronic acid for the treatment of breast cancer patients with bone metastases: results of a randomized phase 3 study. Eur J Cancer Supplements 2009;7(European Journal Cancer supplements):2.

27. Ruggiero S, Dodson T, Fantasia T, et al. American Association of oral and maxillofacial surgeons position paper on medication-related osteonecrosis of the jaw—2014 update. J Oral Maxillofac Surg 2014;72:1938–56.

28. Marx R, Carlson E, Eichstaedt R, et al. Platelet-rich plasma: growth factor enhancement for bone grafts. Oral Surg Oral Med Oral Pathol Oral Radiol Endod 1998;85:638–46.

29. Moghadam HG, Urist MR, Sandor GKB, et al. Successful mandibular reconstruction using a BMP bioimplant. J Craniofac Surg 2001;12(2):119–27.

30. Gerard D, Carlson ER, Gotcher JE, et al. Effects of platelet-rich plasma at the cellular level on healing of autologous bone-grafted mandibular defects in dogs. J Oral Maxillofac Surg 2007;65(4):721–7.

31. Butterfield KJ, Bennett J, Gronowicz G, et al. Effect of platelet-rich plasma with autogenous bone graft for maxillary sinus augmentation in a rabbit model. J Oral Maxillofac Surg 2005;63(3):370–6.

32. Van Hout W, Van der Molen A, Breugem C, et al. Reconstruction of the alveolar cleft: can growth factor-aided tissue engineering replace autologous bone grafting? A literature review and systematic review of results obtained with bone morphogenetic protein-2. Clin Oral Investig 2011;15(3):297–303.

33. Boyne P. Application of bone morphogenetic proteins in the treatment of clinical oral and maxillofacial osseous defects. J Bone Joint Surg Am 2001;83-A-(Suppl 1(Pt 2)):S146–50.

34. Herford AS. rhBMP-2 as an option for reconstructing mandibular continuity defects. J Oral Maxillofac Surg 2009;67(12):2679–84.

35. Kim DH, Han K, Tiel RL, et al. Surgical outcomes of 654 ulnar nerve lesions. J Neurosurg 2003;98: 993–1004.

36. Lohmeyer JA, Kern Y, Schmauss D, et al. Prospective clinical study on digital nerve repair with collagen nerve conduits and review of literature. J Reconstr Microsurg 2014;30(4):227–34.

37. Schmauss D, Finck T, Liodaki E, et al. Is nerve regeneration after reconstruction with collagen nerve conduits terminated after 12 months? the long-term follow-up of two prospective clinical studies. J Reconstr Microsurg 2014;30(8):561–8.

38. Neubrech F, Heider S, Harhaus L, et al. Chitosan nerve tube for primary repair of traumatic sensory nerve lesions of the hand without a gap: study protocol for a randomized controlled trial. Trials 2016; 17:48.

39. Rudes M, Bilić M, Jurlina M, et al. Pectoralis major myocutaneous flap in the reconstructive surgery of

the head and neck–our experience. Coll Antropol 2012;36(Suppl 2):137–42.

40. Vartanian JG, Carvalho AL, Carvalho SM, et al. Pectoralis major and other myofascial/myocutaneous flaps in head and neck cancer reconstruction: experience with 437 cases at a single institution. Head Neck 2004;26(12):1018–23.

41. Milenović A, Virag M, Uglesić V, et al. The pectoralis major flap in head and neck reconstruction: first 500 patients. J Craniomaxillofac Surg 2006; 34(6):340–3.

42. Wilde F, Cornelius CP, Schramm A. Computer-assisted mandibular reconstruction using a patient-specific reconstruction plate fabricated with computer-aided design and manufacturing techniques. Craniomaxillofac Trauma Reconstr 2014; 7(2):158–66.

43. Kääriäinen M, Kuuskeri M, Gremoutis G, et al. Utilization of three-dimensional computer-aided preoperative virtual planning and manufacturing in maxillary and mandibular reconstruction with a microvascular fibula flap. J Reconstr Microsurg 2016;32(2):137–41.

44. Parthasarathy J. 3D modeling, custom implants and its future perspectives in craniofacial surgery. Ann Maxillofac Surg 2014;4(1):9–18.

45. Vannier MW, Marsh JL, Warren JO. Three dimensional CT reconstruction images for craniofacial surgical planning and evaluation. Radiology 1984; 150(1):179–84.

46. Numajiri T, Nakamura H, Sowa Y, et al. Low-cost design and manufacturing of surgical guides for mandibular reconstruction using a fibula. Plast Reconstr Surg Glob Open 2016;4(7):e805.

47. Chang EI, Jenkins MP, Patel SA, et al. Long-term operative outcomes of preoperative computed tomography-guided virtual surgical planning for osteocutaneous free flap mandible reconstruction. Plast Reconstr Surg 2016;137(2):619–23.

48. Snyder CC, Levine GA, Swanson HM, et al. Mandibular lengthening by gradual distraction. Preliminary report. Plast Reconstr Surg 1973;51(5):506–8.

49. McCarthy JG. The role of distraction osteogenesis in the reconstruction of the mandible in unilateral craniofacial microsomia. Clin Plast Surg 1994; 21(4):625–31.

50. Pereira AR, Montezuma N, Oliveira L, et al. Immediate reconstruction of large full-thickness segmental anterior maxillary defect with bone transport. Craniomaxillofac Trauma Reconstr 2016;9(4):305–12.

51. Baek SH, Kim NY, Paeng JY, et al. Trifocal distraction-compression osteosynthesis in conjunction with passive self-ligating brackets for the reconstruction of a large bony defect and multiple missing teeth. Am J Orthod Dentofacial Orthop 2008;133(4): 601–11.

52. Kloukos D, Fudalej P, Sequeira-Byron P, et al. Maxillary distraction osteogenesis versus orthognathic surgery for cleft lip and palate patients. Cochrane Database Syst Rev 2016;(9):CD010403.

Controversies in Microvascular Maxillofacial Reconstruction

Adam P. Fagin, DMD, MD, Daniel Petrisor, DMD, MD, FACS*

KEYWORDS

- Microvascular • Postoperative monitoring • Anticoagulant • Vasoconstrictor • Implantable Doppler

KEY POINTS

- Postoperative monitoring of free flaps with an implantable Doppler probe increases overall flap survival rates and flap salvage rates compared with clinical examination.
- Intraoperative use of vasopressors, ephedrine and phenylephrine, is not associated with an increase in free flap complication rates.
- Postoperative use of norepinephrine or dopamine does not compromise free flap perfusion or increase free flap complication rates, but norepinephrine is associated with less tachycardia.
- The use of anticoagulants, dextran, prostaglandin E_1, aspirin, low-molecular-weight heparin, and unfractionated heparin in the postoperative period does not improve flap survival as compared with no anticoagulant.

INTRODUCTION

The effectiveness and reliability of microvascular reconstruction for large defects in the head and neck is no longer disputed. Many large cohort studies have reported overall success rates greater than 95%.[1–4] However, many controversies still persist in the ideal perioperative management of patients undergoing free tissue transfer. The authors selected three controversial issues that have recently received significant attention in the literature: (1) the optimal method of postoperative monitoring, (2) the use of vasoconstrictors in the perioperative period, and (3) the use of anticoagulants in the postoperative period. Recommendations on each of these controversies based on a review of the current literature are discussed.

POSTOPERATIVE MONITORING
Introduction

Free tissue transfer with microvascular anastomosis is now an established and reliable reconstructive option for major tissue defects. Success rates of large samples are routinely reported more than 95%.[1–4] An integral part of this level of reliability is postoperative monitoring. Take back rates reported in the literature range from 6% to 15% with salvage rates once revision occurs ranging from 46% to 94%.[1–8] The most common cause of flap failure in the early postoperative setting is vascular compromise, typically as a result of venous or arterial thrombosis, compression secondary to hematoma, or kinking of the pedicle. In most cases these mechanical failures are surgically reversible if the compromise is noted

The authors have nothing to disclose.
Department of Oral and Maxillofacial Surgery, Oregon Health & Science University, 3181 Southwest Sam Jackson Park Road, Portland, OR 97239, USA
* Corresponding author.
E-mail address: petrisor@ohsu.edu

oralmaxsurgery.theclinics.com

in a timely fashion and the patient is taken back to the operating room for re-exploration and revision. The time sensitive nature of the issue is why postoperative monitoring is such an important aspect of microvascular reconstruction.

Methods of Monitoring

The original monitoring strategy is the clinical examination, which classically involves several subjective measures including flap color, capillary refill, turgidity, pin pick, and external Doppler. This method also relies heavily on the expertise of the examiner and the ability of the examiner to visualize the flap. In the modern medical system with resident duty hour restrictions, it is no longer feasible to conduct hourly examinations of the flap by physicians at many institutions. This leaves these critical inspections to be primarily performed by nursing staff who then decide to notify the resident, fellow, or attending surgeon if warning signs are present. Additionally, in head and neck reconstruction flaps are often partially or completely buried, which increases the difficulty or prohibits this form of monitoring entirely.

Other forms of monitoring have been proposed, which can fundamentally be broken down into two strategies: monitoring of flow into or out of the pedicle, or monitoring of metabolites or oxygen content of the pedicle itself.[8–12] The most widely used alternative to conventional monitoring is the Cook-Swartz Doppler probe, which is capable of measuring flow through an individual vessel. The device is implanted during surgery and attached to the venous anastomosis, arterial anastomosis, or both. The implantable Doppler helps address the two biggest shortcomings of the clinical examination: it provides an objective measure and it is capable of surveilling buried flaps. As with any device, one of its biggest pitfalls is the potential for it

to malfunction, providing false-positive or false-negative information. The ideal form of postoperative monitoring would be inexpensive, objective, implantable, and reliably performed by a wide range of personnel.

Implantable Doppler

The implantable Cook-Swartz Doppler was first described in 1988 by Swartz and colleagues.[10] It consists of a 20-MHz ultrasonic probe mounted on a silicone cuff. The cuff is adjustable based on vessel size and can accommodate vessels ranging from 1 mm to 4 mm. The cuff is seated onto the desired vessel during surgery and the ultrasonic probe then lies against the vessel wall. A wire attached to the probe then exits the cuff and the patient. This wire is then attached to another disposable wire, which plugs into the ultrasonic device monitor. Removal of the device is done externally by pulling on the implanted wire, which releases from the retained silicone cuff. This can be done anytime during the postoperative period without risk of damaging the vessel or anastomosis. As a result, the inadvertent removal of these probes can occur even when care is taken to secure them, which can lead to an erroneous absence of signal. In the authors experience the inadvertent removal of these devices is prevented by leaving sufficient slack in the primary wire and the application of appropriate dressing to secure the wire postoperatively.

Since its inception many studies have evaluated the effectiveness of monitoring with the Cook-Swartz Doppler.[1–3,5,6] In the last 8 years studies evaluating greater than 150 anastomoses either exclusively in the head and neck[1,3,6] or including the head and neck[2] are summarized in **Table 1**. These studies reported sensitivities between 65% and 100% and specificities between 98%

Table 1
Summary of sensitivity, specificity, re-exploration rate, salvage success rate, and overall flap survival rate for flaps undergoing monitoring with implantable Doppler

Study	# Anastomoses	Probe Location	Sensitivity (%)	Specificity (%)	Re-exploration Rate (%)	Salvage Success Rate (%)	Overall Flap Survival Rate (%)
Guillemaud et al,[3] 2008	369	Arterial/venous	65.80	98.20	12.50	81.60	98.10
Paydar et al,[46] 2014	169	Venous	100	98.70	11.20	94.70	98.20
Schmulder et al,[2] 2011	259	Venous	100	98.70	13.90	87.88	96.14
Wax,[1] 2014	1142	Arterial	87	99	6.10	61	97.60

Data from Refs.[1–3]

and 99%. Re-exploration rates have ranged between 6% and 14% and salvage success rates between 61% and 95% resulting in reported overall flap survival rates between 96% and 98%.

The largest of these trials exclusive to the head and neck was a prospective review of 1142 anastomoses by Wax.[1] When compared with the other reports in **Table 1**, this report seems to be an outlier in two categories: salvage rates 6% compared with 11% to 14%, and salvage success rates 61% compared with 81% to 95%. Importantly, however, these lower salvage rates did not result in a lower overall flap survival rate, reported at 98%. The author of the report hypothesizes that this is because of their use of the implantable Doppler as an intraoperative and postoperative monitor. In their center, the anastomosis is performed before the flap inset, which allows up to 2 hours of intraoperative anastomosis monitoring before leaving the operating room. If there is any alteration in the signal during this time the problem can be evaluated during the initial procedure. In the report, 134 anastomoses (11.7%) demonstrated signal alteration intraoperatively that was addressed before the end of the initial operation. Combining these two categories, Doppler signal alteration resulting in revision before leaving the operation and after leaving the operating room gives a total revision rate of 17.8%, which is closer to the rates of revision in other reports referenced in **Table 1**. Wax considered this an added benefit of performing the anastomosis first with placement of the Doppler probe, which resulted in fewer take backs to the operating room while maintaining a comparable rate of overall flap survival of 98%. This may also help to explain their lower overall salvage rate, 61%, because these complications recognized with intraoperative monitoring were not included in their salvage success rate. One of the major drawbacks of the implantable Doppler is the potential for false positives potentially resulting in unnecessary take backs to the operating room. Wax also reported that in the eight patients who had false-positive absent Doppler signals, all were evaluated with a clinical examination by the attending surgeon, none were reoperated on, and all survived without further complication.

Location of the implantable Doppler probe, on the vein or artery, has been the subject of debate. A logical argument can be made that venous monitoring provides earlier and more sensitive warning because it detects a problem sooner when either the vein or artery becomes compromised. In contrast, arterial monitoring does not alarm until the flap is fully engorged.[2,6] Authors who argue for arterial monitoring report a higher false-

positive rate with venous monitoring. Guillemaud and colleagues[3] reviewed 369 anastomoses monitored by either venous or arterial placement. Thirty-one cases demonstrated altered signal, six of which were false positives, and five of those were noted to be with venous monitoring. Wax[1] also supports arterial Doppler placement in the head and neck given its increased stability because of the inherent difficulty with immobilization of this area in the postoperative period. Recently, this article's main author has used venous couplers with implanted Doppler probes contained within the coupler itself. This provides a more robust connection between the probe and the monitor's wires, which helps to address the biggest downside to venous monitoring. In the author's practice implantable arterial Doppler placement and venous coupler monitoring are routinely performed for up to 7 days postoperatively.

The data presented in **Table 1** support the use of the implantable Doppler probe as an effective method of monitoring in the postoperative period, but how does it compare with the classic clinical examination? A large meta-analysis by Han and colleagues[5] attempted to address this specific question. It included five retrospective studies and a total of 1995 flaps. Of note these studies all included flaps in the head and neck but were not exclusive to the head and neck. The overall flap success rate was significantly greater in the flaps that were monitored by implantable Doppler versus clinical examination (96.8% vs 93.5%; $P = .001$). In addition, the flap salvage rate was significantly greater in the flaps that were monitored by implantable Doppler versus clinical examination (78.9% vs 60.0%; $P = .006$). Also of note, the false-positive rate of the implantable Doppler was reported between 8% and 17% compared with no false positives reported by the clinical examination. This meta-analysis provides strong evidence that implantable Doppler monitoring improves overall flap survival and salvage rates with an acceptable increase in false positives.

The implantable Doppler adds an additional cost to the operation. A Canadian study by Poder and Fortier[7] performed a cost analysis of the implantable Doppler. These authors reported that the Doppler monitoring costs an additional $400 Canadian Dollars (CAD). Their study reported a salvage rate of 81.4% with Doppler monitoring and 60.4% with clinical monitoring. This difference combined with the reported take back rate resulted in a number needed to treat of 50 to prevent one repeat flap operation with the advent of Doppler monitoring. The total cost of the Doppler probes compared with the savings from reducing reoperations secondary to failed flaps priced each Doppler at $120 CAD per patient in nonburied flaps. However, in buried flaps, the authors reported that because of the larger difference in salvage rates of Doppler compared with clinical examination secondary to the limited ability to perform clinical examination in buried flaps, Doppler placement saved $160 CAD per patient. Poder and Fortier[7] also reported that these analyses fail to factor in additional benefits of the Doppler into their cost analysis, such as patient's psychological benefit from not having a repeat operation, ease of monitoring with the probe, and increased success rates being more acceptable to patients in general.

Summary and Recommendations

- Postoperative monitoring with an implantable Doppler increases overall flap survival rates and flap salvage rates compared with clinical examination (IIA)[5]
- An implantable Doppler should be used in combination with a clinical examination by an experienced clinician to limit false positives associated with Doppler probes (IIB)[1]
- Use of the implantable Doppler demonstrates near cost effectiveness in nonburied flaps and cost savings in buried flaps (IIB)[7]
- Anastomosis before complete flap inset combined with Doppler monitoring allows for an intraoperative period of continuous Doppler monitoring to reduce the rates of early take back (V)[1]

VASOPRESSORS IN THE PERIOPERATIVE PERIOD
Introduction

Because of the significant morbidity associated with free flap failure, practitioners have always been cautious of perioperative management that might jeopardize flap survival. The use of vasopressors during the perioperative period has long been a concern because of their potential negative effect on blood flow through the pedicle. This concern has perpetuated itself into common practice, although its original basis was a combination of expert opinion and animal studies.[13,14] A survey of anesthesiologists in the United Kingdom demonstrated the persistent controversy surrounding this issue. Half of the responding anesthesiologists considered vasopressors contraindicated during free tissue transfer.[15] Additionally, half responded they would prefer to treat hypotension with crystalloid infusion rather than vasopressor administration. However, overresuscitation with crystalloid is not without its own

reported risk. In a retrospective study by Haughey and colleagues[16] in 2001, a total of 241 free flap surgeries were retrospectively reviewed and found greater than 7 L of crystalloid administered intraoperatively was associated with major medical complications in a multivariate analysis. Perioperative hypotension is a common problem for these patients during their prolonged surgery and recovery. Often, the preferred treatment of hypotension, in the absence of concern for the flap, is administration of a vasopressor. The following reviews the current evidence regarding vasopressor use in the perioperative setting.

Animal Studies

Some of the earliest studies looking at the effect of systemic and local vasopressors on flap perfusion were conducted in animals. These studies provided conflicting evidence regarding the safety and net effect of vasopressors on flap perfusion. Two studies reported negative effects of vasopressors on flap perfusion. Cordeiro and colleagues[14] in 1997 reported on the effect of systemic phenylephrine, dopamine, and dobutamine in a porcine model of a rectus abdominis musculocutaneous island flap. Phenylephrine was associated with a decrease in flap perfusion. Dopamine did not affect flap perfusion despite a recorded increase in cardiac output. Dobutamine was associated with a concurrent increase in flap perfusion and cardiac output. Of note, in this study no microvascular anastomosis was performed. Godden and colleagues[13] in 2000 reported on the effect of local administration of phenylephrine using a rat model where the femoral artery was divided and microvascularly reconstructed. This study reported an increase in phenylephrine sensitivity on the anastomosed side compared with the control side resulting in decreased perfusion of the flap relative to control. Both studies cautioned against the use of vasopressors in free flaps. In contrast, two studies reported positive effects of vasopressors on flap perfusion in a porcine model using a latissimus dorsi musculocutaneous free flap.[17,18] Banic and colleagues[17] in 1997 reported that a systemic phenylephrine infusion resulted in an increased mean arterial pressure (MAP) with minimal effect on cardiac output or flap perfusion. Erni and colleagues[18] in 1999 reported that systemic phenylephrine produced a 30% increase in MAP with minimal change in heart rate, cardiac output, and flap perfusion. However, local administration of phenylephrine was associated with a 30% decrease in flap perfusion. These mixed results in early animal studies contributed to the controversy surrounding the use of vasopressors with free flaps in the perioperative period.

Intraoperative Human Studies

Recently, two large cohort studies found no adverse effects associated with intraoperative vasopressor use on flap survival or complication rates.[19,20] Monroe and colleagues[19] published two studies in 2010 and 2011, the latter was a larger prospective study of 169 cases. It was appropriately powered to observe a 10% increase in flap failure rate assuming an expected incidence of 5% failure in intraoperative vasopressor and control groups. Intraoperative vasopressor administration was defined as administration of ephedrine or phenylephrine at or after 2 hours before anastomosis. The decision to administer vasopressor was at the discretion of the anesthesia team. Of the 169 patients, 90 received intraoperative vasopressor, and 79 did not. The authors reported no statistically significant increase in early flap failure, or medical or surgical complication rates between the two groups. A second retrospective study of 485 patients by Harris and colleagues[20] in 2012 reproduced similar results. These authors reported an overall incidence of intraoperative vasopressor use of 66% and reported no correlation between its use and complete or partial flap failure or incidence of operative take back.

Additionally, a randomized prospective study by Scholz and colleagues[21] in 2009 observed the effect of intraoperative dobutamine infusion on flap perfusion and systemic hemodynamics immediately after anastomosis. Twenty patients undergoing microvascular reconstruction of the head and neck were randomized to receive a dobutamine infusion of 2, 4, or 6 µg/kg/min. Subjects in the 4 and 6 µg/kg/min groups demonstrated a significant increase in peak and mean flap perfusion, heart rate, and systolic blood pressure; a decrease in systemic vascular resistance; and no significant change in MAP. These studies provide evidence that supports the safety of intraoperative vasopressor use during microvascular free flap surgery.

Postoperative Human Studies

Two recent human studies have observed the effect of various vasopressors on hemodynamics after anastomosis into the head and neck in the immediate postoperative period.[22,23] Eley and colleagues[23] in 2012 observed the effect of four vasopressors (dobutamine, dopexamine, norepinephrine, and epinephrine) at four different concentrations on skin blood flow as measured by laser Doppler. The study enrolled 24 subjects who recently underwent head and neck microvascular reconstruction. Each patient received each of the four drugs at each of the four concentrations for 5 minutes each with a 20-minute washout period in-between. Perfusion of nongrafted skin acted as an internal control for each patient. The authors reported that dopexamine and epinephrine were associated with a decrease in flap perfusion. However, dobutamine and norepinephrine were associated with an increase in flap perfusion, norepinephrine with a greater effect than dobutamine. In addition, dobutamine was associated with undesirable tachycardia. The authors concluded that norepinephrine was the best vasopressor in the postoperative period given its association with the greatest increase on flap perfusion without associated tachycardia. In 2016, Raittinen and colleagues[22] conducted a randomized controlled clinical trial of the effect of dopamine and norepinephrine on lactate/pyruvate ratio as a surrogate for effective flap perfusion. Twenty-seven subjects were recruited who recently underwent head and neck oncologic resection and subsequent microvascular reconstruction and randomized to one of three groups: (1) control, (2) dopamine, or (3) norepinephrine. The control group was given low doses of both vasopressors to maintain a MAP of 60 if necessary and the intervention groups were titrated up on their respective vasopressor to obtain MAPs between 80 and 90 during the initial 72-hour postoperative period. During this time no differences between either of the treatment groups or control group was noted in the lactate/pyruvate ratio suggesting that the vasopressor did not result in a decreased flap perfusion. Additionally, no flap complications were observed in any group. The authors concluded that dopamine and norepinephrine are acceptable vasopressors during the postoperative period and are not associated with evidence of decreased flap perfusion.

Summary and Recommendations

- Intraoperative use of vasopressors, ephedrine and phenylephrine, is not associated with an increase in free flap complication rates (IIB)[19,20,24]
- Postoperative use of norepinephrine or dopamine does not compromise free flap perfusion or increase free flap complication rates, but norepinephrine is associated with less tachycardia (IC)[22,23]
- Postoperative use of norepinephrine may be associated with increased flap perfusion (IIIA)[23]

POSTOPERATIVE ANTICOAGULATION

Introduction

It is well described that one of the most threatening postoperative complications of microvascular reconstructive surgery is thrombotic compromise of the vascular pedicle. In addition, most of these operations are done for oncologic reasons, placing many of these patients in a known hypercoagulable state.[25] As a result, it makes intuitive sense that these patients may benefit from some form of prophylactic, pharmacologic anticoagulation to reduce this risk in the postoperative period. As early as 1978 Ketchman[26] theorized that this anticoagulation had three definable targets: (1) decreasing platelet function (eg, aspirin), (2) decreasing viscosity (eg, dextran), and (3) decreasing the effectiveness of thrombin (eg, heparin). Over the years since this initial idea, the routine use of anticoagulants has become common practice among many microvascular surgeons. A survey-based study in 1997 by Glicksman and colleagues[27] found that 70% of microvascular surgeons routinely used some form of postoperative anticoagulation. Initially, several animal studies demonstrated a potential advantage to postoperative anticoagulation.[28,29] However, a lack of definitive studies has resulted in an absence of a well-defined protocol regarding the application of anticoagulants. More recently, several larger human studies specific to head and neck microvascular reconstruction have failed to show benefit associated with routine postoperative anticoagulation. Some have even demonstrated harm.[30–36] The evidence surrounding the use of these anticoagulants is reviewed in the following sections and summarized in **Table 2**.

Table 2
Summary of trials on postoperative anticoagulation and their major conclusions

Study	Style	# Patients per Anticoagulant	Major Conclusions
Disa et al,[36] 2003	Randomized prospective	• 35 Dextran 40, 48 h • 32 Dextran 40, 120 h • 27 Aspirin	• No difference in overall flap survival between two groups • Dose-dependent increase in cardiac and pulmonary complications with dextran 40
Sun et al,[39] 2003	Retrospective	• 25 Dextran 40 • 30 No anticoagulant	• No difference in overall flap survival between two groups
Ashjian et al,[34] 2007	Prospective	• 260 Aspirin • 245 LMW heparin	• No difference in flap survival or complications rates between two groups
Riva et al,[31] 2012	Retrospective	• 232 PGE1 • 283 Dextran • 836 No anticoagulant	• No overall difference in flap survival or complications difference between three groups
Jayaprasad et al,[30] 2013	Retrospective	• 40 Dextran 40 • 40 No anticoagulant	• No difference in flap survival • Increase in atelectasis in dextran 40 group
Gerressen et al,[32] 2013	Retrospective	• 305 Unfractionated heparin • 101 LMW heparin	• No difference in flap survival rates between the two anticoagulants
Lighthall et al,[33] 2013	Retrospective	• 142 Aspirin • 25 Heparin or LMW heparin • 23 Aspirin + LMW heparin • 184 No anticoagulant	• Increase in revisions in aspirin vs no therapy • Increase in hematoma, infection and medical complication rates with combination therapy vs no anticoagulant
Swartz et al,[38] 2015	Meta-analysis	• 91 Aspirin • 139 Dextran 40 • 218 Unfractionated heparin • 47 LMW heparin • 16 PGE1 • 234 No anticoagulant	• No difference in overall flap survival between anticoagulant groups

Abbreviations: LMW, low molecular weight; PGE1, prostaglandin E_1.
Data from Refs.[30–34,36,38,39]

Dextrans

Dextrans are a group of variously sized polysaccharides that function to reduce erythrocyte aggregation and platelet adhesiveness. Dextran 40 refers to a fractionated subset of dextrans with an average molecular weight of 40 kDa.[37] Several studies have looked at the effect of dextrans in the postoperative period of microvascular head and neck reconstruction, none of which have demonstrated an increase in flap survival or a decrease in medical or surgical complication rate.[30,31,36,38,39] In fact, several trials have demonstrated an increase in medical complications associated with dextran.[30,36] In 2003 Disa and colleagues[36] reported a randomized clinical trial of 100 consecutive patients undergoing microvascular reconstruction in a single institution. Subjects were randomized into three groups: (1) dextran 40 for 48 hours, (2) dextran 40 for 120 hours, or (3) aspirin for 5 days. The authors reported no significant difference in overall flap survival or flap-related complications between aspirin and dextran groups. However, the authors did report a significant increase in postoperative pulmonary complications defined as pulmonary edema, pleural effusion, adult respiratory distress syndrome, or pneumonia and cardiac complications defined as congestive heart failure, arrhythmias, or ischemia confirmed on electrocardiogram or radiograph. In addition, they reported a dose-specific response, with the number of complications greatest in the group that received dextran for 120 hours. Other serious side effects have also been reported with the use of dextran including anaphylaxis, anaphylactoid reactions,[40,41] pseudotumor cerebri, benign intracranial hypertension,[40,42] and renal failure.[43–45] In conclusion, dextrans do not seem to offer any reduction in postoperative complication rates in head and neck microvascular reconstruction and could increase medical complication rates.

Prostaglandin E_1

Prostaglandin E_1 (PGE1) has successfully been used in the treatment of peripheral artery occlusive disease and Raynaud disease. Its success in these realms has led to the hypothesis that it could be useful in the postoperative period of microvascular surgery. PGE1 is thought to reduce microvascular spasm, decrease blood viscosity, and inhibit platelet aggregation.[37] There is limited evidence on use of PGE1 as a postoperative anticoagulant in head and neck reconstruction. The largest study investigating PGE1 was published by Riva and colleagues[31] in 2012. This trial retrospectively reviewed 1068 free flaps: 232 received PGE1 and 836 received no anticoagulant therapy. The authors reported no statistically significant difference in overall flap survival or complication rates between the two groups. However, the authors did note a tendency toward an increase in hematomas in the PGE1 group ($P = .056$). In conclusion, no evidence in human trials exists to support the use PGE1 as a postoperative anticoagulant in head and neck microvascular reconstruction.

Aspirin

Aspirin acetylates and irreversibly inhibits platelet cyclooxygenase, blocking the breakdown of arachadonic acid into thromboxane and prostacyclin. This reduction in thromboxane reduces vasoconstriction and platelet aggregation. Several studies have compared aspirin, 325 mg, with other anticoagulants including low-molecular-weight (LMW) heparin[34] and dextran 40.[36] Neither of these studies showed any significant difference between overall flap survival rates or medical or surgical complications associated with aspirin compared with the respective anticoagulants. However, Lighthall and colleagues[33] conducted a retrospective review of 146 patients who received aspirin and 148 who received no anticoagulant. These authors reported no difference in overall flap survival rates or medical complications between the two groups, but did report an increase in surgical revisions with aspirin compared with no anticoagulant. In conclusion, there is no evidence that aspirin increases overall flap survival rate, and one study found an increase in surgical revision associated with aspirin use compared with no anticoagulant.

Heparin and Low-Molecular-Weight Heparin

Heparin binds antithrombin III and accelerates its deactivation of coagulation factors II and X. In contrast, LMW heparin similarly binds antithrombin III, but preferentially catalyzes the inactivation of factor X. Both serve to impair the clotting cascade. In 2013 a study by Gerressen and colleagues[32] retrospectively reviewed 406 flaps, 305 of which received unfractionated heparin and 101 of which received LMW heparin. These authors reported no significant difference in overall flap survival between the two anticoagulants. Ashjian and colleagues[34] in 2007 conducted a retrospective review comparing aspirin with LMW heparin and demonstrated no significant difference in overall flap survival rate between the two groups. Lighthall and colleagues[33] in 2013 offered a retrospective review of 48 subjects who received LMW heparin or unfractionated heparin and

65 who received a combination of aspirin and heparin and compared these groups to 148 subjects who received no anticoagulation. Again, this study reported no significant difference in flap survival rates with the use of either heparin/LMW heparin or the heparin and aspirin combination group as compared with no anticoagulant. However, the authors did report an increase in hematoma rate, infection rate, and medical complication rate associated with the combination aspirin and LMW heparin group compared with no anticoagulant. In conclusion there is no evidence to support that heparin or LMW heparin increases flap survival rate in the postoperative period.

Postoperative Anticoagulation Meta-analysis

In 2015 Swartz and colleagues[38] conducted a meta-analysis on the most rigorous trials on the use of postoperative anticoagulation in microvascular reconstruction. This study currently provides the highest level of evidence on the topic. Swartz and colleagues solicited and obtained the raw data from four of the previously discussed studies by Disa and colleagues, Gerressen and colleagues, Lighthall and colleagues, and Riva and colleagues. They reanalyzed only the data on radial forearm free flaps to create a more homogenous sample. The final analysis included a total of 754 radial forearm free flaps, which received the following postoperative regimen: 91 aspirin, 139 dextran, 218 heparin, 47 LMW heparin, 16 PGE1, and 234 no anticoagulation. The authors reported no statistically significant difference in overall flap survival between any of the groups. The authors caution that the meta-analysis is only as good as the synthesized data. Three out of four trials were retrospective, which could introduce selection bias because individual surgeons were deciding on a case-by-case basis which flaps they wanted to anticoagulate. It is worth noting that the meta-analysis did not show any significant association of comorbidities, such as smoking, diabetes, or radiation, with any of the anticoagulants. It is also reassuring that the previously mentioned studies and this meta-analysis seem to support the underlying conclusion that postoperative anticoagulation does not confer a significant benefit in overall flap survival.

Summary and Recommendations

- The use of anticoagulants, dextran, PGE1, aspirin, LMW heparin, and unfractionated heparin, does not improve flap survival as compared with no anticoagulant (IIA)[30–34,36,38]
- Dextran should not be used as a postoperative anticoagulant because it has been

associated with increased pulmonary and cardiac complications and has not been shown to have a benefit in flap survival (IIB)[30,36]

REFERENCES

1. Wax MK. The role of the implantable Doppler probe in free flap surgery. Laryngoscope 2014;124(Suppl): S1–12.
2. Schmulder A, Gur E, Zaretski A. Eight-year experience of the Cook-Swartz Doppler in free-flap operations: microsurgical and reexploration results with regard to a wide spectrum of surgeries. Microsurgery 2011;31(1):1–6.
3. Guillemaud JP, Seikaly H, Cote D, et al. The implantable Cook-Swartz Doppler probe for postoperative monitoring in head and neck free flap reconstruction. Arch Otolaryngol Head Neck Surg 2008; 134(7):729–34.
4. de la Torre J, Hedden W, Grant JH, et al. Retrospective review of the internal Doppler probe for intra- and postoperative microvascular surveillance. J Reconstr Microsurg 2003;19(5):287–90.
5. Han ZF, Guo LL, Liu LB, et al. A comparison of the Cook-Swartz Doppler with conventional clinical methods for free flap monitoring: a systematic review and a meta-analysis. Int J Surg 2016;32: 109–15.
6. Paydar KZ, Hansen SL, Chang DS, et al. Implantable venous Doppler monitoring in head and neck free flap reconstruction increases the salvage rate. Plast Reconstr Surg 2010;125(4):1129–34.
7. Poder TG, Fortier PH. Implantable Doppler in monitoring free flaps: a cost-effectiveness analysis based on a systematic review of the literature. Eur Ann Otorhinolaryngol Head Neck Dis 2013;130(2):79–85.
8. Jonas R, Schaal T, Krimmel M, et al. Monitoring in microvascular tissue transfer by measurement of oxygen partial pressure: four years experience with 125 microsurgical transplants. J Craniomaxillofac Surg 2013;41(4):303–9.
9. Hölzle F, Rau A, Loeffelbein DJ, et al. Results of monitoring fasciocutaneous, myocutaneous, osteocutaneous and perforator flaps: 4-year experience with 166 cases. Int J Oral Maxillofac Surg 2010; 39(1):21–8.
10. Swartz WM, Jones NF, Cherup L, et al. Direct monitoring of microvascular anastomoses with the 20-MHz ultrasonic Doppler probe: an experimental and clinical study. Plast Reconstr Surg 1988;81(2): 149–61. Available at: http://www.ncbi.nlm.nih.gov/pubmed/3336646.
11. Hölzle F, Loeffelbein DJ, Nolte D, et al. Free flap monitoring using simultaneous non-invasive laser Doppler flowmetry and tissue spectrophotometry. J Craniomaxillofac Surg 2006;34(1):25–33.

12. Yoshino K, Nara S, Endo M, et al. Intraoral free flap monitoring with a laser Doppler flowmeter. Microsurgery 1997;17(6):337–40.

13. Godden DRP, Little R, Weston A, et al. Catecholamine sensitivity in the rat femoral artery after microvascular anastomosis. Microsurgery 2000;20(5):217–20.

14. Cordeiro PG, Santamaria E, Hu QY, et al. Effects of vasoactive medications on the blood flow of island musculocutaneous flaps in swine. Ann Plast Surg 1997;39(5):524–31.

15. Gooneratne H, Lalabekyan B, Clarke S, et al. Perioperative anaesthetic practice for head and neck free tissue transfer: a UK national survey. Acta Anaesthesiol Scand 2013;57(10):1293–300.

16. Haughey BH, Wilson E, Kluwe L, et al. Free flap reconstruction of the head and neck: analysis of 241 cases. Otolaryngol Head Neck Surg 2001;125(1):10–7.

17. Banic A, Krejci V, Erni D, et al. Effects of extradural anesthesia on microcirculatory blood flow in free latissimus dorsi musculocutaneous flaps in pigs. Plast Reconstr Surg 1997;100(4):945–55 [discussion: 956]. Available at: http://www.ncbi.nlm.nih.gov/pubmed/9290663.

18. Erni D, Banic A, Krejci V, et al. Effects of sodium nitroprusside and phenylephrine on blood flow in free musculocutaneous flaps during general anesthesia. Anesthesiology 1999;47(3):147–55.

19. Monroe MM, Cannady SB, Ghanem TA, et al. Safety of vasopressor use in head and neck microvascular reconstruction: a prospective observational study. Otolaryngol Head Neck Surg 2011;144(6):877–82.

20. Harris L, Goldstein D, Hofer S, et al. Impact of vasopressors on outcomes in head and neck free tissue transfer. Microsurgery 2012;32(1):15–9.

21. Scholz A, Pugh S, Fardy M, et al. The effect of dobutamine on blood flow of free tissue transfer flaps during head and neck reconstructive surgery. Anaesthesia 2009;64(10):1089–93.

22. Raittinen L, Kaariainen MT, Lopez JF, et al. The effect of norepinephrine and dopamine on radial forearm flap partial tissue oxygen pressure and microdialysate metabolite measurements: a randomized controlled trial. Plast Reconstr Surg 2016;137(6):1016E–23E.

23. Eley KA, Young JD, Watt-Smith SR. Epinephrine, norepinephrine, dobutamine, and dopexamine effects on free flap skin blood flow. Plast Reconstr Surg 2012;130(3):564–70.

24. Monroe MM, McClelland J, Swide C, et al. Vasopressor use in free tissue transfer surgery. Otolaryngol Head Neck Surg 2010;142(2):169–73.

25. Anderson JAM, Weitz JI. Hypercoagulable states. Clin Chest Med 2010;31(4):659–73.

26. Ketchman L. Pharmacological alterations in the clotting mechanism: use in microvascular surgery. J Hand Surg Am 1978;3:407.

27. Glicksman A, Ferder M, Casale P, et al. 1457 years of microsurgical experience. Plast Reconstr Surg 1997;100(2):355–63.

28. Buckley RC, Davidson SF, Das SK. The role of various antithrombotic agents in microvascular surgery. Br J Plast Surg 1994;47(1):20–3. Available at: http://www.ncbi.nlm.nih.gov/pubmed/8124561.

29. Salemark L, Wieslander JB, Dougan P, et al. Studies of the antithrombotic effects of dextran 40 following microarterial trauma. Br J Plast Surg 1991;44(1):15–22.

30. Jayaprasad K, Mathew J, Thankappan K, et al. Safety and efficacy of low molecular weight dextran (dextran 40) in head and neck free flap reconstruction. J Reconstr Microsurg 2013;29(7):443–8.

31. Riva FMG, Chen Y-C, Tan N-C, et al. The outcome of prostaglandin-E1 and dextran-40 compared to no antithrombotic therapy in head and neck free tissue transfer: analysis of 1,351 cases in a single center. Microsurgery 2012;32(5):339–43.

32. Gerressen M, Pastaschek CI, Riediger D, et al. Microsurgical free flap reconstructions of head and neck region in 406 cases: a 13-year experience. J Oral Maxillofac Surg 2013;71(3):628–35.

33. Lighthall JG, Cain R, Ghanem TA, et al. Effect of postoperative aspirin on outcomes in microvascular free tissue transfer surgery. Otolaryngol Head Neck Surg 2013;148(1):40–6.

34. Ashjian P, Chen CM, Pusic A, et al. The effect of postoperative anticoagulation on microvascular thrombosis. Ann Plast Surg 2007;59(1):36–40.

35. Chien W, Varvares MA, Hadlock T, et al. Effects of aspirin and low-dose heparin in head and neck reconstruction using microvascular free flaps. Laryngoscope 2005;115(6):973–6.

36. Disa JJ, Polvora VP, Pusic AL, et al. Dextran-related complications in head and neck microsurgery: do the benefits outweigh the risks? A prospective randomized analysis. Plast Reconstr Surg 2003;112(6):1534–9.

37. Askari M, Fisher C, Weniger FG, et al. Anticoagulation therapy in microsurgery: a review. J Hand Surg Am 2006;31(5):836–46.

38. Swartz JE, Aarts MCJ, Swart KMA, et al. The value of postoperative anticoagulants to improve flap survival in the free radial forearm flap: a systematic review and retrospective multicentre analysis. Clin Otolaryngol 2015;40(6):600–9.

39. Sun T-B, Chien S-H, Lee J-T, et al. Is dextran infusion as an antithrombotic agent necessary in microvascular reconstruction of the upper aerodigestive tract? J Reconstr Microsurg 2003;19(7):463–6.

40. Nearman HS, Herman ML. Toxic effects of colloids in the intensive care unit. Crit Care Clin 1991;7(3):713–23. Available at: http://www.ncbi.nlm.nih.gov/pubmed/1713807.

41. van der Klauw MM, Wilson JH, Stricker BH. Drug-associated anaphylaxis: 20 years of reporting in The Netherlands (1974-1994) and review of the literature. Clin Exp Allergy 1996;26(12): 1355–63.

42. Hardin CK, Kirk WC, Pederson WC. Osmotic complications of low-molecular-weight dextran therapy in free flap surgery. Microsurgery 1992;13(1):36–8. Available at: http://www.ncbi.nlm.nih.gov/pubmed/1375307.

43. Ferraboli R, Malheiro PS, Abdulkader RCRM, et al. Anuric acute renal failure caused by dextran 40 administration. Ren Fail 1997;19(2): 303–6.

44. Vos SCB, Hage JJ, Woerdeman LAE, et al. Acute renal failure during dextran-40 antithrombotic prophylaxis: report of two microsurgical cases. Ann Plast Surg 2002;48(2):193–6. Available at: http://www.ncbi.nlm.nih.gov/pubmed/11910227.

45. Zwaveling JH, Meulenbelt J, van Xanten NH, et al. Renal failure associated with the use of dextran-40. Neth J Med 1989;35(5–6):321–6. Available at: http://www.ncbi.nlm.nih.gov/pubmed/2483959.

46. Paydar KZ, Hansen SL, Chang DS, et al. Implantable venous Doppler monitoring in head and neck free flap reconstruction increases the salvage rate. Plastic and Reconstructive Surgery 2010;125(4): 1129–34.

Controversies in Orthognathic Surgery

Daniel E. Perez, DDS[a],*, Aaron Liddell, DMD, MD[b]

KEYWORDS

- Orthognathic surgery • Sequence • Condylar positioning • Virtual planning • Open bites
- Segmental osteotomies • Splint less surgery • Pre/bend plates

KEY POINTS

- Orthognathic surgery remains a mainstay of treatment in the correction of dentofacial deformities.
- Research and technology continue to drive the evolution of current surgical practice.
- The implementation of virtual planning and intraoperative navigation are increasingly becoming mainstay in the day-to-day management of this patient population.
- Clinical studies and patient research must continue in the context of temporomandibular disorders, to establish a standard of care in addition to research-based, directed management.
- With new evidence-based medical practices, the oral and maxillofacial surgeon must increasingly abandon unsubstantiated dogma and antiquated paradigms to deliver long-term, predictable results.

INTRODUCTION

Controversy has accompanied orthognathic surgery since its adaptation for the correction of dentofacial deformities in the 1950s. With the development of less invasive and less morbid osteotomy designs, questions regarding overall osteotomy stability have abounded. Along the lines of stability, the transition from prolonged intermaxillary fixation and wire osteosynthesis to rigid internal fixation has spurred questions regarding the most effective fixation technique, and challenged previously accepted hierarchies of stability, for example: Are bicortical screws superior to lateral border plates for the fixation of the mandibular sagittal osteotomies? How many screws or plates should be used to optimize outcome and stability, while minimizing patient cost and overall health care burden? Is there an ideal technique for seating the condyle in its most anatomic and functionally stable position?

What is the correct sequence to operate bimaxillary cases? These questions represent only the surface of a sea of debate and discussion, as measures have been taken to optimize patient outcome, minimize patient morbidity, and maximize operating room productivity.

Some of these historic questions have been answered; some remain topics of frequent discussion. In addition to osteotomy design and fixation techniques, technology is leading to new paradigms in planning and execution of corrective jaw surgery. Specifically, the application of 3-dimensional imaging technology and virtual surgical planning (VSP) is revolutionizing the way that orthognathic surgery is carried out. With this technology, however, new questions have arisen, which are specific to computer-based surgical planning and technique. Newer paradigms have shifted emphasis away from osteotomy design, and focused on the possibility of negating the

a Oral and Maxillofacial Surgery, University of Texas Health Science Center at San Antonio, 8210 Floyd Curl Drive MC 8124, San Antonio, Texas 78229-3900, USA; b Colorado Oral and Maxillofacial Surgery, 400 S Colorado Boulevard, STE 450, Denver, CO 80246, USA
* Corresponding author.
E-mail address: perezd5@uthscsa.edu

Oral Maxillofacial Surg Clin N Am 29 (2017) 425–440
http://dx.doi.org/10.1016/j.coms.2017.07.008
1042-3699/17/© 2017 Elsevier Inc. All rights reserved.

need for positioning splints, ushering in an era where prebent, patient-specific plates may be the new norm. Questions that have prevailed as technique has evolved include the following:

1. What is the proper sequence to operate a bi-maxillary case?
2. Are segmental osteotomies safe, stable, or necessary, and if so, what are the indications and limitations?
3. Is there an ideal fixation technique and configuration in orthognathic surgery?
4. Is there an ideal technique for seating the mandibular condyle that will optimize jaw function and minimize the risk for early or delayed relapse?
5. What is the best way to close an anterior open bite (AOB)? Is counterclockwise rotation of the mandible in apertognathia stable?

As technology has evolved, and accelerated treatment paradigms have proven stable, new questions have presented, including:

1. How does VSP compare with more "conventional" hinge-articulator based planning?
2. What is the predictability of splintless surgery, using prebent, custom designed plates?
3. Is there an indication for a "surgery first" model, and if so, is it as predictable as the more conventional model of decompensation, surgery, and dental finishing model?
4. What is the etiology of mandibular condylar resorption as it relates to orthognathic surgery, and are there measures that can be taken to prevent or treat it?

With these considerations in mind, the authors' aim is to provide a concise review of "classical" and current controversies that have prevailed in orthognathic surgery, and to address these questions, where possible, with the most recent evidence-based treatment paradigms.

SEQUENCING: WHICH JAW SHOULD GO FIRST?

The question of sequencing in the context of bimaxillary surgery has prevailed since the introduction of rigid internal fixation. In the years preceding rigid internal fixation, where wire osteosythesis was mainstream, rigid stability of the mandible, if done first, was not feasible. In this context, maxillary surgery was completed and stabilized, followed by the mandibular osteotomies. The mandible was then wired to the maxilla in the final occlusion, with a subsequent period of maxillomandibular fixation (MMF).[1,2]

With the introduction of rigid internal fixation, however, the option of completing the mandibular osteotomies first, rigidly fixating the mandibular segments, and finishing with repositioning of the osteotomized maxilla into final position is now possible. Buckley and colleagues[3] were among the first to describe the sequencing of this technique, which has since been optimized in the execution of bimaxillary surgery. Numerous publications have addressed indications and advantages of one technique versus the other; however, no consensus has been reached, in terms of whether one method provides superior results to the other.[1,2,4,5]

Circumstances where mandible-first surgery can be beneficial include bimaxillary surgery cases where a multipiece maxillary osteotomy is indicated to optimize the maxillary occlusal plane and normalize transverse occlusal relations. By performing the mandibular osteotomies first, followed by rigid mandibular fixation, the segmented maxilla can be wired into a single final splint, then to the stably fixated mandible, negating the need for the "splint within a splint" paradigm, which is required when the maxilla is completed first. In this instance, only the vertical repositioning of the maxillomandibular complex remains to be measured intraoperatively (**Fig. 1**).

In addition to segmental maxillary osteotomies, cases in which the clinical situation calls for large maxillomandibular advancements (obstructive sleep apnea) or significant counterclockwise rotations of the skeletofacial complex are typically easier to carry out when the mandibular osteotomies are completed first. The advantage in these situations is splint stability. When the mandible is

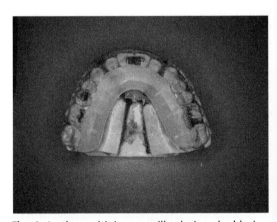

Fig. 1. In the multipiece maxilla during double jaw surgery, performing the mandible first significantly simplifies model surgery because the segmented maxilla can be wired into a single final splint, then to the stably fixated mandible, negating the need for the "splint within a splint" paradigm.

done first, there is more dental contact in the intermediate position, which renders the intermediate splint easier to fit and generally more stable, requiring less acrylic bulk.

In the case of significant counterclockwise rotation, a relatively small posterior open bite is created in the intermediate position, and is facilitated by the mandibular osteotomies (**Fig. 2**). This posterior open bite is readily closed by performing a maxillary osteotomy and differentially disimpacting the posterior maxilla, which is then wired into intermaxillary fixation with the fixated mandibular dentition. Again, this technique minimizes the splint bulk (especially anterior) that would be encountered if the maxilla was done first, and simplifies the intermediate splint position.[5]

Another situation where mandible-first planning and surgery might be considered is one wherein it is difficult to coerce a patient into centric relation (frequently seen in severe skeletal class II malocclusion). When planning surgery conventionally, if the facebow transfer and model surgery is completed with a "postured" mandibular position, the maxilla will be underprojected when wired to the mandible in a nonpostured state, as is seen on the operating room table when a patient has clinical effects of nondepolarizing paralytics (**Fig. 3**). In these cases, doing the mandible first ensures adequate anterior projection of the skeletofacial complex, as long as the mandible is

moved into an intermediate position relative to the uncut maxilla, and the condyles are adequate seated in the intermediate occlusion, coincident with what was planned in the laboratory.

Perhaps the best example when one should consider operating the mandible first is when performing concomitant temporomandibular joint (TMJ) and orthognathic surgery and the TMJ surgery is done first, followed by the orthognathic component. Here, the mandible must be performed before the maxillary osteotomy because of the change of the condylar position that accompanies the joint surgery.

Finally, classic model surgery (non-VSP) for mandible-first cases is significantly less involved than the mutiplane, multivector model surgery that is involved with maxilla-first surgery. When planning mandible-first cases, movements can be accomplished without the use of a conventional model surgery platform, requiring only a few key skeletal and occlusal measurements or landmarks (usually including the first molars, the central incisors, and bony pogonion; **Fig. 4**).[6] It should be noted, however a big clockwise rotation *of the occlusal plane*, operating on the maxilla first makes the intermediate splint thinner and easier to handle in surgery (**Fig. 5**). It is important to emphasize that properly planned and executed either sequence can provide accurate positioning of the jaws.

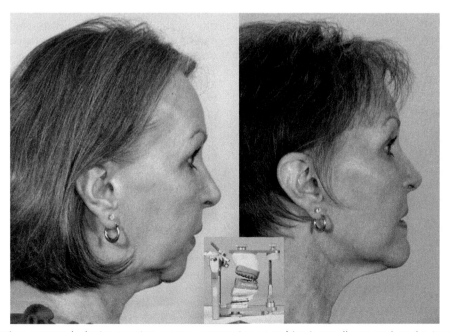

Fig. 2. During counterclockwise rotation moves, a posterior open bite is usually created at the intermediate stage. Notice the greater pogonion projection obtained from rotating the occlusal plane before and after surgery.

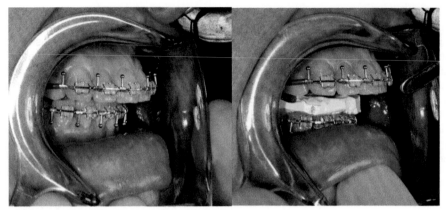

Fig. 3. Before and after nondepolarizing paralytics have been given. Notice the green clinical bite registration obtained with the patient awake no longer fits when the patient is fully relaxed. If the maxilla is done first, this will translate in an inaccurate intermediate position.

SEGMENTAL OSTEOTOMIES

The possibility of maxillary segmentalization was realized by Cohn-Stock, as early as 1921. Various modifications were used through the early to mid 1900s by the likes of Wassmund, Axhausen, Wunderer, and Kole.[7] Bell's studies of maxillary revascularization truly revolutionized the techniques of maxillary osteotomies, and brought to light the possibility of stability and predictably of the segmentalized Le Fort 1. Since that time, however, discussion has persisted, pertaining to whether segmentalization of the maxilla is safe and provides long-term stability. Multiple articles have provided sound evidence that, when done correctly, the segmented maxillary osteotomy is not only useful and stable, but also not detrimental to the patient.[8] Posnick and associates,[9] in 2016, studied 262 subjects who had undergone a variety of maxillary osteotomies. Specifically, these investigators addressed the incidence of complications after surgery, including direct injury to dental root structure, pulpal injuries, gingival/periodontal compromise, the need for hardware removal, the incidence of wound infection, aseptic (avascular) necrosis, fibrous union, and oronasal fistula formation/persistence. They found no associations between the type of Le Fort I osteotomy (single piece, 2 piece, or 3 piece) and the occurrence of specific perioperative complications.[9]

The most common indication for maxillary segmentalization is the presence of a transverse discrepancy in the maxilla, which is greater than can be stably corrected with conventional orthodontic treatment, usually more than 5 to 6 mm.[7] The second classic indication is related to a tooth mass/size discrepancy, were class I canine relationships cannot be achieved owing to an unrecognized or untreated Bolton discrepancy.[10] In these cases, segmentalization optimizes arch–form and interarch alignment, and minimizes the need for orthodontic compromise, when finishing cases (**Fig. 6**).

Freeman and colleagues[11] studied a sample of 157 patients who presented for orthodontic treatment. 97 of 157 patients (61.7%) had an anterior ratio greater than the Bolton norm of 77.2. In light of these considerations, it becomes critical that these tooth–mass discrepancies are noticed early in treatment, and correction be planned into the surgical movement and correction. To overcome these tooth–size discrepancies, the orthodontist might need to increase the maxillary arch perimeter by opening spaces distal to the lateral incisors, or shorten the mandibular arch-length by slenderizing the mandibular incisors.[10] If this is

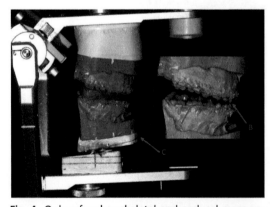

Fig. 4. Only a few key skeletal and occlusal measurements/landmarks (usually including the first molars [A], the central incisors [B], and bony pogonion [C]) are necessary to position the mandible in the intermediate stage.

A   **B**

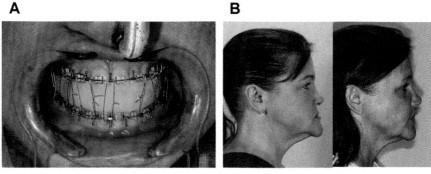

Fig. 5. (*A*) During a clockwise rotation when the mandible is done first, a big intermediate splint may be intrusive. (*B*) Notice how pogonion moves posteriorly and the midface increases its projection.

not done, attempting to reposition the casts into a solid class I canine relationship during the model surgery can become problematic and sometimes impossible; the surgeon is left with the challenge of creating a space between the lateral incisor and canine that can later be built up with composite or porcelain veneers (**Fig. 7**).

Although maxillary expansions are done frequently in orthognathic surgery, one needs to remember the limitations of it, and recall that the incidence of relapse in this move is the highest reported in the literature.[12] Still, Phillips and colleagues[13] reported a series of 32 patients who had transverse expansion using Le Fort I osteotomies and his group of patients was used by Chamberland and Proffit subsequently to compare it to a group of surgically assisted rapid palatal expansion study patients of their own. They found that (1) the mean difference in transverse relapse across the first molars in the 2 groups was not statistically significant, and (2) the mean transverse relapse across the canines was greater for the surgically assisted rapid palatal expansion group, noting the difference was statistically significant. Kretschmer and colleagues[14] concluded that "surgical expansion of the maxilla through segmental osteotomies provides stable results at the skeletal base." However, they documented significant dental relapse once the orthodontic appliances were removed. One can ask the orthodontist to avoid tipping the molars and "over-verticalization" of the incisors through extrusion mechanics to try to minimize dental relapse.[9] Communication between the surgeon and treating orthodontists becomes paramount in these cases so that minimal or no expansion is attempted with the archwire before surgery. Additionally, preparing to hold the surgical expansion once the splint is removed with a transpalatal arch or bolstering appliance should be communicated before removal of the surgical splint.[9]

RIGID FIXATION CONFIGURATION

The sagittal split ramus osteotomy, as described by Obwegeser, with its myriad modifications, is now a standard in the armamentarium used in oral and maxillofacial surgery to address mandibular growth or posttraumatic discrepancies.[15,16] As previously noted, before rigid internal fixation, patients required a period of MMF because bone stabilization was achieved by means of wire osteosynthesis. Since the introduction of plates and screw fixation, a variety of configurations can now be used to promote bone healing through rigid internal fixation without the need for concomitant MMF. However, animal studies, such as those undertaken by Ellis and Goallo,[17] have shown that inadequate securing of the segments through appropriate fixation practices can lead to distal segment displacement, nonunion or fibrous union, and initiate early relapse.

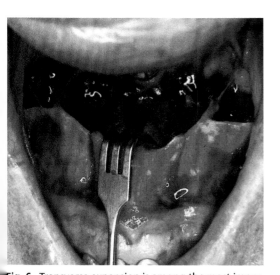

Fig. 6. Transverse expansion is among the most important indications for a segmented maxilla.

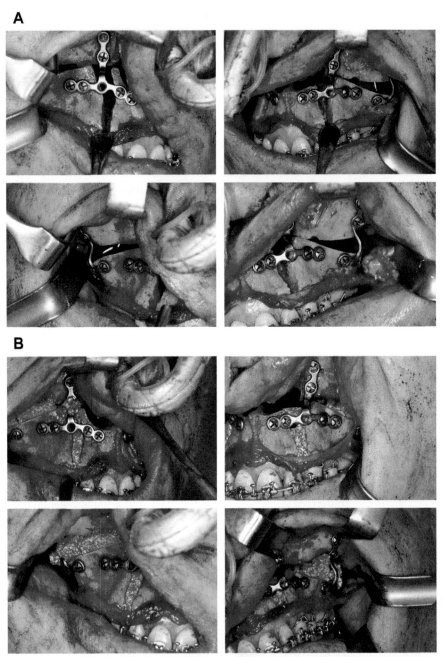

Fig. 7. (*A*) Bolton's discrepancy requiring segmented surgery for opening of space between laterals and canines to obtain adequate class 1 occlusion. (*B*) Notice the bone graft in the gap.

Accordingly, debate remains as to which is the best fixation modality for stabilizing a sagittal split ramus osteotomy and many surgeons base their fixation practice methods on their own clinical experience. Looking at principles of osteosynthesis, the ideal internal fixation method should obtain maximum rigidity between osseous segments while exerting minimal stress on the surrounding hard tissues to facilitate proper healing.[15–17] Fixation techniques should also be economical, biocompatible, and negate the need for additional surgery.

One of the possible benefits of using a plate is using it as a "handle" to manipulate the proximal segment in position without the need of a clamp to hold the segments together. Also, a bad or unplanned lingual split is inconsequential if a plate is used to stabilize the segments (**Fig. 8**).

In 2012, Sato and associates[16] published a finite element analysis comparing the mechanical stress in a 5-mm mandibular advancement with a variety of hardware using 5 different techniques: 3 linear 60° screw arrangement; 3 linear 90° screw arrangement; 3 inverted L screw arrangement; 1 conventional miniplate; and 1 locking miniplate with 4 monocortical screws. They applied a continuous load until 3 mm of intersegmental displacement was reached and found a lower mechanical stress rate in both the bone and in the fixation system with the inverted L arrangement, followed by the linear 90° and linear 60° arrangements. The locking miniplate and screw system presented lower maximum principal stress and better stress distribution compared with the conventional system. Under the conditions tested, the inverted L bicortical screw arrangement provided the most favorable stress dissipation behavior.[16] These results have been corroborated by a variety of studies by multiple practitioners.[16–21]

Further analysis of these studies raises the question of the benefit of lateral body plate and screw fixation. The benefit of using lateral body plate and screw fixation comes in securing and positioning the proximal segment passively. When using passively bent plate and screw fixation along the lateral mandibular body, less torque is exerted on the condylar head(s) and seating of the proximal segment(s) can be done more passively.[16] This realization of the effects of condylar torque and relapse using nonpassive bicortical screw or lag screw techniques has led many experienced practitioners

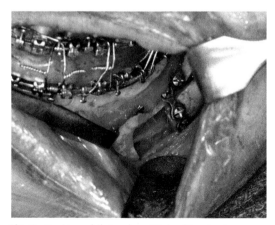

Fig. 8. During a bilateral sagittal split osteotomy, using a plate in the front facilitates the seating of the condylar segment. It also makes a possible lingual plate fracture inconsequential.

away from bicortical/lag screw fixation. A logical step would be to switch to a locking system, which in theory would facilitate passivity of condylar seating, while distributing load over the plate and screws.

Noting the potential benefits of plate and screw fixation, Joss and colleagues[20], in 2008, published a systematic review on stability after bilateral sagittal split osteotomy advancement surgery comparing different rigid internal fixation systems. Their conclusions were that bicortical screws of titanium, stainless steel, or bioresorbable material show little difference regarding skeletal stability compared with miniplates in the short term, but when looking long term they found more studies with larger relapse rates in patients treated with bicortical screws instead of miniplates. The etiology of relapse is multifactorial, involving the proper seating of the condyles, the amount of advancement, the soft tissue and muscles, the mandibular plane angle, the remaining growth and remodeling, the skill of the surgeon, and preoperative age.[20]

CONDYLE POSITION DURING ORTHOGNATHIC SURGERY

Since 1976, when Leonard first reported the use of a condylar positioning device, there have been many reports in the literature of techniques and devices used to position the condyle during orthognathic surgery.[22] These reports and this pointed interest has come as a direct consequence of the use of rigid internal fixation and the associated torqueing of the condyle-baring proximal segment, which has been attributed as an etiologic factor in postoperative relapse and condylar resorption. Ultimately, over time, each surgeon adapts his or her own technique for repositioning the proximal segment. To date, no consensus exists on what is the most effective and reproducible way of doing this today.[22]

Ellis in 1994 argued that our ability to reproduce condyle position, even in the absence of surgery, is greatly affected by the state of consciousness, position of the patient, and tone of the masticatory muscles. He reports that multiple studies have shown that changes in the position of the condyle can and do occur with a variety of orthognathic surgical corrections. The question herein is, does our ability to reproduce condylar position matter?[22,23]

Today, very little scientific data show whether condylar positioning devices can place the condyle in the desired location or if that is critical for the ultimate success of the operation. Most articles that describe the use of such devices make the assumption that they will be effective.[22] Most surgeons rely on the haptics or "experience" associated with manual repositioning after sagittal split osteotomy to obtain the best mandibular proximal segment relationship with the condylar fossa. To our knowledge, no conclusive scientific evidence exists today to support the use of condylar positioning devices during orthognathic surgery.

In 1986, Epker and Wylie[24] suggested 3 reasons for accurately controlling the mandibular proximal segment: to ensure stability, reduce detrimental effects to the TMJ, and improve masticatory function. The relationship between condylar position and the stability of mandibular advancement is well-known. Distracting the condyle from the fossa during surgery causes an immediate skeletal relapse, and posterior repositioning of the condyle has been shown to induce condylar resorption, resulting in late relapse.[22–24]

A variety of terminology has been attributed to intraoperative malpositioning of the mandibular condyles. Reyneke and Ferretti[25] have written extensively on clinical presentations associated with aberrantly seated condyles. During surgery, one can experience condylar displacement after releasing the patient from MMF. If the occlusion immediately changes, the mandible will not passively fit into the splint, noting a tendency to "fall back", deviating towards the side where the condyle was not seated appropriately. Reyneke and Ferretti[25] referred to this as "condylar sag." Condylar sag is readily identified, and easily corrected, but requires removal of the fixation hardware on the side(s) of the aberrant condylar position, repositioning of the condyle, and passive replacement of the fixation appliance(s). In these cases, the surgeon must be critical with their work until the preplanned, passive occlusion is achieved. If this is not done and "elastics" are used to correct the problem, there is a high probability of failure and suboptimal occlusal outcomes.[22–29]

In addition to immediate relapse, as seen on the operating table in the context of condylar sag, relapse arise when condylar changes occur secondary to pressure resorption, over a long period of time. This change is related to torque placed distally on the proximal segment, which causes pressure changes along the medial condylar pole(s). Ultimately, condylar remodeling leads to delayed condylar seating, and associated occlusal relapse. In many instances, however, the adaptive capacity of the TMJ likely masks inaccuracy in condylar positioning, and occlusal relapse does not manifest. There is no question the TMJ has incredible capacity to adapt, even in the absence of orthognathic surgical movements. This adaptation is probably what makes orthognathic surgery possible and predictable.[30]

It is our opinion that, instead of focusing on which condylar positioning device works best, clinical judgment should guide each practitioner. One should attempt to passively position the proximal segment, eliminating any interference the planned surgical moves may have created. A thorough study of the surgical plan will ensure that the practitioner is anticipating aberrant contact points, and have appropriate measures to address any factor that may lead to a lack of passivity of condylar seating. Additionally, the surgeon should ensure that the condyle–disc relationship is healthy and stable before operating and be thoughtful in osteotomy design and selection when planning each individual case.

ANTERIOR OPEN BITE TREATMENT

The correction of the AOB malocclusion is one of the most difficult and most debated malocclusions that the oral and maxillofacial surgeon encounters. Frequently, after an initially successful correction of the vertical dimension by a combined orthodontic and orthognathic surgical treatment, patients exhibit a decrease in clinical overbite, increased overjet, or the reappearance of an AOB. Relapse of an AOB may occur because of various factors, such as tongue size or posture, an unfavorable growth pattern, orofacial musculature, respiratory problems, careless orthodontic preparation, dental movements, and condylar resorption after orthognathic surgery.[31,32]

According to Proffit and colleagues,[33] AOBs are not particularly common. Population studies suggest a prevalence of approximately 2.9% in the adult Caucasian American population.[33] In pediatric (skeletally immature) patients, AOBs are usually treated orthodontically with appliances aimed at growth modification, showing mixed outcomes. Historically, treatment of AOB in the skeletally mature patient involved posterior maxillary impaction and autorotation of the mandible.[32,33] This movement was done to decrease relapse potential, but more specifically because rigid internal fixation was not readily available. In terms of facial esthetics, however, these movements typically result in an unpleasant esthetic profile, noting a lack of ability to correct high mandibular and occlusal plan angles (and in many cases, worsening this relationship; **Fig. 9**).

In 2013, Solano-Hernández and colleagues[32] found that overbite changes after surgical management show significant variation, with relapse

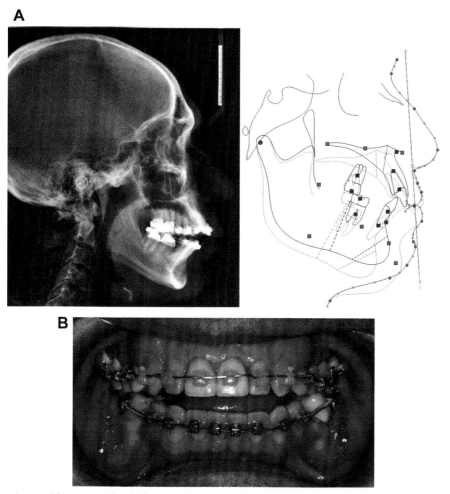

Fig. 9. In patients with steep occlusal planes and anterior open bites, a proposed maxillary posterior impaction usually worsens the profile and is detrimental for the patient's cosmetic outcome.

rates of 16% (opening of bite of >2 mm) in patients followed long term after Le Fort I osteotomies. They noted a relapse rate of 13% in patients closed with sagittal split ramus osteotomy and counterclockwise rotation, followed short term. They did not note significant long-term changes after bimaxillary surgery. They concluded that vertical relapse is a characteristic in a certain number of patients after combined orthodontic/surgical treatment, regardless of the type of surgery used. This is observed clinically, noting an opening of the bite (dentally) and an increase in the mandibular plane and intermaxillary angles (skeletally) during long-term follow-up. Long-term skeletal relapse seems to be more common after bimaxillary surgery. Greenlee and colleagues[34] in 2011 published a meta-analysis looking at stability of treating AOBs. They found that success rates were greater than 75% with both surgical and nonsurgical treatment of AOB. They noted

however, a lack of within-study control, and significant variability among studies.

Today, we know that AOBs can be managed surgically with 1 or 2 jaw procedures. When closing open bites surgically, there can be a tendency toward relapse; however, with adequate planning, long-term stability and successful outcomes are possible. Care must be taken to identify condylar resorption as a possible causes of relapse. Communication with the orthodontist during decompensation must be undertaken to prevent preoperative extrusion of incisors, which is known to be inherently unstable and relapse prone. Dentoalveolar growth and patient age must also be considered, because these factors are a known source of relapse. Finally, newer orthodontic-only options with temporary anchorage devices (TADs) or skeletal fixation plates are becoming popular in closing AOBs.[31] One must keep in mind that mild to moderate skeletal AOBs can be treated with TAD and skeletal fixation plates without orthognathic surgery. True molar intrusion of up to 4 mm has been reported causing anterior rotation of the mandible and a significant reduction in anterior face height. Although promising, growth modification techniques with TAD and miniplates require long-term follow-up studies.[31–34]

VIRTUAL SURGICAL PLANNING AND SPLINTLESS SURGERY

With technologic advancements, newer methods for planning and executing surgery have become available. More recently, it seems that the era of plaster models and long hours in the laboratory fabricating and polishing guide splints is coming to an end, as VSP becomes more mainstream for surgical planning and splint fabrication. As noted by proponents of VSP, some patients with complex problems undergo surgical treatment with suboptimal results despite well-planned operations by experienced surgeons in the conventional model.[35–37] Surgeons' reliance on 2-dimensional imaging for treatment planning of a 3-dimensional problem makes it difficult to assess the intraoperative position, projection, and symmetry of repositioned or deformed skeletal anatomy.

Although analytical model surgery using plaster casts mounted on a semiadjustable articulator is effective for most orthognathic surgical cases, deformities of pitch, roll, and yaw are difficult to correct predictably, even in experienced hands.[35] With that in mind, the demand for accuracy has driven the development of computer-assisted planning and splint fabrication.

Computer-aided orthognathic surgery can be divided into 3 basic categories: (1) computer-aided preoperative planning, (2) intraoperative navigation, and (3) intraoperative computed tomography or MRI.[35] Very complex dentofacial deformities especially the asymmetric cases can be planned using computer-assisted surgical simulation (**Fig. 10**). Virtually fabricated splints are milled for use at the time of surgery, as described previously, which allows for optimal maxillomandibular repositioning in all 3 planes of space. This technique can be further augmented by combining it with the use of a stereolithographic model to prebend reconstruction plates and/or the construction of custom guide stents to accurately design osteotomies or shape bone grafts.[36,38–40]

Intraoperative navigation can be used as an additional tool during the implementation of the treatment plan to achieve the most accurate results possible by assessing the vertical, horizontal, and sagittal jaw and tooth relationships in real time.[41] Navigation surgery in the mandible is more difficult because it is a moving bone; therefore, it requires that the sensor frame is mounted onto the mandible, which can be cumbersome and sensitive to the relative movements of the mandible, which in turn undermines the accuracy of the intraoperative navigation. Today we do not have an excellent method for navigation of the mandibular osteotomy.[40]

Intraoperative computed tomography scanning provides an option for checking position and cuts with linear measurements in "real time" and is an option for complex reconstructive procedures. Although this technique probably has greater efficacy for posttraumatic reconstruction, and in particular orbital reconstruction, complex osteotomy design, and segment positioning, in the context of orthognathic surgery, can be optimized using intraoperative computed tomography imaging.[37,41,42]

Kwon and colleagues[43] reported that use of conventional, noncomputer fabricated splints for maxillary osteotomies resulted in a mean ± standard deviation accuracy of 1.17 ± 0.74 mm. They compared the accuracy of surgery using 3-dimensional printed splints derived from virtual plans, and found it to be 0.95 ± 0.58 mm. Kraeima and coworkers[44] in 2016 reported on the use of patient-specific computer-aided design (CAD)–computer-aided manufacturing (CAM) drilling guides and osteosynthesis plates for maxillary positioning and fixation. Postoperative analysis showed a mean ± standard deviation of 1.3 ± 1.4 mm from the preoperative plan. They did noticed that moves that would cause interferences (maxillary impactions) can be difficult because it is not easy to simulate the exact axis of the hinge of the mandibular condyle. They concluded that the main advantages of their method are positioning of the maxilla independent of the condyle or mandible, and the fact that extraoral reference points are not necessary.[44]

Today, most methods used for planning and splint fabrication have been validated and have reported as being at least as accurate as conventional orthognathic surgery planning.[37] The major benefit is evident in the asymmetric patient, where subtle skeletal deformities, which are difficult to appreciate, clinically, can be identified and corrected. However, are we ready to move forward in an era of splintless surgery, relying exclusively on cutting guides, prefabricated plates, and intraoperative navigation? The evidence remains unclear and the technology too new to recommend use on a daily basis.

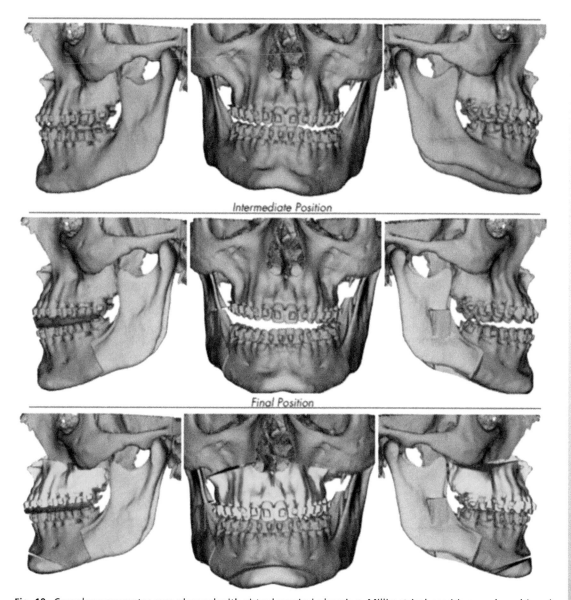

Intermediate Position

Final Position

Fig. 10. Complex asymmetry case planned with virtual surgical planning. Millimetrical precision can be achieved using 3-dimensional analysis and planning tools.

SURGERY-FIRST TREATMENT MODEL

The request to accelerate treatment in our patient population is increasingly evident. From immediate implant placement and loading to interdental osteotomies aimed at expediting dental movement during orthodontic treatment, the push for more rapid, definitive treatment modalities dominates treatment today. Although preoperative orthodontic treatment has been accepted as a necessary process for stable surgical correction in the traditional orthognathic approach, recent advances in the application of

miniscrews and in the preoperative simulation of orthodontic management using dental models have shown that it is possible to perform a surgery-first approach without the need for preoperative dentoalveolar decompensation. The above, then, brings into play 2 questions, namely, (1) Is this a reliable method? And (2) What are indications for the use of this approach to treatment?

With an average preoperative decompensation time of 12 to 15 months and postoperative orthodontic finishing time of 6 to 12 months, the average orthognathic surgery case can require 18 to

36 months of patient commitment to enable treatment. This consideration, alone, is a powerful argument against the decision to pursue combined surgical and orthodontic treatment for many patients.

Preoperative orthodontic treatment is thought to be required for the correction of dental compensation, and to facilitate arch alignment, maxillary, and mandibular arch coordination, and the leveling of accentuated occlusal plane discrepancies. If one decides to obviate this and proceed with surgery first, followed by orthodontic finishing, 2 possible outcomes can occur: (1) longer total treatment time owing to unstable occlusion that requires more orthodontics than normal, or (2) a shorter total treatment time owing to faster dental adaptation process or a regionally accelerated phenomenon, or by facilitating natural compensation during postoperative orthodontic treatment.

Some studies support that surgery-first offers an alternative to the orthodontics-first (conventional technique) approach for correction of maxillofacial deformity with a final outcome, in the way of facial esthetics, dental occlusion, and stability, similar when using orthodontics-first and surgery-first approaches.[45,46]

Peiró-Guijarro and colleagues,[47] in a systematic review, compared 295 patients that underwent the "surgery-first" approach versus 164 patients who underwent a conventional approach. On average, these "surgery-first" patients completed their treatment in approximately 14.2 months, roughly 6 months shorter than those (n = 164) who were treated with the conventional approach (mean, 20.16 months). The ages of the patients ranged from 16 to 36 years at the time of treatment. The most prevalent type of malocclusion treated was a skeletal class III occlusion (84.7% of surgery-first patients).[47] This study, among others, suggests that a surgery-first approach allows for a shorter total treatment time when compared with a conventional approach to orthognathic surgery in patients with a dentofacial deformity requiring surgical and orthodontic correction. This systematic review supports this primarily in class III malocclusion with limited dentoalveolar compensation.

Despite the increasing popularity of the surgery-first approach, there are contraindications to this model, including cases wherein the amount of decompensation required is difficult to build into the surgical occlusion, in addition to severe craniofacial deformities, where decompensation and arch form development helps to guide definitive surgical planning. In addition, caution should be exercised in patients with severe crowding or severe vertical discrepancies (**Fig. 11**).

TEMPOROMANDIBULAR DISORDERS AND ORTHOGNATHIC SURGERY

Temporomandibular disorders (TMD) is a broad term, with varying implications in corrective jaw surgery. There are specific subclasses or TMDs that can directly cause a dentofacial deformity

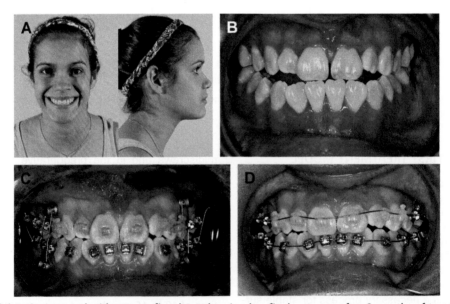

Fig. 11. (*A*) Patient treated with surgery first, here showing her final outcome after 6 months of treatment. (*B*) Preoperative position. (*C*) Intraoperative position. (*D*) At 2 weeks postoperative. (*E*) At 2 months postoperative. (*F*) At 6 months postoperative and debonded. (*G*) Before and after. (*H*) Before and after.

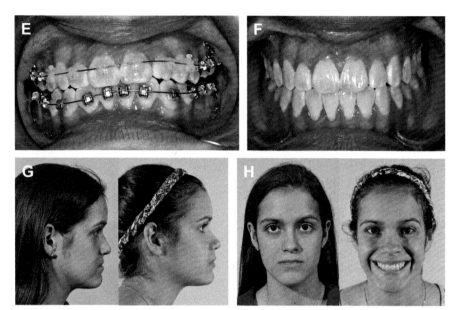

Fig. 11. (*continued*)

and, if left untreated, result in a suboptimal outcome. These include active condylar hyperplasia, idiopathic/progressive condylar resorption, and chronic dislocation and TMJ ankylosis. We believe that, to facilitate successful surgical outcomes, these types of TMDs should be addressed before, or concomitantly with, the orthognathic surgical correction. Along those lines, our experience suggest that failure to address these joint maladies significantly increases the probability of postoperative relapse and, ultimately, failure rates.[48] The literature is not always clear in terms of the most effective modality of identification of active disease in the context of TMJ pathologic entities. Along those lines, we do not advocate ignoring or treating these pathologic conditions with orthognathic surgery alone during states of active disease.

Controversy has persisted, both within the orthodontic and surgical specialties alike, of how to best manage TMDs in the orthognathic surgery patient population. Common sense dictates that a healthy and stable TMJ should perform better during and after orthognathic surgery than a joint that, for example, has evidence of an unstable internal derangement, including open or closed locking, or persistent arthralgia. However, most papers today suggest that a pre-existing TMD usually improves with the orthognathic correction in both class II and III patients. Although this phenomenon is well-documented, the mechanism by which this occurs remains unclear.[49–51]

After orthognathic surgical correction for class II and class III malocclusions, specifically, certain factors associated with the etiology of TMD improve. Included among these are fewer obstructive interferences, better masticatory efficiency, muscular/occlusal balance, less centric occlusion to centric relation discrepancy, and improvement in patient appearance and self-esteem. These factors, when corrected, help to explain why there is an improvement in the overall functionality and stability of the TMD. These findings, however, do not suggest that every TMD is cured by orthognathic surgery. Accordingly, careful patient assessment must to be conducted by the clinician before planning any surgical correction, and early and long-term patient observation must become routine clinical practice, to intervene early in the context of postoperative relapse or growth tendencies.[52,53]

Included in the management of TMDs and associated dentofacial deformities, concomitant orthognathic surgery and total joint replacement increasingly shows clinical predictability, and long-term stability. Progressive, medication-refractory arthritides, idiopathic/progressive condylar resorption, congenital defects (ie, hemifacial macrosomia), and idiopathic and posttraumatic ankyloses are just a few among a growing list of indications for joint replacement. Although haunted by a history of material failure and associated compromised patient outcomes, new materials and patient-fitted custom alloplastic implants designed in the context of virtual bimaxillary movements are showing minimal morbidity, greater long-term stability, and substantial functional improvements.

SUMMARY

Orthognathic surgery remains a mainstay of treatment in the correction of dentofacial deformities. Research and technology continue to drive the evolution of current surgical practice. Included in this is the implementation of virtual planning and intraoperative navigation, which are increasingly becoming mainstay in the day-to-day management of this patient population. Clinical studies and patient research must continue in the context of temporomandibular disorders, to establish a standard of care in addition to research-based, directed management in patient with TMDs. With new evidence-based medical practices, the oral and maxillofacial surgeon must increasingly abandon unsubstantiated dogma and antiquated paradigms, so as to deliver long-term, predictable results in our patient populations.

REFERENCES

1. Perez D, Ellis E. Implications of sequencing in simultaneous maxillary and mandibular orthognathic surgery. Atlas Oral Maxillofac Surg Clin North Am 2016;24(1):45–53.
2. Borba AM, Borges PS. Mandible-first sequence in bimaxillary orthognathic surgery: a systematic review. Int J Oral Maxillofac Surg 2016;45:472–5.
3. Buckley MJ, Tucker MR, Fredette SA. An alternate approach for staging simultaneous maxillary and mandibular osteotomies. Int J Adult Orthodon Orthognath Surg 1987;2:75.
4. Beziat JL, Babic B, Ferreira S, et al. Justification for the mandibular maxillary order in bimaxillary osteotomy. Rev Stomatol Chir Maxillofac 2009; 110:323.
5. Posnick JC. Sequencing of orthognathic procedures: step-by-step approach. In: Posnick JC, editor. Orthognathic surgery: principles and practice. St Louis (MO): Elsevier; 2014. p. 441–74.
6. Cottrell DA, Wolford LM. Altered orthognathic surgical sequencing and a modified approach to model surgery. J Oral Maxillofac Surg 1994;52:1010.
7. Fonseca, Marciani and Turvey. Oral and maxillofacial surgery. 2nd edition. vol. 3. Saunders, Elsevier; 2009. p. 1145–2980.
8. Chow J, Hägg U, Tideman H. The stability of segmentalized Le Fort I Osteotomies with miniplate fixation in patients with maxillary hypoplasia. J Oral Maxillofac Surg 1995;53:1407–12.
9. Posnick JC, Adachie A, Choi E. Segmental maxillary osteotomies in conjunction with bimaxillary orthognathic surgery: indications –safety – outcome. J Oral Maxillofac Surg 2016;74:1422–40.
10. Hanna A, Ellis E 3rd. Tooth size discrepancy in patients requiring mandibular advancement surgery. J Oral Maxillofac Surg 2016;74:2481–6.
11. Freeman JE, Maskeroni AJ, Lorton L. Frequency of Bolton toothsize discrepancies among orthodontic patients. Am J Orthod Dentofacial Orthop 1996; 110:24.
12. Chamberland S, Proffit WR. Closer look at the stability of surgically assisted rapid palatal expansion. J Oral Maxillofac Surg 1895;66:2008.
13. Phillips C, Medland WH, Fields HW Jr, et al. Stability of surgical maxillary expansion. Int J Adult Orthodon Orthognath Surg 1992;7:139.
14. Kretschmer G, Baciut C, Dinu M, et al. Dietz: the influence of expansion on intraoperative bone blood flow in multisegmental maxillary osteotomies: an experimental study. Int J Oral Maxillofac Surg 2010;39:282–6.
15. Luhr H-G. The significance of condylar position using rigid fixation in orthognathic surgery. Clin Plast Surg 1989;16:147.
16. Sato FRL, Asprino L, Consani S, et al. Comparative biomechanical and photoelastic evaluation of different fixation techniques of sagittal split ramus osteotomy in mandibular advancement. J Oral Maxillofac Surg 2010;68:160e166.
17. Ellis E III, Goallo J. Relapse following mandibular advancement with dental plus skeletal maxillomandibular fixation. J Oral Maxillofac Surg 1986;44:509–15.
18. Reyneke JP, Johnston T, Van der Linden WJ. Screw osteosynthesis compared with wire osteosynthesis in advancement genioplasty: a retrospective study of skeletal stability. Br J Oral Surg 1997;35:352.
19. Joss CU, Thüer UW. Stability of hard tissue profile after mandibular setback in sagittal split osteotomies: a longitudinal and long-term follow-up study. Eur J Orthod 2008;30:16.
20. Joss CU, Vassalli IM. Stability after bilateral sagittal split osteotomy setback surgery with rigid internal fixation: a systematic review. J Oral Maxillofac Surg 2008;66:1634–43.
21. Van Sickels JE, Richardson DA. Stability of orthognathic surgery: a review of rigid fixation. Br J Oral Maxillofac Surg 1996;34:279–85.
22. Ellis E III. Condylar positioning devices for orthognathic surgery: are they necessary? J Oral Maxillofac Surg 1994;52:536–52.
23. Costa F, Robiony M, Toro C, et al. Condylar positioning devices for orthognathic surgery: a literature review. Oral Surg Oral Med Oral Pathol Oral Radiol Endod 2008;106:179–90.

24. Epker BN, Wylie GA. Control of the condylar-proximal mandibular segments after sagittal split osteotomies to advance the mandible. Oral Surg Oral Med Oral Pathol Oral Radiol Endod 1986;62: 613–7.

25. Reyneke J, Ferretti C. Intraoperative diagnosis of condylar sag after bilateral sagittal split ramus osteotomy. Br J Oral Maxillofac Surg 2002;40: 285–92.

26. Fernández Sanromán J, Gómez González JM, del Hoyo JA. Relationship between condylar position, dentofacial deformity and temporomandibular joint dysfunction: an MRI and CT prospective study. J Craniomaxillofac Surg 1998;26(1):35–42.

27. Kim YK, Yun PY, Ahn JY, et al. Changes in the temporomandibular joint disc position after orthognathic surgery. Oral Surg Oral Med Oral Pathol Oral Radiol Endod 2009;108(1):15–21.

28. Rotskoff KS, Herbosa EG, Villa P. Maintenance of condyle proximal segment position in orthognathic surgery. J Oral Maxillofac Surg 1991;49:2.

29. Saka B, Petsch I, Hingst V, et al. The influence of pre-and intraoperative positioning of the condyle in the centre of the articular fossa on the position of the disc in orthognathic surgery. A magnetic resonance study. Br J Oral Maxillofac Surg 2004;42: 120–6.

30. Arnett GW, Tamborello JA. Progressive class II development: female idiopathic condylar resorption. Oral Maxillofac Surg Clin North Am 1990;2:699.

31. Turkkahraman H, Sarioglu M. Are temporary anchorage devices truly effective in the treatment of skeletal open bites? Eur J Dent 2016;10(4): 447–53.

32. Solano-Hernández B, Antonarakis GS, Scolozzi P, et al. Combined orthodontic and orthognathic surgical treatment for the correction of skeletal anterior open-bite malocclusion: a systematic review on vertical stability. J Oral Maxillofac Surg 2013; 71(1):98–109.

33. Proffit WR, Fields HW, Moray LJ. Prevalence of malocclusion and orthodontic treatment need in the United States: estimates from the NHANES III survey. Int J Adult Orthodon Orthognath Surg 1998;13:97.

34. Greenlee GM, Huang GJ, Chen SS, et al. Stability of treatment for anterior open-bite malocclusion: a meta-analysis. Am J Orthod Dentofacial Orthop 2011;139(2):154–69.

35. Bell RB. Computer planning and intraoperative navigation in cranio-maxillofacial surgery. Oral Maxillofac Surg Clin North Am 2010;22:135–56.

36. Polley JW, Figueroa AA. Orthognathic positioning system: intraoperative system to transfer virtual surgical plan to operating field during orthognathic surgery. J Oral Maxillofac Surg 2013;71: 911–20.

37. Xia JJ, Shevchenko L, Gateno J, et al. Outcome study of computer-aided surgical simulation in the treatment of patients with craniomaxillofacial deformities. J Oral Maxillofac Surg 2011;69: 2014.

38. Lutz JC, Nicolau S, Agnus V, et al. A novel navigation system for maxillary positioning in orthognathic surgery: preclinical evaluation. J Craniomaxillofac Surg 2015;43:1723–30.

39. Mazzoni S, Badiali G, Lancellotti L, et al. Simulation-guided navigation: a new approach to improve intraoperative three-dimensional reproducibility during orthognathic surgery. J Craniofac Surg 2010;21: 1698–705.

40. Bell RB. Computer planning and intraoperative navigation in orthognathic surgery. J Oral Maxillofac Surg 2011;69:592.

41. Mischkowski RA, Zinser MJ, Ritter L, et al. Intraoperative navigation in the maxillofacial area based on 3D imaging obtained by a cone-bean device. Int J Oral Maxillofac Surg 2007;36:687.

42. Baker S, Goldstein JA, Seruya M. Outcomes in computer-assisted surgical simulation for orthognathic surgery. J Craniofac Surg 2012;23:509.

43. Kwon TG, Choi JW, Kyung HM, et al. Accuracy of maxillary repositioning in two-jaw surgery with conventional articulator model surgery versus virtual model surgery. Int J Oral Maxillofac Surg 2014; 43(6):732–8.

44. Kraeima J, Jansma J, Schepers RH. Splintless surgery: does patient-specific CAD-CAM osteosynthesis improve accuracy of Le Fort I osteotomy. Br J Oral Maxillofac Surg 2016;54(10): 1085–9.

45. Huang CS, Hsu SS, Chen YR. Systematic review of the surgery-first approach in orthognathic surgery. Biomed J 2014;37:184–90.

46. Hernandez-Alfaro F, Guijarro-Martinez R, Peiro-Guijarro MA. Surgery first in orthognathic surgery: what have we learned? A comprehensive workflow based on 45 consecutive cases. J Oral Maxillofac Surg 2014;72:376–90.

47. Peiró-Guijarro MA, Guijarro-Martínez R, Hernández-Alfaro F. Surgery first in orthognathic surgery: a systematic review of the literature. Am J Orthod Dentofacial Orthop 2016;149(4): 448–62.

48. Wolford LM, Reiche-Fischel O, Mehra P. Changes in temporomandibular joint dysfunction after orthognathic surgery. J Oral Maxillofac Surg 2003;61: 655–60.

49. Abrahamsson C, Henrikson T, Nilner M, et al. TMD before and after correction of dentofacial deformities by orthodontic and orthognathic treatment. Int J Oral Maxillofac Surg 2013;42(6):752–8.

50. Al-Riyami S, Moles DR, Cunningham SJ. Orthognathic treatment and temporomandibular disorders:

a systematic review. Part 1. A new quality-assessment technique and analysis of study characteristics and classifications. Am J Orthod Dentofacial Orthop 2009;136(5):624.e1-15 [discussion: 624–5].

51. Al-Riyami S, Cunningham SJ, Moles DR. Orthognathic treatment and temporomandibular disorders: a systematic review. Part 2. Signs and symptoms and meta-analyses. Am J Orthod Dentofacial Orthop 2009;136(5):626.e1-16 [discussion: 626–7].

52. Al-Moraissi EA, Wolford LM, Perez D, et al. Does orthognathic surgery cause or cure temporomandibular disorders? a systematic review and meta-analysis. J Oral Maxillofac Surg 2017;75(9):1835–47.

53. Cascone P, Di Paolo C, Leonardi R, et al. Temporomandibular disorders and orthognathic surgery. J Craniofac Surg 2008;19(3):687–92.

Controversies in Facial Cosmetic Surgery

Armando Retana, DDS, MD

KEYWORDS

- Blepharoplasty • Genioplasty • Alloplastic chin augmentation • Facial cosmetic surgery
- Controversy

KEY POINTS

- Facial cosmetic surgery is performed by a variety of surgeons with different surgical backgrounds.
- New facial cosmetic surgery techniques are described constantly to meet with the expectations of patients who demand less invasive procedures and less recovery time.
- Current trends in lower eyelid surgery call for periorbital fat repositioning rather than excision of fat.
- Controversies still exist in chin augmentations because some surgeons prefer to perform an osseous genioplasty and other surgeons prefer to use an alloplastic chin implant.

INTRODUCTION

Facial cosmetic surgery techniques have been described since the early twentieth century. Every year, more contemporary techniques are described in the literature in an effort to address the limitations or to minimize the risks of more traditional facial cosmetic techniques. In addition, there are multiple surgical specialties that perform facial cosmetic surgery. Both of those factors, combined with the increased demands of facial cosmetic patients seeking the least invasive procedure with minimal recovery time that can address their chief complaint in a predictable fashion, contribute to some of the controversies. There are controversies in almost all the cosmetic surgeries that are performed in the head and neck region, but their scientific discussion is difficult because many of these surgeries are performed mainly based on the level of experience and not necessarily based on the level of scientific evidence. As an example, many facelift modifications have been described in the literature and it is fair to assume that not every facial cosmetic surgeon performs the same facelift procedure. Therefore, this article does not discuss every modification or controversy in facial cosmetic surgery but, instead, 2 topics in facial cosmetic surgery of which every oral and maxillofacial surgeon should be aware.

LOWER BLEPHAROPLASTY: TO TAKE OUT PERIORBITAL FAT OR TO REPOSITION IT?

For many years, facial cosmetic surgeons have searched for the best, most reliable, and predictable technique that provides aesthetic rejuvenation of the lower eyelid and its transition to the cheek (**Fig. 1**). The traditional treatment of bulging lower eyelid fat has been resection of fat.[1] However, new trends are pointing toward decreasing the removal of tissue and favoring tissue repositioning,[2–10] but it is still controversial because each surgical technique comes with several advantages and disadvantages.

When evaluating a patient for lower eyelid surgery, the preoperative evaluation should include a careful examination of the patient's medical history and ophthalmic history, along with a visual examination. It should also take into account the position of the eyebrow, the presence of upper eyelid ptosis, lower eyelid margin position, and the projection of the cheek. Upper eyelid surgery in which skin is removed and medial orbital fat is excised is a procedure that is reliable and has

Private Practice, Capital Center for Oral and Maxillofacial Surgery, 2311 M Street NW, Suite 200, Washington, DC 20037, USA
E-mail address: aretana@ccomfs.com

Oral Maxillofacial Surg Clin N Am 29 (2017) 441–446
http://dx.doi.org/10.1016/j.coms.2017.07.002
1042-3699/17/© 2017 Elsevier Inc. All rights reserved.

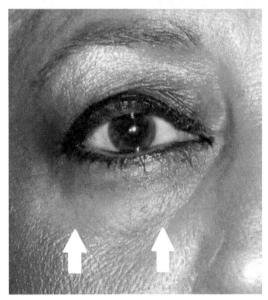

Fig. 1. The tear trough deformity, also known as the nasojugal groove, is the natural depression that extends inferolaterally from the medial canthus of the eye (*white arrows*). Laterally, it demarcates the lid-cheek junction.

consistent results. Lower eyelid blepharoplasty is a bit more controversial.

One of the reasons why the topic is thought to be controversial is because healing after lower eyelid surgery can be unpredictable in nature. This has allowed some surgeons to adopt a more conservative approach to lower blepharoplasty.

In 1995, Hamra[10] described the release of the arcus marginalis to reposition the herniated fat pads over the entire orbital rim by securing it to the periosteum. In 2000, Goldberg[7] described repositioning the fat in a subperiosteal plane to decrease the change of a visible demarcation. In 2003, Kawamoto and Bradley[11] suggested there was better filling of the nasojugal groove when the fat was repositioned in a supraperiosteal plane.

Other less invasive approaches to ablate the tear trough deformity have been described. Coleman[12,13] described fat grafting the periorbital area to camouflage the defect and Trepsat[14] described a combination of periorbital fat grafting and transconjunctival blepharoplasty (**Fig. 2**A).

Several surgeons consider resection of the excess skin if a skin pinch test with forceps warrants it. This is performed via a subciliary incision. A more aggressive technique involves a skin-muscle flap in which the skin and the underlying orbicularis oculi muscle fibers are excised. At that point, the periorbital fat can be excised via small incisions in the septum. This, however, may lead to lower eyelid malposition and muscle denervation due to violation of the middle lamella, a complication known as ectropion (**Fig. 3**).

The main aesthetic concerns that are addressed with a lower blepharoplasty include pseudoherniation of periorbital fat, excess skin, and a certain degree of skin laxity. A good technique that can be used in younger individuals with minimal skin laxity is a transconjunctival approach that allows fat excision via a retroseptal dissection, which has the advantage of keeping the middle lamella intact (**Fig. 4**). The skin can then be treated with either laser skin resurfacing or a chemical peel and fat grafting of the cheek to allow for a smooth transition at the tear trough region. As previously mentioned, lower eyelid excess skin can also be addressed with a conservative pinch excision rather than laser resurfacing or a chemical peel (1–2 coats of 30% trichloroacetic acid). The

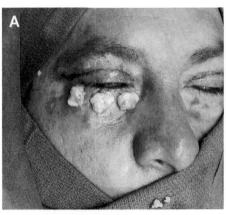
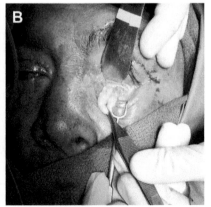

Fig. 2. Transconjunctival blepharoplasty with periorbital fat excision (*A*) versus a transconjunctival blepharoplasty showing medial fat pat repositioning over the arcus marginalis (*B*). (*Courtesy of* Angelo Cuzalina, MD, DDS, Tulsa Surgical Arts, Tulsa, Oklahoma, USA.)

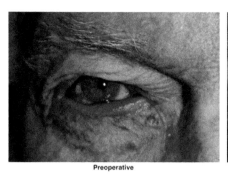 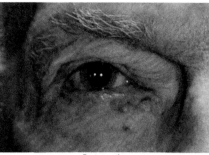

Preoperative   Postoperative

Fig. 3. Before (*left*) and after (*right*) right lower eyelid ectropion repair with retractor reinsertion and lateral tarsal strip. This 82-year-old man noted tearing and foreign body sensation in the right eye. A lower eyelid retractor reinsertion and lateral tarsal strip was performed to restore the eyelid to its native state. (*From* Korn BS, Kikkawa DO. Ectropion repair by retractor reinsertion and lateral tarsal strip. In: Video atlas of oculofacial plastic and reconstructive surgery. 2nd edition. Philadelphia: Elsevier; 2017. p. 176–181. Figure 25-10; with permission.)

disadvantage of this cheek fat grafting technique is that fat grafting is not as predictable in its healing, which can lead to bumpy irregularities that are hard to treat or it may create a facial asymmetry if 1 side responds differently than the other. Complications such as fat thromboembolism can occur that can lead to blindness or cavernous sinus thrombosis. Those complications could be avoided by the use of blunt cannulas, and minimizing the pressure of the syringe when injecting in the periorbital region.

The more contemporary techniques in lower blepharoplasty call for transposition of the periorbital fat to redrape over the arcus marginalis to fill the lid or cheek junction[7] (see **Fig. 2**B). The advantage of this technique is that it takes the periorbital fat out of the retroseptal position to be used as a pedicle and a vascularized fat graft to fill the tear trough deformity and infraorbital hollows without the need to harvest fat from a distant site. The major downside of this technique is the difficultly of handling the fat and reliably securing the fat in its new position. Securing the fat may require a suture onto the underlying periosteum or a bolster dressing on the skin. Some patients may not like the appearance of a bolster dressing

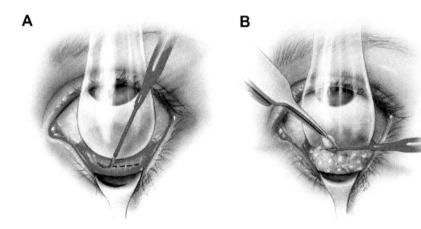

Fig. 4. Transconjunctival blepharoplasty. Lower eyelid dissection. The dissection is begun centrally, to avoid the inferior oblique muscle, and performed in layered fashion through the conjunctiva and lower eyelid retractors (*A*). A cotton-tip applicator is used to ballot the conjunctiva and lid retractors inferiorly and allow the fat pads to reposition anteriorly (*B*). Once the fat pads are identified, gentle posterior pressure on the globe with the Jaeger retractor is applied to allow the fat pads to prolapse forward. Each fat pad is gently teased anteriorly with forceps. Only a moderate amount of fat should be excised from each fat pad. (*From* Marshak H, Dresner SC. Transconjunctival lower blepharoplasty. In: Azizzadeh B, Murphy MR, Johnson CM, editors. Master techniques in facial rejuvenation. Philadelphia: Elsevier; 2007. p. 89–98. Figure 6-6; with permission.)

on their face in the postoperative period, which makes this technique less attractive for some surgeons.

Other treatment considerations include the need for lateral canthal support to address any preexisting lower eyelid laxity, which can lead to severe lid malposition.[15] A lateral canthopexy with or without a tarsal strip procedure can be performed in those patients with lid laxity that is determined to be moderate (3–6 mm lid distraction) or severe (>6 mm of lid distraction).

Summary

Lower blepharoplasty is a common procedure performed by facial cosmetic surgeons from a variety of surgical backgrounds. It has the potential to make a significant difference in facial rejuvenation, but it is associated with several complications. Unlike upper blepharoplasty, it is among most controversial topics in facial cosmetic surgery and many different techniques have been described in the current literature. All of those techniques have advantages and disadvantages that should be considered when performing a lower blepharoplasty procedure. The surgeon should be able to perform all of the previously mentioned techniques and to try to avoid treating every lower eyelid case in the same fashion. The surgeon should be have knowledge of and be able to deal with all possible complications that are associated with lower eyelid surgery.

THE CHIN: WHAT IS THE BEST OPTION FOR CHIN AUGMENTATION, AN OSSEOUS GENIOPLASTY OR A CHIN IMPLANT?

Obwegeser[16] was the first to describe the details of bony chin surgery back in 1957. However, it was Converse and Wood-Smith,[17] in 1964, who popularized the sliding genioplasty. They described the horizontal osteotomy of the mandible to reposition the chin anteriorly. Alloplastic materials became popular in the 1980s and continue to gain popularity. Both osseous genioplasty and the use of alloplastic chin implants continue to be common procedures in the armamentarium of many facial cosmetic surgeons worldwide from multiple surgical backgrounds. The biggest advantage of an osseous genioplasty is the ability to treat almost all chin deformities, including microgenia, macrogenia, and chin asymmetries.[16]

One advantage of the osseous genioplasty is that it avoids the use of alloplastic materials that are associated with increased cost and complications from having a foreign body in situ for a long period of time. Another advantage of this procedure is that it is the treatment of choice for those

patients who exhibit a short lower facial height with increased projection of their chin soft tissues. That type of patient usually has a deep mentolabial grove that will only be deepened by the placement of a chin implant. Thus, they are better treated with a genioplasty that is moved mainly in a caudal direction to increase the lower facial height.

When assessing the lower facial third, a clinician must take into account the patient's gender and height. Limiting the evaluation to the chin or even just the face is a mistake that is made by many. A methodical evaluation must include the sex of the patient, their stature, the harmony of their bite, facial thirds evaluation, the proportions of the lower facial third components (upper lip, lower lip and chin), the relationship of the chin to the nose, the relationship of the upper and lower lip, the amount of incisor show, the depth of the labiomandibular fold (marionette lines), the presence of lower lip eversion, the height and depth of the labiomental fold, chin pad thickness, and evaluation of the soft tissues of the chin at rest and during smile.

Controversy

Perhaps the controversy in this area is because a surgeon is going to perform the procedure that he or she is comfortable executing. This is most likely going to be the procedure they learned in their surgical training. For instance, oral and maxillofacial surgeons are very comfortable performing osseous genioplasties, whereas plastic surgeons are more comfortable doing alloplastic chin implants. One should not perform the same procedure on every patient who has an aesthetic need in the lower facial third, just because that is the way one was trained to do it. Instead, one should try to tailor the surgical approach to the specific needs to the patient after listing to the patient's chief complaint, completing a physical evaluation, and having a discussion with the patient about all risks, benefits, alternatives, and limitations.

Advantages and Disadvantages of Osseous Genioplasty

Both an osseous genioplasty and a chin implant have their advantages and disadvantages (**Box 1**). The main advantages of a genioplasty are the use of the patient's own tissue, which avoids the use of an alloplastic implant; the scar is intraoral; and the patient gets a genioglossus advancement, which could potentially help prevent the development of sleep apnea. This procedure, however, has fallen out of favor by some surgeons because of several disadvantages that are associated with it. It involves more soft tissue

Box 1	
Osseous genioplasty compared with alloplastic chin implants placed via a submental approach	
Advantages	**Disadvantages**
Use of patient's own tissue	Extensive tissue dissection
No implant required, less cost	More invasive
No skin incisions	Bone edges might be palpable
Genioglossus advancement	Neurosensory changes are common
	Technique-sensitive
	Plate and screws palpability or exposure
	Increased surgery time
	Floor of mouth hematoma
	Mentalis muscle strain

Box 2	
Alloplastic chin implants place via a submental approach when compared with osseous genioplasty	
Advantages	**Disadvantages**
Less soft tissue dissection	More cost
Less invasive	Foreign body
Less severe initial neurosensory deficit	Implant displacement
Short procedure time	Implant mobility
Low complication rate	Bone resorption if no fixation used
Reversible	Skin incision

dissection. The mental nerve must be identified to make an osteotomy 5 to 6 mm inferior to the mental foramen, which makes short-term and long-term nerve numbness a common postoperative morbidity. Genioplasty has a higher incidence of neurosensory deficit when compared with alloplastic chin implants, with almost all cases reporting immediate neurosensory deficit. There is a possibility of mentalis muscle strain and for the metal plates and screws to become palpable and/or exposed. A genioplasty is extremely technique-sensitive and, if not done correctly, the edges of the osteotomy could become palpable. When taking into account efficiency, a genioplasty is more time-consuming than the placement of an alloplastic implant, which is an influential factor for those surgeons who practice in the private practice setting.

Because of the extensive dissection required to perform a genioplasty, there is a life-threatening complication that could compromise the airway postoperatively, which is a floor of mouth hematoma. Moreover, healing of the bony segment depends the blood supply to all of its components. Thus, resorption of repositioned bony segment could happen, which may yield a distorted look to the chin.

Advantages and Disadvantages of Alloplastic Chin Augmentation

Chin augmentation with alloplastic material comes with several advantages and disadvantages when compared with a genioplasty procedure (**Box 2**). The surgical approach and fixation techniques for chin augmentation are controversial among facial cosmetic surgeons. Some surgeons advocate for the intraoral approach and others prefer the submental incision approach. To secure the implants to periosteum, some surgeons do not use any fixation, others use sutures, and others use titanium screws.

The intraoral incision hides the scar in the mucosa of the oral cavity but the soft tissue dissection could be extensive. Intraoral scars may not be visible but may be bothersome to the patient if unfavorable healing takes place. To minimize dissection of the oral mucosa, a vertical incision could be made between the mentalis muscles, but this may limit visualization of the mental nerves. With the intraoral approach, bilateral mental nerves should be visualized and the implant should be screwed in place because the implant pocket is usually over-dissected with this approach. The number of screws used varies between 1, 2, and even 3. The objective is to stabilize the implant to prevent any rotation or movement. It is thought that the micromovement of the implant is a major factor that contributes to bone resorption by the alloplastic implant over the anterior portion of the mandible. When making the incision and closing in a layered fashion, the surgeon must keep in mind that reapproximation of the mentalis muscles is essential to prevent postoperative mentalis straining. A good cuff of muscle must be kept on both sides of the incision and well reapproximated to prevent this hard-to-treat postoperative complication.

The other surgical alternative for placement of an alloplastic chin implant is the submental approach. A 2 to 3 cm incision is placed just posterior to the natural submental crease, minimal soft tissue dissection is performed until the inferior-anterior portion of the mandible is reached, a periosteal elevator is then used to dissect the soft tissues along the inferior border of the mandible bilaterally without the need to dissect the mental nerve in most individuals. Older patients might have a mental foreman that can be positioned closer to the inferior border of the mandible, in which case the nerves might be encountered. Posterior dissection is performed slightly beyond the dimension of the implant. Some of the advantages of this approach are as follows. The entire procedure is not as time-consuming as an osseous genioplasty or as the placement of an alloplastic chin implant via an intraoral approach. The layered closure includes reapproximation of the deep subcutaneous tissues and the skin edges. It does not require transection or reapproximation of the mentalis muscles. The submental approach also provides the opportunity to release the mandibular ligaments in older patients, if necessary. The submental scar is usually well tolerated and the risk of implant exposure and colonization with oral bacteria is lessened. In addition, it is a great approach to perform if the patient is already undergoing a rhytidectomy, a platysmaplasty, or neck liposuction.

Additional Considerations

Preoperative clinical evaluation and discussion with the patient are both very important in determining the best surgical approach and surgical technique. Patients who have a stable bite but exhibit clinical signs of microgenia would benefit from a quick and simple procedure such as an alloplastic chin implant to give their chin more projection. Patients with a short facial height and microgenia would most likely benefit from a sliding genioplasty that would bring the chin anteriorly and caudally to not only address the lack of projection but also to lengthen the lower facial third for a more balanced facial profile. However, the latter patient would also benefit from the placement of a vertical tilt silicone implant, which could achieve similar results.

SUMMARY

Osseous genioplasty and alloplastic chin implants are 2 acceptable treatments for lower facial third rejuvenation. Both techniques are predictable, safe, reproducible, and carry a low complication rate. The technique to be used should address the chief complaint of the patient in a safe fashion and should have the lowest complication rate in the hands of the surgeon that is performing it. Informed consent in which all risks, benefits, alternatives, and limitations to the technique are considered should be part of the preoperative work up, which could help the surgeon choose which technique to use.

REFERENCES

1. Castanares S. Blepharoplasty for herniated intraorbital fat: anatomical basis for a new approach. Plast Reconstr Surg 1951;8:46–58.
2. Barton FE Jr, Ha R, Awada M. Fat extrusion and septal reset in patients with the tear trough triad: a critical appraisal. Plast Reconstr Surg 2004;113:2115–21 [discussion: 2122–3].
3. Hamra ST. The zygorbicular dissection in composite rhytidectomy: an ideal midface plane. Plast Reconstr Surg 1998;102:1646–57.
4. Camirand A, Doucet J, Harris J. Eyelid aging: the historical evolution of its management. Aesthetic Plast Surg 2005;29:65–73.
5. de la Plaza R, Arroyo JM. A new technique for the treatment of palpebral bags. Plast Reconstr Surg 1988;81:677–87.
6. Eder H. Importance of fat conservation in lower blepharoplasty. Aesthetic Plast Surg 1997;21:168–74.
7. Goldberg RA. Transconjunctival orbital fat repositioning: transposition of orbital fat pedicles into a subperiosteal pocket. Plast Reconstr Surg 2000;105:743–8 [discussion: 749–51].
8. Hamra ST. The role of orbital fat preservation in facial aesthetic surgery: a new concept. Clin Plast Surg 1996;23:17–28.
9. Huang T. Reduction of lower palpebral bulge by plicating attenuated orbital septa: a technical modification in cosmetic blepharoplasty. Plast Reconstr Surg 2000;105:2552–8 [discussion: 2559–60].
10. Hamra ST. Arcus marginalis release and orbital fat preservation in midface rejuvenation. Plast Reconstr Surg 1995;96:354–62.
11. Kawamoto HK, Bradley JP. The tear "TROUF" procedure: transconjunctival repositioning of orbital unipedicled fat. Plast Reconstr Surg 2003;112:1903–7 [discussion: 1908–9].
12. Coleman SR. Structural fat grafts: the ideal filler. Clin Plast Surg 2001;28:111–9.
13. Coleman SR. The technique of the periorbital lipo infiltration. Oper Tech Plast Reconstr Surg 1994;1:120–6.
14. Trepsat F. Periorbital rejuvenation combining fat grafting and blepharoplasties. Aesthetic Plast Surg 2003;27:243–53.
15. Muzaffar AR, Menderlson BC, Adams WP Jr. Surgical anatomy of the ligamentous attachments of the lower lid and canthus. Plast Reconstr Surg 2002;110:873.
16. Obwegeser TR. The surgical correction of mandibular prognathism and retrognathia with consideration of genioplasty. I. Surgical procedures to correct mandibular prognathism and reshaping of the chin. Oral Surg Oral Med Oral Pathol 1957;10:677.
17. Converse JM, Wood-Smith D. Horizontal osteotomy of the mandible. Plast Reconstr Surg 1964;34:464.

Current Controversies in Metopic Suture Craniosynostosis

Michael S. Jaskolka, DDS, MD

KEYWORDS

- Metopic craniosynostosis • Trigonocephaly • Metopic ridge • Neurodevelopment • Endoscopic
- Virtual surgical planning

KEY POINTS

- The diagnosis of metopic craniosynostosis may be challenging as the metopic suture fuses physiologically during the infant period.
- Metopic craniosynostosis frequently occurs in combination with other abnormalities or syndromes.
- Patients generally perform within intellectual norms but are at a higher risk of cognitive, speech, language and behavioral problems.
- The main goal of surgical treatment is the correction of the "trigonocephalic" craniofacial dysmorphology.
- Anterior cranial vault expansion with fronto-orbital advancement and endoscopic suturectomy with post-operative cranial orthotic treatment are the most common techniques. Long-term study is necessary to determine which is the most appropriate treatment.

 Video content accompanies this article at http://www.oralmaxsurgery.theclinics.com.

INTRODUCTION

Metopic craniosynostosis is being reported with an increasing incidence and is now the second most common type of isolated suture craniosynostosis. Numerous areas of controversy exist in the workup and management, including defining the diagnosis in the less severe phenotype, the association with neurodevelopmental delay, the impact of surgical treatment, and the applicability of various techniques and their timing on outcomes.

BACKGROUND AND GENERAL CONCEPTS

The cranium is composed of numerous plates of bone that are formed through an intramembranous process. Interspaced between these plates are the sutures, which are dural reflections with a mesenchymal and neural crest origin (**Fig. 1**).

Craniosynostosis is defined as the premature fusion of 1 or more of the cranial sutures.[1] In general, this occurs during the gestational period and presents as congenital absence of the suture. Craniosynostosis is a defining feature of the craniofacial dysostosis syndromes (ie, Crouzon, Apert, Pfeiffer, Saethre-Chotzen, Carpenter) but more commonly is encountered as an isolated finding (~85%) that is limited to a single major suture (70%).[2] The incidence of craniosynostosis is approximately 1 per 2000 live births. Sagittal craniosynostosis is the most common, followed by metopic, unilateral coronal, and lambdoid types.

Isolated suture craniosynostosis is classified by the specific missing suture (eg, metopic) and each type is associated with a unique pattern of growth and resulting characteristic shape (eg, trigonocephaly) These types are shown in **Fig. 2**.

Department of Maxillofacial Surgery, New Hanover Regional Medical Center, 2131 South 17th Street, Wilmington, NC 28401, USA
E-mail address: michael.jaskolka@nhrmc.org

Oral Maxillofacial Surg Clin N Am 29 (2017) 447–463
http://dx.doi.org/10.1016/j.coms.2017.07.003
1042-3699/17/© 2017 Elsevier Inc. All rights reserved.

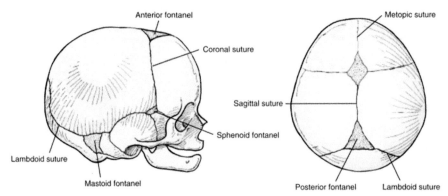

Fig. 1. During infancy, the cranial vault sutures remain open to allow for normal brain growth. Major cranial vault sutures include the metopic, right and left coronal, sagittal, and right and left lambdoid. (*From* Ruiz RL, Ritter AM, Turvey TA, et al. Nonsyndromic craniosynostosis: diagnosis and contemporary surgical management. Oral Maxillofacial Surg Clin North Am 16:448, 2004; with permission.)

The absence of a cranial suture leads to restricted perpendicular growth and increased parallel growth.[3] Delashaw and colleagues[4] published a set of 4 additional principles that further describe the abnormal and compensatory growth patterns that more accurately describe the development of specific skull shapes.

The normal skull grows in a propulsive fashion secondary to brain growth. There is compensatory appositional bone growth at the cranial suture complex as well as endocranial resorption and ectocranial deposition. The overall form of the skull is determined by the brain and likely influenced by the cranial base through dural attachments.[5]

The definitive cause of craniosynostosis is unknown. Associations with genetic abnormalities, intrauterine constraint, metabolic disorders and environmental factors have all been identified. There is a genetic predisposition that is affected by epigenetic and environmental factors leading to phenotypic expression. The biological origin and signaling pathways are postulated to involve fibroblast growth factor receptors, transforming

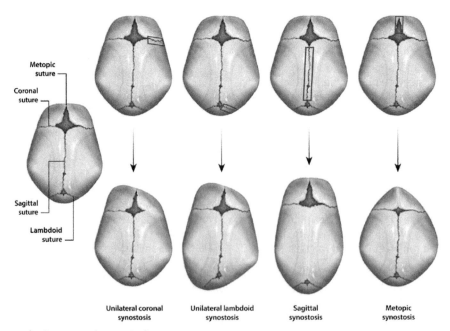

Fig. 2. Types of primary craniosynostosis.

growth factor beta, bone morphogenetic protein, and Wnt signaling pathways. Investigation of the molecular and cellular microenvironment of the cranial suture complex continues to advance through the use of murine and rabbit models. In general, there is agreement that there is a localized abnormality in the dura that regulates sutural fusion.[6–8]

Pathophysiology

The traditional concept is of propulsive brain growth pushing against a restricted skull with a reduced intracranial volume resulting in increased intracranial pressure (ICP) with subsequent risk of neurologic injury.[9]

Numerous challenges have become apparent related to the application of this concept to patients with single-suture craniosynostosis. The literature is fraught with limited sample sizes, comingling of patient populations (syndromic, nonsyndromic, multisuture, different suture types), disagreement over reference standards for cranial volume and ICP, and difficulty of accurate neurodevelopmental testing in infants.

Indications for Surgical Treatment

The indications for surgical treatment of isolated suture craniosynostosis are 2-fold: a concern for prevention or limitation of neurodevelopmental injury and correction of abnormal morphology.

Surgical Treatment

The surgical treatment of isolated suture craniosynostosis began with strip craniectomy for release of the microcephalic skull to provide relief of intracranial hypertension and treat mental delay.[10,11]

The evolution of craniofacial surgery was marked by the development of techniques for surgical access, osteotomy design, autogenous bone grafting, internal fixation, and instrumentation. These techniques were refined, consolidated, and popularized by Dr Paul Tessier.[12] As the specialty of craniofacial surgery was disseminated, these techniques were applied to the cranial vault by numerous surgeons and led to a shift in surgical approach to the treatment of craniosynostosis. The new focus was the excision of the fused suture, the removal of the affected areas of the skull and orbits, immediate reconstruction for expansion of the skull, and normalization of the cranial and orbital shape.

METOPIC CRANIOSYNOSTOSIS

Metopic craniosynostosis results in a trigonocephalic configuration of the skull. The details of the dysmorphology include a triangular-shaped forehead, an absent metopic suture, a prominent metopic ridge, orbital hypotelorism, ethmoidal hypoplasia, retruded lateral orbital rims, a narrow bitemporal dimension, and expanded biparietal dimension.[13–15]

The metopic suture is unique relative to the other major sutures in that it is the only suture that has been shown to close physiologically as early as 3 months of age, and almost always by 9 months.[16,17] Fusion has been shown to start at the nasion and progress toward the anterior fontanelle.[18] Physiologic closure is frequently associated with ridging over the metopic suture.

Incidence of Metopic Craniosynostosis

Metopic craniosynostosis has traditionally been cited to occur with an incidence of 1 per 15,000 live births with a male to female ratio of 3.3:1.[19] An increasing incidence more closely approaching 1 per 5000 has been reported.[15] A pan-European study including 7 craniofacial centers indicated a current incidence of 23% of isolated suture craniosynostosis,[20] whereas other publications from North America report an incidence as high as 27% and 31%.[21,22] Multiple explanations are proposed, including increasing maternal and paternal age, changes in prenatal folic acid consumption, an increase in syndrome-associated subtypes, and a possible correlation with uterine constraint and other deformational conditions.[23] The most concerning possible explanation is overdiagnosis and treatment related to the potentially subjective assessment of the mild and moderate phenotypes.[14,24]

Type of Metopic Craniosynostosis

There seem to be 2 categories of metopic craniosynostosis: the first is isolated, whereas the second is associated with other anomalies or syndromes. In a sample of 237 patients, 78% (184) had isolated synostosis, whereas 22% (53) had additional abnormalities. Of this second group, 75% (40) were noted to have additional abnormalities, whereas 25% (13) had a known syndrome. A family history was reported in 5.6%.[19] This concept is further supported by Kini and colleagues,[25] who reported a 17-year review of 110 patients with metopic craniosynostosis with a 34.6% rate of additional abnormalities or syndromic diagnosis. There is a strong association with maternal valproic acid exposure and numerous studies supporting the concept of intrauterine constraint. A higher association with environmental contribution as well as submicroscopic chromosomal abnormalities in midline craniosynostosis types has been noted as well.[2]

NEURODEVELOPMENTAL CONSIDERATIONS
Cranial Volume

Metopic craniosynostosis has been shown to involve normal or supranormal cranial volume.[26–28] These values may be questioned because of the methodology of measurement and calculation, but more so because of their comparison with historical reference standards that were abstracted from limited and biased samples.[29–31] Current high-resolution computed tomography (CT) and postimage processing are now being used to accurately measure intracranial volume[32,33] and generate new standard data sets.[34] Questions still remain regarding their validity and application,[35,36] but the concept that patients with isolated metopic suture craniosynostosis have overall reduced cranial volume is likely incorrect. Some investigators suggest that the answer may not be static because volume may be lower at birth but normalizes over the first year of life.[37]

Shape

Contemporary CT-based data are able to specifically address the cranial shape and interaction with regional volume. Although overall intracranial volume is likely comparable with unaffected controls, the frontal volume (anterior to the coronal sutures) is reduced in terms of absolute measurements as well as the proportion of the total cranial volume.[33]

Deformation Versus Malformation

The concept of constricted anterior cranial volume suggests deformational changes to the brain secondary to skull shape. Intrinsic malformation of the brain is a contrasting but not necessarily exclusive concept because metopic synostosis is associated with an increased incidence of brain abnormalities. MRI analysis reveals both cortical and subcortical brain dysmorphology that cannot be completely explained by the abnormal cranial shape.[38] Other structural abnormalities include smaller frontal lobes, widened precentral sulci, frontal subdural space distention, increased ventricular

size, and corpus callosum and cerebellar anomalies.[39,40] Brain volume in preoperative and postoperative patients with metopic craniosynostosis compared with controls seems to be similar in the gray matter, white matter, and regional and total volume.[40]

Intracranial Pressure

The concern for increased ICP associated with craniosynostosis is frequently cited. Most occurrences are in patients with multisuture or syndromic forms. In consideration of patients with isolated suture metopic craniosynostosis, the largest challenge is the limited number of sampled patients, the general discussion related to reference standards for ICP in infants and children, and the various methodologies for measurement.[41]

The classic study by Renier and colleagues[42] reported high ICP (>15 mm Hg) in 14% of patients with single-suture craniosynostosis and 47% of patients with multiple sutures involved. There were 5 patients with metopic craniosynostosis and none of them showed increased ICP. A more recent report by the same group reported on 51 patients with isolated suture craniosynostosis with high ICP (>15 mm Hg) in 2 patients (4%), both of whom had sagittal suture involvement. There were 4 patients with metopic craniosynostosis included in the study group.[9] A combined summary of their additional data set included 31 patients with metopic craniosynostosis and reported high ICP in 2 (6%).[43]

There is a conflicting theme found in the literature of a higher rate of increased ICP in metopic craniosynostosis, most notably in older patients. As part of the development of a protocol for the use of ICP in a surgical decision-making protocol, 33% (3 of 9) of patients with metopic craniosynostosis were shown to have increased ICP (>15 mm Hg).[44] In a report by the same group, 33% (4 of 12) with metopic craniosynostosis that were not operated because of cosmesis alone were noted to have increased ICP (>15 mm Hg).[45] The implications of these reports are uncertain because of vague inclusion criteria and selection bias without controls. Even higher rates of increased ICP are reported in 79% (44 of 56) of patients between the ages of 2 and 8 years with mild trigonocephaly who presented with neurodevelopmental concerns.[46] This literature has multiple shortcomings, the most significant of which are the questionable diagnosis of metopic craniosynostosis, the brief measurement of ICP under anesthesia, and selection bias without controls.

Ultimately the risk of increased ICP in patients with metopic synostosis is likely extremely small and there continues to be limited understanding of the impact of these findings on neurodevelopment.

Other Considerations

Other factors, such as upper airways obstruction and venous hypertension, have been considered in their impact on the intracranial environment but relate primarily to multisuture and syndromic craniosynostosis.[41] Although cerebrospinal fluid (CSF) abnormalities (production, collection, and absorption) are also considered, a retrospective review of 1447 patients affected by nonsyndromic craniosynostosis showed the occurrence of hydrocephalus with the same frequency as in the normal population.[47] Interestingly, abnormalities in frontal cerebral blood flow may correlate with frontal constriction and have been shown to improve following surgical expansion.[33,48,49]

Developmental Delay

Numerous historical publications report a high incidence of mental delay in patients with metopic craniosynostosis; comingling of various patient populations and different means of assessment confound these findings.[50–52] Normal mental development was reported in a small group of metopic patients before (7 patients) and after (4 patients) surgery.[53] The need for long-term evaluation was raised by retrospective reviews of 32 and 37 patients respectively, showing a higher risk (47% and 57%) of cognitive, speech, and behavioral issues in older children.[54,55] There is recognition of the potential for additional abnormal findings as children enter school and undergo a higher social and developmental burden.

As testing has become more focused and standardized, and patients are being followed in a more longitudinal fashion, patients seem to perform within intellectual norms but are at a higher risk of cognitive, speech, language, and behavioral problems.[56,57]

Impact of Severity of Phenotype on Developmental Delay

Correlation between the severity of the phenotype and risk of neurodevelopmental delay may help to support the recommendation for or against surgery. A significant challenge encountered in the literature is caused by the variability in which severity is quantified. In combination with small and comingled study samples without matched controls and incomplete longitudinal patient participation, each study has limited power and ability to identify significant differences.

Preoperative developmental assessment in a series of 22 patients aged 3.6 to 25 months was compared with a grouped clinical and radiographic severity classification scheme without any overall correlation.[58] Postoperative speech and language development at 3 and 5 years was measured in a series of 20 infants, including those with other extracranial abnormalities, and was compared with preoperative evaluation of several CT-based angular and linear measurements. A 30% delay was noted (compared with a 6% baseline in the United Kingdom population) without any statistical correlation with the severity of the preoperative phenotype.[59] A questionnaire was used to evaluate the developmental, educational, and behavioral domains in a group of 63 patients. Seventy percent of the patients were treated surgically at a mean of 1 year of age, whereas the other 30% were deemed to have a mild deformity and followed. There was no statistical difference between the two groups.[60] A subset of the Infant Learning Project reviewed 49 infants with metopic craniosynostosis. Preoperative CT scans were evaluated with the Trigonocephaly Severity Indices (craniosynostosis severity index)[61] and the subjects underwent preoperative and postoperative (18 and 36 months) neurodevelopmental testing. There was no association between phenotypic severity and outcomes.[57] A recent study has taken a neurophysiologic approach to this question. Auditory stimulated evoked potentials were measured and compared with severity of trigonocephaly as measured by the endocranial angle. They were shown to be reduced in the severe phenotype compared with a moderate phenotype and control group. The clinical significance of these findings has yet to be determined.[62]

In summary, there seems to be a risk of neurodevelopmental delay in metopic craniosynostosis but the underlying pathophysiology is not well understood. There may be both extrinsic (cranial) and intrinsic (cerebral) variables that are not clearly related to ICP and are independent of the phenotypic severity.

DIAGNOSIS OF METOPIC CRANIOSYNOSTOSIS

Severe trigonocephaly is pathognomonic for metopic craniosynostosis, allowing the diagnosis to be made by history and physical examination.[22] Patients with craniosynostosis have a craniofacial dysmorphology at birth that does not improve. Those with physiologic closure and metopic ridging develop the abnormal findings during the first year of life as the metopic suture closes. The diagnosis becomes more challenging when patients present with a less severe or atypical phenotype with metopic ridging. This condition is compounded by delayed referral and inaccurate history provided by families.[14]

Because of the nature of the metopic suture and the potential for physiologic closure, the diagnosis of metopic craniosynostosis cannot always be made based on the absence of the metopic suture, which generates a subjective evaluation: where does isolated metopic ridging end and metopic craniosynostosis begin?

Additional Methods to Aid in Diagnosis

CT characteristics of the metopic suture are suggested to be helpful in distinguishing between metopic ridging and craniosynostosis. Increased thickness with an ectocranial ridge is most commonly seen in craniosynostosis. An endocranial spur was not seen in any cases of metopic craniosynostosis, whereas an endocranial notch (omega or W shaped) was associated with a diagnosis of metopic synostosis in 93% of the 30-patient sample surgically treated with metopic craniosynostosis compared with a 76-patient control group. The metopic notch was only present in patients with metopic craniosynostosis[18] (Fig. 3).

A standardized clinical and radiographic evaluation has been suggested to assist in differentiating between metopic craniosynostosis and isolated metopic ridging. Clinical findings included narrow forehead, hypotelorism, epicanthal folds, biparietal widening, metopic ridge, raised brows, and lateral orbital hypoplasia/pterional constriction. CT findings include closed metopic suture with a ridge, pulled anterior fontanelle, straight lateral frontal bone that is posteriorly displaced and tangential to the midorbit or medial to the midorbit, upsloping lateral orbital rim, interorbital narrowing, and narrowing of the upper orbital width[14] (Figs. 4 and 5).

A retrospective review of 258 patients with metopic abnormalities showed a significant "gray zone" in which an ambiguous diagnosis was given to 34% of patients by a multispecialty panel reviewing photographs alone. The presence of 3 or more radiographic characteristics had a high correlation with the diagnosis of metopic craniosynostosis: no children with clinical or photographic diagnosis of metopic ridging had 3 or more CT findings.[14]

Computed Tomography–based Measurements

The use of CT-based measurements serves the purpose of aiding in diagnosis and classification of severity. However, the literature is full of individual protocols for the selection of points, angles, planes, proportions, and indices without any standardization, leading to significant selection bias.[17,50,61,63,64]

Three-dimensional (3D) CT–based shape analysis is likely to be more useful but is currently in its infancy. These techniques are likely to have the same limitations as noted earlier unless a standard is widely adopted. Presently, the complexity of this type of analysis is a barrier to clinical application. In the interim, a relevant approach has been the correlation between shape analysis and

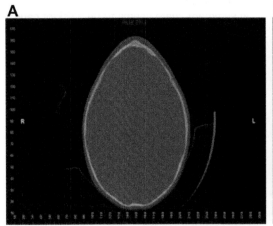
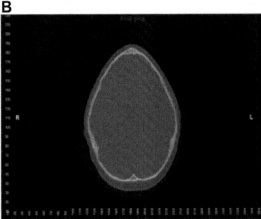

Fig. 3. (*A*) Axial CT demonstrating a narrow endocranial metopic notch in a patient with metopic craniosynostosis. (*B*) Axial CT demonstrating a wide endocranial metopic notch in a patient with metopic craniosynostosis.

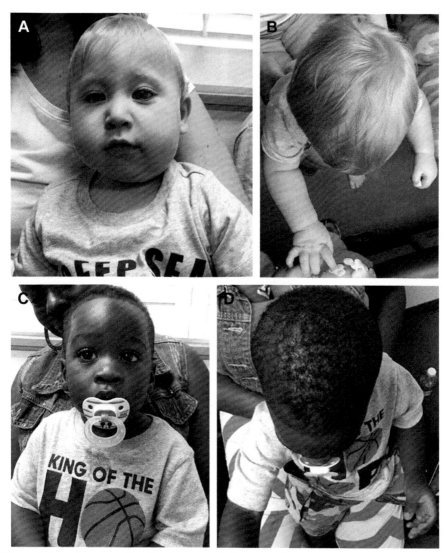

Fig. 4. (*A*) Frontal view, demonstrating the characteristic features of a patient with metopic craniosynostosis. (*B*) Bird's eye view, demonstrating the characteristic features of a patient with metopic craniosynostosis. (*C*) Frontal view, demonstrating a patient with a prominent metopic ridge and bitemporal narrowing without other signs of metopic craniosynostosis. (*D*) Bird's eye view, demonstrating a patient with a prominent metopic ridge and bitemporal narrowing without other signs of metopic craniosynostosis.

the interfrontal divergence angle, which is easily applied[24,65] (**Fig. 6**).

A further effort to correlate a break point greater than or equal to 118° for recommending surgical intervention has been suggested based on expert review of patients in the gray zone.[66]

Although these are significant efforts and useful tools for research, metopic craniosynostosis and resulting trigonocephaly is a 3D condition that presents along a phenotypic spectrum; there are no simple radiographic measurement that can confirm the diagnosis and determine treatment.[67,68]

TREATMENT OF METOPIC SUTURE CRANIOSYNOSTOSIS
Indications and Goals

The indication for the treatment of metopic cranio-synostosis is the craniofacial 3D dysmorphology and trigonocephaly. The goal is normalization of the appearance and prevention of the psychosocial impact of a craniofacial difference. Although surgical reconstruction has been shown to be generally safe, any intervention should only be undertaken if necessary. Controversy presents when considering the mild and moderate phenotypes: what is a cosmetically acceptable level of

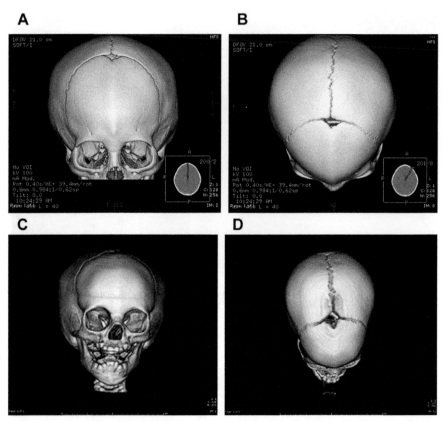

Fig. 5. (*A*) CT reconstruction, frontal view, demonstrating the characteristic features of a patient with metopic craniosynostosis. (*B*) 3D CT reconstruction, bird's eye view, demonstrating the characteristic features of a patient with metopic craniosynostosis. (*C*) 3D CT reconstruction, frontal view, demonstrating a patient with a prominent metopic ridge and bitemporal narrowing without other signs of metopic craniosynostosis. (*D*) 3D CT reconstruction, bird's eye view, demonstrating a patient with a prominent metopic ridge and bitemporal narrowing without other signs of metopic craniosynostosis.

craniofacial dysmorphology and who should make this decision? Although there is research investigating objective methods to delineate which patients should undergo surgery, at this time the treatment decision is best made in an open and honest discussion regarding the risks and benefits of surgery between the surgeon and family.

The other potential indication for surgical treatment is the prevention or limitation of neurodevelopmental injury: does surgical treatment of metopic craniosynostosis have any impact on neurodevelopment? There continue to be supporters of the premise that cranial vault expansion prevents, limits, or even treats neurodevelopmental delay in patients with metopic craniosynostosis,[46,48] but this has yet to be convincingly shown in the literature.[69] As such, there is likely no role for surgical treatment of patients with mild deformities or isolated metopic ridges.

Surgical Techniques

Metopic craniosynostosis is currently treated surgically with 2 primary techniques; endoscopy-assisted suturectomy followed by postoperative cranial orthotic therapy, or fronto-orbital advancement combined with anterior cranial vault reconstruction. Regardless of the approach, the goals are the same: the correction of the trigonocephalic deformity through the lateral and superior expansion of the frontal bones, correction of the pterional and frontozygomatic restriction, improvement in the lateral and superior orbital rim projection and hypotelorism, and improved contour of the forehead.

At this time, open surgical reconstruction has a longer history and has been proved to be safe and reliable. The drawbacks to this approach include a larger incision, longer surgical time, the likely need for blood transfusion, a longer hospitalization, increased overall health care costs, and a risk of relapse.[70] Supporters of this technique argue that properly executed incisions are well

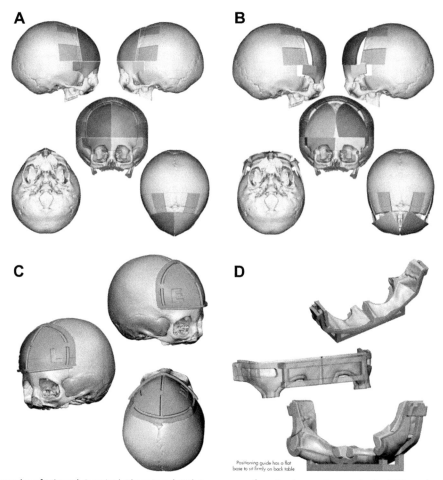

Fig. 6. Example of Virtual Surgical Planning (VSP) in a case of metopic craniosynostosis. Although used in the past, VSP is currently only employed in cases of severe or atypical dysmorphology. (*A*) Virtual osteotomy planning. (*B*) Virtual repositioning of osteotomized segments. (*C*) Design of frontal cutting guide. Mark along route highlighted in green for osteotomies. Mark blue letters for final positioning. (*D*) Design of orbital bandeau reconstruction guide.

hidden, surgical times are reasonable with experienced surgeons, relapse can be minimized by completing surgery at a later age and with overcorrection, blood transfusions are safe in the current medical era and can be minimized with the use of transfusion-sparing strategies, and hospitalization is only 1 to 2 days longer.[71] The increased expense is negligible in terms of overall health care expenditure and is worth the improved predictability and quality of outcomes.

Endoscopy-assisted suturectomy followed by postoperative cranial orthotic wear is a more recent intervention that has been extended from the treatment of sagittal craniosynostosis and scaphocephaly.[72–75] The drawbacks to this approach include the necessity for earlier surgery, which may be related to worse long-term neurodevelopmental outcomes secondary to anesthesia exposure;[76] blood transfusions are often still required; postoperative helmet therapy is the determination of the outcome and requires compliance; and long-term results are not yet available regarding the predictability and quality of outcomes.

Mortality is extremely low for both interventions.[71,77,78] Although short-term morbidity is generally increased in the open approach, the need for extended postoperative cranial orthotic wear is a burden associated with the endoscopy-assisted approach. Selection of intervention strategy is currently based on surgeon preference and family acceptance but is likely to be driven by long-term outcomes in the future.

Surgical Outcomes

The long-term cosmetic outcome of the surgical treatment of metopic craniosynostosis is the most relevant metric. The literature is limited by short-term follow-up in most studies with a clear bias shown by the correlation between length of follow-up and worsening aesthetic results.[79] It is inherently difficult to quantify the highly subjective nature of cosmesis.

The most frequently cited measurement tool is a classification system based on the need for subsequent surgery.[80] This system is conceptually valid, but the need for additional surgery may be related to a postoperative complication (ie, infection, dural tear/CSF leak), reconstruction because of inadequate bone healing, or revision because of scaring or an unsatisfactory result. There is the potential for disparity between surgeon and family impression, leading to unclear indications for revision. As surgery moves toward patient-centered and family-centered outcomes, it is the patient and family satisfaction that are likely to be most important.

Objective measurement strategies continue to evolve and provide a supportive role in documenting outcomes and stability by comparison with preoperative and matched reference cohorts. The most prominent techniques include anthropometry,[81] CT, and 3D photogrammetry. Discussion exists regarding the most relevant anatomic landmarks and the ability to reproducibly track their change over time. CT-based techniques are more precise and are moving toward shape analysis, but there is significant controversy over the need for CT evaluation, even for preoperative evaluation, in consideration of the lifetime oncologic risk.[22,82] Three-dimensional photogrammetry has been shown to be reliable[83] and interchangeable with CT.[84]

Type and Timing of Surgical Treatment and Impact on Appearance

The variables that most affect the outcome of the surgical treatment of metopic craniosynostosis are the type of surgical technique and timing of intervention. In practice, these are interrelated because most surgeons limit the use of endoscopic techniques to those presenting before the age of 4 months.

The relevant issues when considering the timing of cranial vault reconstruction (aside from perioperative morbidity/mortality) largely relate to the pliability of the cranium, the ability to support fixation, the timing of reossification of the cranium, and the healing of bone defects.

Many individual techniques for open cranial reconstruction have been published for metopic craniosynostosis. In general, they are variations on a theme of fronto-orbital advancement and lateral expansion combined with anterior cranial vault expansion. There are many minor modifications in osteotomy design, reshaping, reconstruction, and fixation, without any clear objective advantage of one technique compared with another. There seems to be an evolving consensus in the more recent literature that later (>6 months) open cranial reconstruction may lead to less recapitulation of the presenting deformity and a lower risk of total reoperation.[71,85–88] Although surgery at an older age may be associated with a higher rate of secondary repair of cranial defects, this can be managed with primary split-thickness cranial bone grafting.[89,90] Cranial growth is potentially reduced[71,91] but the significance of this finding is unclear, especially when surgery is completed at a later age with overcorrection.

Endoscopic techniques for the treatment of metopic craniosynostosis range from suturectomy to more complicated hybrid procedures.[92] In general, early treatment (>4 months) is advocated and involves a single incision anterior to the fontanelle with midline resection of the suture down through the nasofrontal junction, with or without additional osteotomies anterior to the coronal sutures.[72,74,93,94] There is reliance on the propulsive growth of the brain, which is guided by a postoperative cranial orthotic. Most of the current literature is weakened by limited sample sizes and/or short-term follow-up (1 year). A retrospective review comparing open and endoscopic techniques from the same institution shows equivalent morphologic results at 1 year[95] but only time will show whether these are maintained.

Type and Timing of Surgical Treatment and Impact on Development

Surgical treatment of metopic craniosynostosis is unlikely to have a positive impact on neurodevelopmental delay. Both treated and untreated cohorts show similar outcomes irrespective of intervention, timing, or technique.[53,56,60] Regardless of treatment, patients should be followed for the early diagnosis of delays and referred for therapy.[96]

THE AUTHOR'S APPROACH TO THE MANAGEMENT OF METOPIC CRANIOSYNOSTOSIS

A significant amount of effort is spent on community outreach and the education of primary care providers. Early referral is encouraged without the ordering of radiographic imaging (either plain films or CT scans). A detailed history and physical examination is undertaken at the first visit, including anthropomorphic measurements, and clinical photographs from 6 views (anterior, posterior, left, right, worm's eye, and bird's eye). A standardized examination checklist is used. Three-dimensional photogrammetry is also used and craniofacial surface measurements are obtained.

Diagnosis is usually made at the first visit. If the diagnosis is in question, a CT scan is obtained and evaluated for supportive findings (ie, metopic notch and significant interfrontal angle). If the diagnosis remains in question, patients are reevaluated at 3-month intervals to follow cranial growth. In general, these patients have either a significant metopic ridge or mild trigonocephaly. They are also followed for the detection of neurodevelopmental delay and referral for early intervention services.

Once the diagnosis is made 2 options are provided. Endoscopic suturectomy with postoperative cranial orthotic treatment is offered up to the age of 4 months. Patients see an orthotist before surgery and the helmet is delivered within the first week of surgery. Families are informed that the orthotic may be prescribed for up to 1 year. If open cranial reconstruction is selected, it is performed at approximately 9 months of age and visits are scheduled every 2 to 3 months before surgery to follow cranial growth and neurodevelopment.

A confirmatory CT scan is obtained before surgical treatment and in-office 3D-printed skull models are used as an educational tool for families, as well as for preoperative planning (Video 1). Virtual surgical planning has been used in the treatment of metopic craniosynostosis (**Fig. 6**), but is currently only employed in cases of severe or atypical dysmorphology.

Preoperative erythropoietin is prescribed for 3 consecutive weeks before surgery. Preoperative ophthalmologic examination as well as neurodevelopmental testing is completed for all patients.

Endoscopic repair is performed in a similar fashion to published protocols.[72,74,94] A small horizontal incision is made posterior to the hairline and a 1-cm strip including the metopic suture is removed from the anterior fontanelle to the nasofrontal junction. Additional osteotomies are made to weaken the frontal bones depending on their rigidity and severity of the trigonocephaly.

Open reconstruction is performed in a similar fashion to published techniques[97] with a tailored approach for each patient based on the presenting deformity (**Fig. 7**). A posterior sinusoidal coronal incision is made and flaps elevated. Bifrontal craniotomy is completed anteriorly to the coronal suture and split along the metopic ridge. The orbital bandeau is removed and segmented in the midline as well as lateral to the orbital rims. Barrel staves are completed posteriorly to the point of greatest width of the skull and out-fractured to create a smooth contour to the anterior cranial vault following reconstruction. Split-thickness bone grafts are harvested from the inner table of the frontal bones. A segment of full-thickness bone is also removed from one of the barrel staves. The bandeau is reassembled with resorbable fixation in an overcontoured fashion. The bandeau is widened in the midline and stabilized with a segment of full-thickness cranium and endocranial fixation. The lateral Tenon extensions are reassembled with ectocranial fixation. Polydioxanone suture is used to stabilize the bandeau at the lateral orbital rims and the nasion. The bandeau is repositioned anteriorly as well as tipped using the nasion as the point of rotation. Additional onlay grafting is often performed to further enhance and overcorrect the brow position (**Fig. 8**). The frontal bones are then rearranged to match the contour of the bandeau. They often require reshaping with a bone bender as well as rotation to provide the appropriate vertical forehead contour and expansion. They are stabilized with resorbable fixation. All of the bone defects are reconstructed with split-thickness cranial bone grafts to stabilize the reconstruction in an overcorrected position. The coronal incision is closed with resorbable suture. No drains are placed. A tranexamic acid drip is used throughout the procedure and discontinued while the scalp is being closed. Virtually all patients receive transfused blood. A dexmedetomidine drip is initiated at the end of the procedure and used in conjunction with ketorolac and acetaminophen to minimize postoperative narcotic usage. The average length of hospitalization is 3.5 days.

Postoperative ophthalmologic examination is completed 6 months following surgery. Postoperative neurodevelopmental testing is completed at 6 and 18 months as well as 5 years following surgery, with referral for early intervention services as appropriate. CT scan evaluation is completed only if clinically indicated. Patients are followed with anthropometric measurements and 3D photogrammetry at 3 months, 6 months, and then annually following surgery (**Fig. 7**).

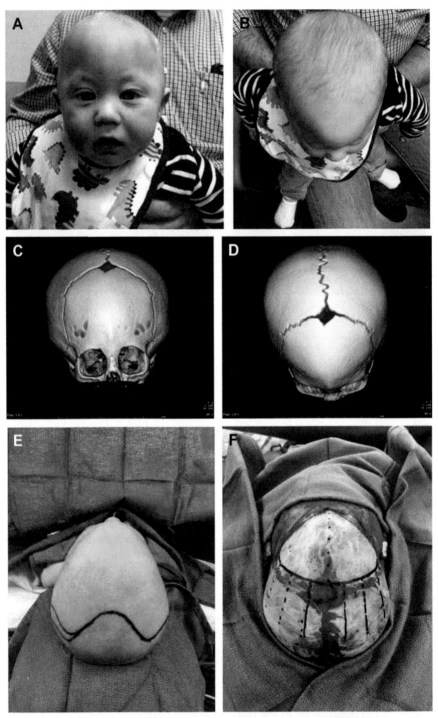

Fig. 7. Case example of a typical patient with metopic craniosynostosis undergoing correction of trigonocephaly through normalization of the configuration of the orbital bandeau and anterior half of the cranial vault. (*A*) Preoperative frontal photograph. (*B*) Preoperative bird's eye photograph. (*C*) 3D CT reconstruction, frontal view. (*D*) 3D CT reconstruction, bird's eye view. (*E*) Intraoperative bird's eye photograph demonstrating the posterior position of the sinusoidal coronal incision. (*F*) Intraoperative bird's eye photograph demonstrating the surgical markings including extended posterior barrel staves to the temporal parietal prominence that are used to weaken and facilitate improved contour posterio to the bifronal craniotomy.

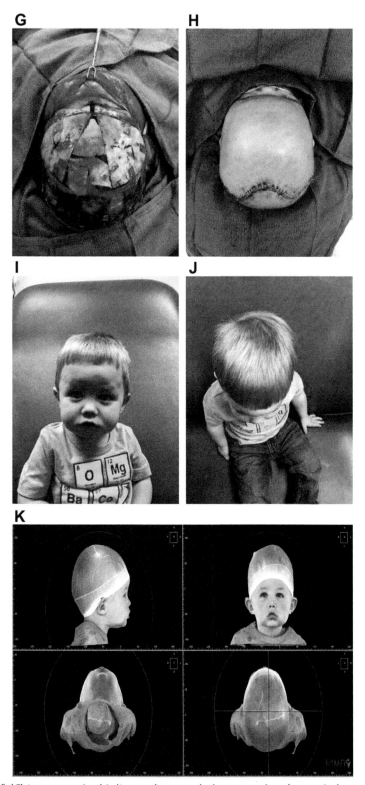

Fig. 7. (*continued*) (*G*) Intraoperative bird's eye photograph demonstrating the surgical correction and primary reconstruction of all skull defects with autogenous cranial bone and resorbable fixation. (*H*) Intraoperative bird's eye photograph demonstrating the surgical overcorrection. (*I*) Postoperative frontal photograph, 9 months following surgery. (*J*) Postoperative bird's eye photograph, 9 months following surgery. (*K*) 3D surface imaging used for objectivee peri-operative and long term evaluation.

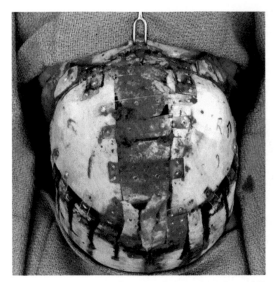

Fig. 8. Intraoperative photograph demonstrating additional onlay bone grafting used to increase the projection of the lateral half of the superior orbital rims.

SUPPLEMENTARY DATA

Supplementary data related to this article can be found at http://dx.doi.org/10.1016/j.coms. 2017.07.003.

REFERENCES

1. Otto AW. Lehrbuch der pathologischen anatomie. Berlin: Rucher; 1830.
2. Lattanzi W, Bukvic N, Barba M, et al. Genetic basis of single-suture synostoses: genes, chromosomes and clinical implications. Childs Nerv Syst 2012;28: 1301–10.
3. Virchow R. Uber den Cretinismus, namentlich in Franken, und uber pathologische Schadelformen. Verh Phys Med Ges (Wurzburg) 1851;2:230–56.
4. Delashaw JB, Persing JA, Broaddus WC, et al. Cranial vault growth in craniosynostosis. J Neurosurg 1989;70(2):159–65.
5. Moss ML, Young RW. A functional approach to craniology. Am J Phys Anthropol 1960;18:281–92.
6. Roth DA, Bradley JP, Levine JP, et al. Studies in cranial suture biology: part II. Role of the dura in cranial suture fusion. Plast Reconstr Surg 1996; 97(4):693–9.
7. Opperman LA, Rawlins JT. The extracellular matrix environment in suture morphogenesis and growth. Cells Tissues Organs 2005;181(3–4):127–35.
8. Cooper GM, Durham EL, Cray JJ Jr, et al. Tissue interactions between craniosynostotic dura mater and bone. J Craniofac Surg 2012;23(3):919–24.
9. Gault DT, Renier D, Marchac D, et al. Intracranial pressure and intracranial volume in children with craniosynostosis. Plast Reconstr Surg 1992;90(3): 377–81.
10. Lannelongue M. De la craniectomie dans la microcephalie. Compte Rendu Acad Sci 1890;110: 1382.
11. Lane LC. Pioneer craniectomy for relief of mental imbecility due to premature sutural closure and microcephalus. JAMA 1892;18:49.
12. Ghali MGZ, Srinivasan VM, Jea A, et al. Craniosynostosis surgery: the legacy of Paul Tessier. Neurosurg Focus 2014;36(4):E17.
13. Posnick JC, Lin KY, Chen P, et al. Metopic synostosis: quantitative assessment of presenting deformity and surgical results based on CT scans. Plast Reconstr Surg 1994;93(1):16–24.
14. Birgfeld CB, Saltzman BS, Hing AV, et al. Making the diagnosis: metopic ridge versus metopic craniosynostosis. J Craniofac Surg 2013;24(1):178–85.
15. van der Meulen J. Metopic synostosis. Childs Nerv Syst 2012;28:1359–67.
16. Vu HL, Panchal J, Parker EE, et al. The timing of physiologic closure of the metopic suture: a review of 159 patients using reconstructed 3D CT scans of the craniofacial region. J Craniofac Surg 2001; 12(6):527–32.
17. Pindrik J, Molenda J, Uribe-Cardenas R, et al. Normative ranges of anthropometric cranial indices and metopic suture closure during infancy. J Neurosurg Pediatr 2016;25(6):667–73.
18. Weinzweig J, Kirschner RE, Farley A, et al. Metopic synostosis: defining the temporal sequence of normal suture fusion and differentiating it from synostosis on the basis of computed tomography images. Plast Reconstr Surg 2003; 112(5):1211–8.
19. Lajeunie E, Le Merver M, Marchac D. Syndromal and nonsyndromal primary trigonocephaly: analysis of a series of 237 patients. Am J Med Genet 1998; 75:211.
20. van der Meulen J, van der Hulst R, van Adrichem L, et al. The increase of metopic synostosis: a panEuropean observation. J Craniofac Surg 2009; 20(2):283–6.
21. Selber J, Reid RR, Chike-Obi CJ, et al. The changing epidemiologic spectrum of singlesuture synostoses. Plast Reconstr Surg 2008; 122(2):527–33.
22. Fearon JA, Singh DJ, Beals SP, et al. The diagnosis and treatment of single-sutural synostoses: are computed tomographic scans necessary? Plast Reconstr Surg 2007;120(5):1327–31.
23. Fisher DC, Kornrumpf BP, Couture D, et al. Increased incidence of metopic suture abnormalities in children with positional plagiocephaly. J Craniofac Surg 2011;22(1):89–95.
24. Wood BC, Mendoza CS, Oh AK, et al. What's in a name? Accurately diagnosing metopic

craniosynostosis using a computational approach. Plast Reconstr Surg 2016;137(1):205–13.

25. Kini U, Hurst JA, Byren JC, et al. Etiological heterogeneity and clinical characteristics of metopic synostosis: evidence from a tertiary craniofacial unit. Am J Med Genet A 2010;152A(6):1383–9.

26. Gault DT, Renier D, Marchac D, et al. Intracranial volume in children with craniosynostosis. J Craniofac Surg 1990;1(1):1–3.

27. Posnick JC, Armstrong D, Bite U. Metopic and sagittal synostosis: intracranial volume measurements prior to and after cranio-orbital reshaping in childhood. Plast Reconstr Surg 1995;96(2): 299–309.

28. Marsh J. Metopic and sagittal synostosis: intracranial volume measurements prior to and after cranio-orbital reshaping in childhood – discussion. Plast Reconstr Surg 1995;96(2):310–5.

29. Lichtenberg R. Radiographic du crane de 226 enfants normaux de la naissance a 8 ans. Impressions digit-formes. Capacite: angles et indices [Thesis]. University of Paris; 1960.

30. Blinkov SM, Glezer I. The human brain in figures and tables; a quantitative handbook. New York: Basic Books; 1968.

31. Dekaban AS. Tables of cranial and orbital measurements, cranial volume and derived indexes in males and females from 7 days to 20 years of age. Ann Neurol 1977;2:485–532.

32. Wikberg E, Bernhardt P, Maltese G, et al. A new computer tool for systematic evaluation of intracranial volume and its capacity to evaluate the result of the operation for metopic synostosis. J Plast Surg Hand Surg 2012;46(6):393–8.

33. Maltese G, Tarnow P, Wikberg E, et al. Intracranial volume before and after surgical treatment for isolated metopic synostosis. J Craniofac Surg 2014; 25:262–6.

34. Abbott A, Netherway DJ, Niemann D, et al. CT-determined intracranial volume for a normal population. J Craniofac Surg 2000;11:211–23.

35. Anderson PJ, Netherway DJ, Abbott A, et al. Intracranial volume measurement of metopic craniosynostosis. J Craniofac Surg 2004;15(6):1014–6.

36. Kolar JC, Salyer KE. Intracranial volume measurement of metopic craniosynostosis – discussion. J Craniofac Surg 2004;15(6):1017–8.

37. Sgouros S, D Hockley A, H Goldin J, et al. Intracranial volume change in craniosynostosis. J Neurosurg 1999;91(4):617–25.

38. Aldridge K, Marsh JL, Govier D, et al. Central nervous system phenotypes in craniosynostosis. J Anat 2002;201(1):31–9.

39. Kapp-Simon KA, Speltz ML, Cunningham ML, et al. Neurodevelopment of children with single suture craniosynostosis: a review. Childs Nerv Syst 2007; 23(3):269–81.

40. Aldridge K, Collett BR, Wallace ER, et al. Structural brain differences in school-age children with and without single-suture craniosynostosis. J Neurosurg Pediatr 2017;19(4):479–89.

41. Tamburrini G, Caldarelli M, Massimi L, et al. Intracranial pressure monitoring in children with single suture and complex craniosynostosis: a review. Childs Nerv Syst 2005;21(10):913–21.

42. Renier D, Sainte-Rose C, Marchac D, et al. Intracranial pressure in craniostenosis. J Neurosurg 1982; 57(3):370–7.

43. Renier D, Marchac D. Longitudinal assessment of mental development in infants with nonsyndromic craniosynostosis with and without cranial release and reconstruction – discussion. Plast Reconstr Surg 1993;92(5):840–1.

44. Thompson DN, Harkness W, Jones B, et al. Subdural intracranial pressure monitoring in craniosynostosis: its role in surgical management. Childs Nerv Syst 1995;11(5):269–75.

45. Thompson DNP, Malcolm GP, Jones BM, et al. Intracranial pressure in single suture craniosynostosis. Pediatr Neurosurg 1995;22:235–40.

46. Shimoji T, Tomiyama N. Mild trigonocephaly and intracranial pressure: report of 56 patients. Childs Nerv Syst 2004;20(10):749–56.

47. Cinalli G, Sainte-Rose C, Kollar EM, et al. Hydrocephalus and craniosynostosis. J Neurosurg 1998; 88(2):209–14.

48. Shimoji T, Shimabukuro S, Sugama S, et al. Mild trigonocephaly with clinical symptoms: analysis of surgical results in 65 patients. Childs Nerv Syst 2002; 18(5):215–24.

49. Fearon JA. Evidence-based medicine: craniosynostosis. Plast Reconstr Surg 2014;133(5):1261–75.

50. Oi S, Matsumoto S. Trigonocephaly (metopic synostosis). Clinical, surgical and anatomical concepts. Childs Nerv Syst 1987;3(5):259–65.

51. Bottero L, Lajeunie E, Arnaud E, et al. Functional outcome after surgery for trigonocephaly. Plast Reconstr Surg 1998;102(4):952–8.

52. Posnick J. Functional outcome after surgery for trigonocephaly – discussion. Plast Reconstr Surg 1998; 102(4):959–60.

53. Kapp-Simon KA, Figueroa A, Jocher CA, et al. Longitudinal assessment of mental development in infants with nonsyndromic craniosynostosis with and without cranial release and reconstruction. Plast Reconstr Surg 1993;92(5):831–9.

54. Sidoti EJ Jr, Marsh JL, Marty-Grames L, et al. Long-term studies of metopic synostosis: frequency of cognitive impairment and behavioral disturbances. Plast Reconstr Surg 1996;97(2):276–81.

55. Becker DB, Petersen JD, Kane AA, et al. Speech, cognitive, and behavioral outcomes in nonsyndromic craniosynostosis. Plast Reconstr Surg 2005;116(2): 400–7.

56. Starr JR, Kapp-Simon KA, Cloonan YK, et al. Presurgical and postsurgical assessment of the neurodevelopment of infants with single-suture craniosynostosis: comparison with controls. J Neurosurg 2007;107(2 Suppl):103–10.

57. Starr JR, Lin HJ, Ruiz-Correa S, et al. Little evidence of association between severity of trigonocephaly and cognitive development in infants with single-suture metopic synostosis. Neurosurgery 2010;67: 408–15 [discussion: 415].

58. Warschausky S, Angobaldo J, Kewman D, et al. Early development of infants with untreated metopic craniosynostosis. Plast Reconstr Surg 2005;115(6): 1518–23.

59. Mendonca DA, White N, West E, et al. Is there a relationship between the severity of metopic synostosis and speech and language impairments? J Craniofac Surg 2009;20(1):85–8 [discussion: 89].

60. Kelleher MO, Murray DJ, McGillivary A, et al. Behavioral, developmental, and educational problems in children with nonsyndromic trigonocephaly. J Neurosurg 2006;105(5 Suppl):382–4.

61. Ruiz-Correa S, Starr JR, Lin HJ, et al. New severity indices for quantifying single suture metopic craniosynostosis. Neurosurgery 2008;63(2):318–24 [discussion: 324–5].

62. Yang JF, Brooks ED, Hashim PW, et al. The severity of deformity in metopic craniosynostosis is correlated with the degree of neurologic dysfunction. Plast Reconstr Surg 2017;139(2):442–7.

63. Beckett JS, Chadha P, Persing JA, et al. Classification of trigonocephaly in metopic synostosis. Plast Reconstr Surg 2012;130:442e–7e.

64. Wang JY, Dorafshar AH, Liu A, et al. The metopic index: an anthropometric index for the quantitative assessment of trigonocephaly from metopic synostosis. J Neurosurg Pediatr 2016; 18(3):275–80.

65. Kellogg R, Allori AC, Rogers GF, et al. Interfrontal angle for characterization of trigonocephaly: part 1: development and validation of a tool for diagnosis of metopic synostosis. J Craniofac Surg 2012; 23(3):799–804.

66. Anolik RA, Allori AC, Pourtaheri N, et al. Objective assessment of the interfrontal angle for severity grading and operative decision-making in metopic synostosis. Plast Reconstr Surg 2016;137(5): 1548–55.

67. Fearon JA. What's in a name? Accurately diagnosing metopic craniosynostosis using a computational approach – discussion. Plast Reconstr Surg 2016; 137(1):214–5.

68. Shimoji T, Tominaga D, Shimoji K, et al. Analysis of pre- and post-operative symptoms of patients with mild trigonocephaly using several developmental and psychological tests. Childs Nerv Syst 2015; 31(3):433–40.

69. Ijichi S, Ijichi N, Ishida A, et al. Ethical fallacies, tricky ambiguities, and the misinterpretation of the outcomes in the cranioplasty for mild trigonocephaly. Childs Nerv Syst 2015;31(7):1009–12.

70. Chan JW, Stewart CL, Stalder MW, et al. Endoscope-assisted versus open repair of craniosynostosis: a comparison of perioperative cost and risk. J Craniofac Surg 2013;24(1):170–4.

71. Fearon JA, Ruotolo RA, Kolar JC. Single sutural craniosynostoses: surgical outcomes and long-term growth. Plast Reconstr Surg 2009;123(2):635–42.

72. Jimenez DF, Barone CM. Early treatment of anterior calvarial craniosynostosis using endoscopic-assisted minimally invasive techniques. Childs Nerv Syst 2007;23:1411–9.

73. Keshavarzi S, Hayden MG, Ben-Haim S, et al. Variations of endoscopic and open repair of metopic craniosynostosis. J Craniofac Surg 2009; 20(5):1439–44.

74. Hinojosa J. Endoscopic-assisted treatment of trigonocephaly. Childs Nerv Syst 2012;28:1381–7.

75. Erşahin Y. Endoscope-assisted repair of metopic synostosis. Childs Nerv Syst 2013;29(12):2195–9.

76. Backeljauw B, Holland SK, Altaye M, et al. Cognition and brain structure following early childhood surgery with anesthesia. Pediatrics 2015;136(1):e1–12.

77. Czerwinski M, Hopper RA, Gruss J, et al. Major morbidity and mortality rates in craniofacial surgery: an analysis of 8101 major procedures. Plast Reconstr Surg 2010;126(1):181–6.

78. Tahiri Y, Paliga JT, Wes AM, et al. Perioperative complications associated with intracranial procedures in patients with nonsyndromic single-suture craniosynostosis. J Craniofac Surg 2015;26(1): 118–23.

79. Wes AM, Paliga JT, Goldstein JA, et al. An evaluation of complications, revisions, and long-term aesthetic outcomes in nonsyndromic metopic craniosynostosis. Plast Reconstr Surg 2014;133(6):1453–64.

80. Whitaker LA, Bartlett SP, Schut L, et al. Craniosynostosis: an analysis of the timing, treatment, and complications in 164 consecutive patients. Plast Reconstr Surg 1987;80:195–212.

81. Kolar JC, Salter EM. Preoperative anthropometric dysmorphology in metopic synostosis. Am J Phys Anthropol 1997;103(3):341–51.

82. Engel M, Castrillon-Oberndorfer G, Hoffmann J, et al. Value of preoperative imaging in the diagnostics of isolated metopic suture synostosis: a risk-benefit analysis. J Plast Reconstr Aesthet Surg 2012;65:1246–51.

83. McKay DR, Davidge KM, Williams SK, et al. Measuring cranial vault volume with three-dimensional photography: a method of measurement comparable to the gold standard. J Craniofac Surg 2010;21(5):1419–22.

84. Mendonca DA, Naidoo SD, Skolnick G, et al. Comparative study of cranial anthropometric

measurement by traditional calipers to computed to-mography and three-dimensional photogrammetry. J Craniofac Surg 2013;24(4):1106–10.

85. Seruya M, Oh AK, Boyajian MJ, et al. Long-term outcomes of primary craniofacial reconstruction for craniosynostosis: a 12-year experience. Plast Reconstr Surg 2011;127(6):2397–406.

86. Engel M, Thiele OC, Mühling J, et al. Trigonocephaly: results after surgical correction of nonsyndromatic isolated metopic suture synostosis in 54 cases. J Craniomaxillofac Surg 2012;40(4):347–53.

87. Utria AF, Lopez J, Cho RS, et al. Timing of cranial vault remodeling in nonsyndromic craniosynostosis: a single-institution 30-year experience. J Neurosurg Pediatr 2016;18(5):629–34.

88. Layliev J, Gill R, Spear M, et al. The optimal timing for primary cranial vault reconstruction in nonsyndromic craniosynostosis. J Craniofac Surg 2016; 27(6):1445–52.

89. Steinbok P, Seal SK, Courtemanche DJ. Split calvarial bone grafting in patients less than 1 year of age: technical note and use in craniofacial surgery for craniosynostosis. Childs Nerv Syst 2011;27(7): 1149–52.

90. Vercler CJ, Sugg KB, Buchman SR. Split cranial bone grafting in children younger than 3 years old: debunking a surgical myth. Plast Reconstr Surg 2014;133(6):822e–7e.

91. Metzler P, Zemann W, Jacobsen C, et al. Cranial vault growth patterns of plagiocephaly and trigonocephaly patients following fronto-orbital advancement: a long-term anthropometric outcome assessment. J Craniomaxillofac Surg 2013;41(6): e98–103.

92. Cohen SR, Pryor L, Mittermiller PA, et al. Nonsyndromic craniosynostosis: current treatment options. Plast Surg Nurs 2008;28(2):79–91.

93. Proctor MR. Endoscopic cranial suture release for the treatment of craniosynostosis–is it the future? J Craniofac Surg 2012;23(1):225–8.

94. Gociman B, Agko M, Blagg R, et al. Endoscopic-assisted correction of metopic synostosis. J Craniofac Surg 2013;24:763–8.

95. Nguyen DC, Patel KB, Skolnick GB, et al. Are endoscopic and open treatments of metopic synostosis equivalent in treating trigonocephaly and hypotelorism? J Craniofac Surg 2015;26(1): 129–34.

96. Kunz M, Lehner M, Heger A, et al. Neurodevelopmental and esthetic results in children after surgical correction of metopic suture synostosis: a single institutional experience. Childs Nerv Syst 2014;30: 1075–82.

97. Posnick JC. Trigonocephaly: metopic synostosis. In: Jeff Posnick, editor. Craniofacial and maxillofacial surgery in children and young adults. 1st edition. Philadelphia: Saunders; 2000. p. 162–98.

FURTHER READING

Simpkins H, Schoaf F, Katz J, et al. An acute granular lymphoid leukemia: a case report. Hum Pathol 1987;18:93–9.

Controversies in the Management of Oral and Maxillofacial Infections

 CrossMark

Daniel Taub, DDS, MD*, Andrew Yampolsky, DDS, MD,
Robert Diecidue, DMD, MD, MBA, MPH, Lionel Gold, DDS

KEYWORDS

- Infection • Deep neck space infection • Abscess • Cellulitis • Biofilm • Head and neck infection
- Antibiotics • Imaging

KEY POINTS

- Although the general principles of infection management have not changed, there have been modifications in the timing of treatment sequences as well as treatment techniques.
- Numerous prospective and retrospective studies have been performed confirming the utility of computed tomography (CT) scanning in the diagnosis of these infections, as well as corroborating the thoroughness nature of clinical examinations.
- Contrast-enhanced CT is the most practical imaging modality for severe oral and maxillofacial infections, but ultrasound also can be used in selected circumstances.
- Surgical drainage should focus on areas of defined collections whereas cellulitis and less severe infections can often be treated medically using appropriately selected antibiotics.

INTRODUCTION

The management and treatment of odontogenic infection, and its frequent extension into the head and neck, remains an important segment of oral and maxillofacial surgical practice. This area of maxillofacial expertise, historically and widely recognized by the medical community, is essential to the hospital referral system.

Although the general principles of infection management have not changed, there have been modifications in the timing of treatment sequences as well as treatment techniques, influenced by the development of diagnostic methods and advances in bacterial genetics and antibiotic usage. Thus, a review of treatment considerations and controversies is warranted, and is the purpose of this article. The following issues of diagnosis and treatment are explained and discussed.

TOPICS OF CONTROVERSY

- Diagnosis
  - Clinical examination
  - Use of computed tomography (CT)
  - Use of MRI
  - Use of ultrasound
  - Correlation with presence of drainable collection
- Treatment
  - Role of conservative management
  - Interventional radiology–guided drainage
  - Microbiota and antibiotic selection
  - Antibiotic resistance
  - Role of biofilms
  - Irrigation
  - Use of steroids
  - Airway management
  - Early versus late tracheostomy

Department of Oral and Maxillofacial Surgery, Sidney Kimmel Medical College, Thomas Jefferson University, 909 Walnut Street, Philadelphia, PA 19106, USA
* Corresponding author.
E-mail address: Daniel.Taub@jefferson.edu

Oral Maxillofacial Surg Clin N Am 29 (2017) 465–473
http://dx.doi.org/10.1016/j.coms.2017.06.004
1042-3699/17/© 2017 Elsevier Inc. All rights reserved.

oralmaxsurgery.theclinics.com

IS CONTRAST-ENHANCED COMPUTED TOMOGRAPHY IMAGING MORE ACCURATE THAN CLINICAL EXAMINATION ALONE?

In relatively recent decades (1930s–1950s) deep neck infection was diagnosed by clinical presentation, physical examination, and surgical exploration, with, or more often without, plain film imaging.[1] The introduction of CT has provided an excellent modality for the diagnosis of potential life-threatening infections.[1,2] Nonetheless, there has been debate in the literature regarding the value of CT scanning.[1–5]

Proponents of physical examination as the sole diagnostic criterion have argued that a trained clinician can accurately distinguish between a drainable collection and cellulitis, and the time required to obtain a CT scan may result in an unnecessary and harmful delay to timely treatment. Radiographic criteria for the identification of abscess in a contrast-enhanced CT include "discrete low attenuation areas within a soft tissue inflammatory mass with an enhancing peripheral rim." Most investigators state that homogeneous hypodensities without rim enhancement are less likely to correlate with discrete areas that require drainage[1] (**Fig. 1**).

Numerous prospective and retrospective studies have been performed confirming the utility of CT scanning in the diagnosis of these infections, as well as corroborating the thoroughness nature of clinical examinations.[1] Although individual study

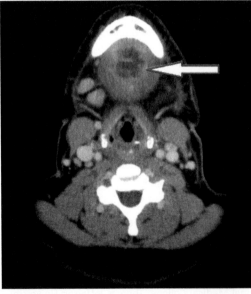

Fig. 1. A representative contrast-enhanced CT image, demonstrating the classic appearance of a hypodensity with peripheral rim enhancement (*arrow*). Such lesions have a strong correlation with a drainable abscess cavity when surgically accessed.

results vary, the majority opinion suggests that the sensitivity and specificity of a contrast-enhanced CT scan is far superior to stand-alone clinical examination. One commonly cited prospective study suggests the accuracy of contrast CT in the detection of a drainable fluid collection is 77% accurate compared with 63% for physical examination only.[1] When clinical examination and CT scan were combined, the accuracy improved to 89%, thus confirming the utility of assessing several diagnostic modalities in concert.[1]

The authors believe that despite early controversy, they and the literature clearly support the use of contrast-enhanced CT imaging in the diagnosis of deep neck space infection. Our practice experience and guidelines rely on ready access to adequate imaging and that diagnostic imaging is indicated in most instances, unless there is possibility or probability of an impending airway blockage.

IS THERE A ROLE FOR THE USE OF MRI IN THE DIAGNOSIS OF DEEP NECK SPACE INFECTIONS?

Having already established the utility of imaging to aid in the diagnosis of deep neck infections, one must now ask the question "Which of the many available imaging modalities is most useful?" MRI has several potentially beneficial advantages over CT imaging. MRI has a superb ability to differentiate soft tissue pathology from surrounding tissues and can often differentiate soft tissue structures not readily discerned on CT imaging. MRI is also said to result in less image degradation from dental restorations as well as ossified structures.[6] Furthermore, by not using iodinated gadolinium compounds for contrast enhancement, MRI may carry an additional advantage for patients who have impaired renal function or have a history of reactions to iodinated contrast agents.[7]

The primary disadvantages of MRI relate to the prolonged acquisition time and cost. Modern CT scanners are capable of acquiring imaging within minutes, whereas MR scans are far more prolonged. This increases the chances of motion artifacts, decompensation of unstable patients, and may be a contraindication for patients suffering from severe anxiety. Furthermore, implants with ferromagnetic properties may be displaced during image acquisition, resulting in iatrogenic harm. These properties make MRI impractical for most typical head and neck infections, CT imaging provides adequate diagnostic information.[7]

However, there are cases in which MRI modalities offer a distinct advantage. MRI is superior to CT to demonstrate bone marrow alterations, particularly bone marrow edema in T2-weighted imaging, thus showing increases in sensitivity in the diagnosis of osteomyelitis. In addition, neuro-ophthalmological complications of head and neck infections, such as cavernous sinus thrombosis, are best visualized using MRI techniques.[7,8]

IS THERE A ROLE FOR ULTRASOUND IN THE DIAGNOSIS OF HEAD AND NECK INFECTIONS?

Although CT imaging remains the most frequently used modality to assess head and neck infection, one should not ignore the diagnostic values of adjunctive imaging techniques, such as ultrasound imaging. Clinical research in ultrasound for medical purposes began in Germany in the1940s. Development continued in many countries following World War II, and resulted in the production of commercially available units in the 1960s. Since then, this technology has been embraced by the general medical community as an effective, safe, and cost-effective diagnostic modality.[9]

Despite the widespread adoption of ultrasound imaging for the diagnosis of head and neck infection, there have been only sporadic studies reported in the oral and maxillofacial surgery literature. More recently, however, there has been wide interest and publications reported in the otolaryngology literature that describe ultrasound imaging modalities useful for the diagnosis of peritonsillar abscess.[4,10–12] Although peritonsillar abscesses have a different pathophysiologic mechanism than infections due to odontogenic origin, they share anatomic and diagnostic similarities.[13] The otolaryngology literature will serve as an example to demonstrate the use of ultrasound to diagnose deep neck space infection secondary to odontogenic origin.

Several ultrasound techniques are described. A classic technique describes a small-diameter elongated probe suitable for intraoral use that can be easily used to examine the oral cavity medial to the mandible and the lateral tonsillar pillars. If trismus is present, a transcervical probe may be used to visualize the lateral pharyngeal, masticator, and submandibular spaces. Doppler flow modes may allow the operator to distinguish between blood vessels and abscess collections.[10–12,14,15] Studies that compare the utility of ultrasound diagnosis of peritonsillar and parapharyngeal infections with CT diagnosis vary in their findings; however, the sensitivity and specificity of identifying a drainable collection appears to be similar. Both modalities are more reliable than clinical diagnosis alone.[4]

We believe that ultrasound imaging in select patient populations should be considered for deep neck space infection diagnosis, especially in children and pregnant women for whom we should limit radiation exposure, and those unable to tolerate a contrast administration and thus would have limited diagnostic information from a non–contrast-enhanced CT.

The technical execution and gain of ultrasound data are usually performed by a technician, and frequently repeated (for confirmation) by the radiologist. In either instance, anatomic knowledge of the oral cavity and deep neck space is critical to correct imaging and interpretation. Thus, the diagnostic value of the procedure is dependent on the experience and expertise of the ultrasound department. Because we are not aware of ultrasound in oral and maxillofacial surgery resident programs, the surgeon must rely on the radiologist's interpretation. Parenthetically, we believe such training should be instituted in all programs.

IS THERE A ROLE FOR CONSERVATIVE MANAGEMENT OF HEAD AND NECK INFECTIONS?

In 1836, a German physician - Wilhelm Frederick von Ludwig described a severe acute infection affecting the "mouth, throat, neck, submandibular and parotid regions." The description goes on in graphic language "a gangrenous odor develops, the lungs become affected and death ensues… cellular tissue and muscles around and under the jaw and posterior portion of the throat are found to be gangrenous."[16] Such imagery of the severity and potential mortality of deep neck space infections are instilled in most oral and maxillofacial surgery trainees. As a result the traditional management of deep neck space infections has been aggressive and surgically oriented. Concepts such as dependent drainage and the incision of unaffected spaces to change the oxygen tension have been advocated.

We are now aware that Ludwig angina, as it has become known, although a severe bilateral form of a deep neck space infection, is in fact treatable with mortality that has decreased from close to 100% when the condition was first described, to less than 5%.[17] The difference in mortality is in large part a consequence of the advent of effective antimicrobial therapy. In the current era, broad-spectrum antibiotics provide excellent empiric coverage for most odontogenic infections. As a result, it may be useful to reconsider the dictum that all infectious swelling in the head and neck requires aggressive and prompt incision and drainage.[18–20] (As a saying goes, "never let the sun set on pus.")

An evolving body of evidence in the otolaryngology literature recommends fashioning treatment based on CT and clinical findings. CT and ultrasound findings allow one to distinguish between discrete abscess formations and cellulitis with a high positive predictive value. Patients without discreet abscess formation are thought to respond favorably to treatment with antibiotics and corticosteroids alone. In fact, even small collections have been reported to respond to antibiotics without additional surgical intervention.[18–20]

Most deep neck space infections treated by otolaryngologists have a different etiology and microflora than deep neck infections treated by oral and maxillofacial surgeons. Parapharyngeal abscess commonly arises from peritonsillar abscess, trauma, foreign bodies, and idiopathic causes. However, oral and maxillofacial surgeons routinely treat odontogenic infection that has a different bacterial pathogenesis. Consequently, the oral and maxillofacial surgical treatment algorithm will be similar but different.

1. Control of infection source: if it is necessary to extract teeth that are the cause of a severe deep neck space infection, the patient may be already under anesthesia in the operating room.
2. Literature that supports conservative management cites a 10% to 15% treatment failure rate that requires surgical intervention. In this instance, we recommend that incision and drainage is performed at the time of the tooth extraction to decrease the risk of a second general anesthetic.[18,20]
3. We believe there is enough evidence in the literature to support the use of preoperative imaging to guide surgical planning:
   a. Limit surgical incision and drainage to spaces that have identifiable purulent collections.[21,22]
   b. Cellulitis often can be managed medically after eliminating the source of infection.[18,20]

IS THERE A ROLE FOR INTERVENTIONAL RADIOLOGY–GUIDED DRAINAGE OF HEAD AND NECK INFECTIONS?

Interventional radiology (IR)-guided drainage is a technique often used to access fluid collections in anatomically difficult locations in the chest, abdomen, and pelvis. The advent of this technique has significantly reduced the need for invasive open surgery in such patients.[23] Parenthetically, IR approaches have shown great usefulness in the retrieval of minimally invasive biopsies in the head and neck region, such as the retropharyngeal

space, the temporomandibular joint (TMJ) and central nervous system.[24] As established, there is evidence to support the treatment of deep neck space infections with less aggressive surgery. Is there then a role for treating difficult to access deep neck infections with the aid of our IR colleagues?

Several studies have demonstrated the utility of image-guided aspiration in the management of retropharyngeal collections, many, depending on cephalocaudal location in the neck, would be difficult to access otherwise.[25,26] Thus, we believe it would be appropriate to use such techniques on a case-by-case basis, particularly when approaching the collection may be morbid surgically, and there has been a limited response to antibiotic therapy.

WHAT IS THE BACTERIAL FLORA OF HEAD AND NECK INFECTIONS?

Antibiotics provide an essential role in the management of deep neck space infection. An understanding of the microbiology associated with head and neck infection and antibiotic susceptibility profiles are highly important in the management of potentially life-threatening infection. Because most deep neck infection treated by oral and maxillofacial surgeons are pathologically odontogenic in origin, bacterial cultures show predominantly oral flora. The oral cavity is the entrance to the aerodigestive tract; a unique complex of anatomical microenvironments that have featured a bacterial ecosystem. The mucosal surfaces, gingival sulci, periodontal pockets, enamel surfaces, and pulpal tissue have unique microbial profiles that contribute to polymicrobial infections.[27,28]

Numerous studies have characterized the bacterial profiles of oral infection, and although there are differences among studies, which may be due to differences in study populations, infection severity, and culture techniques, there are some general trends:

- The infections are polymicrobial; it is theorized that the pathogens within an odontogenic infection are interdependent upon one another, with a complex interplay of commensalism between different organisms.[27–29]
- Most commonly mixed aerobic and anaerobic growth[27–30]
  ○ Some studies show predominant anaerobic growth
  ○ Very few studies show predominant aerobic growth

- Gram (+) cocci and gram (−) bacilli tend to predominate[27–29]
- Streptococci are the most common aerobes isolated, Staphylococci are less frequent[27–29]
  - Alpha hemolytic streptococci are the most common group among the aerobes
  - Beta hemolytic streptococci are less frequent
- Anaerobic streptococci are the most common anaerobic isolates[27–29]
- Bacteroides are less common[27–29]

One group of bacteria that requires special interest is *Streptococcus milleri*, that are microaerophilic bacteria within the *Streptococcus viridans* group. There are several different species that have demonstrated similar clinical behavior and have been associated with increased virulence and abscess formation, including morbidity and death. Within this group, the species *Streptococcus constellatus* has been associated with the formation of satellite abscesses and a more aggressive disease process. Interestingly, animal models have demonstrated that *S constellatus* works synergistically with other bacteria commonly present in odontogenic infections, such as *Fusobacterium nucleatum*.[31–35]

The increasing antibiotic resistance is fueled by the overuse of antibiotic therapy, as well as the widespread improper use by the medical and dental community. It is necessary to note that although we can reference recent studies to estimate relative percentages of resistance, clinically this is highly variable and dependent on the patient population as well as the facility in which the treatment is performed. Thus, it is important to reference institutional nomograms and consider culture-guided therapy in cases resistant to initial therapy. It also has been demonstrated in several studies that some patients who have eventually demonstrated bacterial culture resistance to the prescribed antibiotics, still proceeded to full recovery. This is thought to be evidence of a polymicrobial interdependence of infections, in which sensitivity to particular bacteria may render the entire complex less virulent.[27–29]

The common antibiotics used for deep neck space infections of odontogenic origin are penicillin based, clindamycin, and metronidazole (Flagyl). Estimates of penicillin and clindamycin resistance vary but 20% is often sited. Thus, there should be a low threshold to transition to a penicillin with a B-lactamase inhibitor, or with the addition of Flagyl to expand the anaerobic spectrum. It may be observed also that resistance to cephalosporins and fluoroquinolones is less common and provides additional options.[27–29]

WHAT IS THE ROLE OF BIOFILMS IN MAXILLOFACIAL HARDWARE INFECTIONS? DOES THE HARDWARE HAVE TO BE REMOVED?

Advances in implantable biomaterials over the past several decades have greatly increased the use of alloplastic materials in reconstructive maxillofacial surgery. As a result, chronic bacterial infection and the role of bacterial biofilms has become important. We now know that bacterial colonies can exist in 2 states: planktonic and sessile. The sessile state is physiologically distinct from the planktonic state in which bacteria are free floating in the body and much less resistant to our body's defense mechanisms.[36–38]

Alloplastic implants that are commonly used in maxillofacial surgery include ceramics, acrylic, porous polyethylene, and titanium. These alloplasts are poorly vascularized and provide a substrate surface to bacteria that is isolated from the body's immunologic defense mechanisms. The bacteria, *Staphylococcus aureus*, for example forms a sessile community that is attached to both the implant surface and adjacent bacteria. An extracellular matrix is created by staphylococci, which consists of a polymer of beta-1,6-linked N-acetylglucosamine. This matrix restricts access to the immune system and can be corrected only by surgical debridement. A mechanism known as "quorum sensing" allows bacteria to communicate and alter their gene expression dependent on population density of a specific bacteria within a colony. Thus, bacteria can assume an entirely different phenotype dependent on a complex interplay of environment and interbacterial signaling of a polymicrobial colony. In addition, the high-density bacterial population present in biofilms significantly contributes to the spread of antibiotic resistance secondary to an increase in horizontal transfer of novel genes.[37–40]

Perhaps most relevant to the oral and maxillofacial surgeon is the potential addition of a biofilm to failure of alloplastic total joint reconstruction. The head and neck is a highly vascular area and thus less likely to be affected by chronic infection and bacterial colonization encountered in orthopedic surgery. Further, most fixation hardware can be removed safely following a period of bone healing should infection occur. However, alloplastic TMJ reconstruction is an exception and a chronic site of infection or development of a biofilm on the implanted hardware can have disastrous consequences. Contaminated prosthetic devices typically produce cultures that are consistent with the human body's normal flora. The most commonly cited bacteria include *Staphylococcus epidermidis*, *S aureus*, *Pseudomonas aeruginosa*, and the *Enterococcus* species. It is probable that the alloplastic implant is contaminated during handling and insertion of the prosthesis. Consequently, many investigators recommend stringent sterile technique during TMJ replacement surgery.[37,41] These include the following:

- Thorough surgical site preparation
- Preparation of the external auditory canal
- Stringent sterile technique
- Minimal surgical manipulation of alloplast and operative site
- Repeat antiseptic preparation of the surgical area following oral contamination
- Avoid contact with parotid tissue that may contain bacterial pathogens

Management and salvage of contaminated hardware may be difficult. Mercuri[37] and Wolford and colleagues[41] advocate similar protocols for the management of a chronically infected and bacterially colonized joint prosthesis. They recommend removal of the prosthesis, placement of an antibiotic-eluding spacer followed by a peripherally inserted central catheter (PICC) line with administration of broad-spectrum intravenous antibiotics and subsequent placement of a new prosthesis. Unfortunately, there is no reliable protocol within our literature for salvaging a prosthesis that has already become colonized by a biofilm.[37,41]

Research into the prevention and treatment of biofilm formation is important. Potential avenues of development include implantable devices with antimicrobial coatings that prevent and disrupt the adhesion of microbes. In addition, so-called "quorum-quenching" antimicrobial agents offer an important area of research that attempts to interrupt communication between individual members of a harmful biofilm and thus decrease its resilience.[42]

IS IT SAFE TO USE CORTICOSTEROIDS IN THE MANAGEMENT OF DEEP NECK SPACE INFECTIONS?

Corticosteroids are a well-investigated and essential class of hormones, endogenously produced by the adrenal cortex, that regulate a wide range of physiologic processes, including stress response, glycemic balance, vascular repair, inflammation, and immune response. Corticosteroids are frequently administered following dentoalveolar and maxillofacial surgery to decrease postoperative edema, improve patient comfort, and thus hasten recovery time.[43,44]

One of the major sources of morbidity in deep neck space infections is the mass effect produced by edema causing airway obstruction. In addition, surgical management of the infection also may result in increased swelling around the airway, necessitating prolonged intubation or tracheostomy. Inflammation and spasm of the muscles of mastication may result in severe trismus, which also compromises the ability to successfully intubate the patient.

Some have expressed concern that the use of corticosteroids during an infection may worsen outcomes secondary to the immunosuppressive nature of corticosteroids. This concern has not been supported in the literature. The otolaryngology literature in a recent relevant meta-analysis reported that the combined use of antibiotics and corticosteroids was found to have synergistic effects. Corticosteroid groups had statistically significant clinical improvement relative to control groups in multiple parameters including the following:

- Reduced pain
- Decreased trismus
- Normalization of body temperature
- Decreased hospital stay

The literature supports the use of corticosteroids as an adjunctive treatment in the management of deep neck space infections; however, there is no agreed upon administration regimen. One regimen is as follows: methylprednisolone 2–3 mg/kg (maximum 250 mg) × 1 dose.[43,44]

IS IT IMPORTANT TO IRRIGATE DRAINS PLACED IN DEEP NECK COLLECTIONS?

"Dilution is the solution to pollution," is an adage often quoted by surgeons. One of the many duties of the diligent oral and maxillofacial surgery intern is to carefully irrigate the drains of patients with deep neck space infection who are admitted to their service. This process is repeated several times a day, and any break from clinic duty should be spent performing this required wound care. This was the doctrine taught in residency. However, as with many tenets, it does not fully stand up to scrutiny. Drain irrigation can be time-consuming, uncomfortable to the patient, and also may have the potential to seed skin flora deep into a fascial space with another flora. In view of such concerns, a literature review was performed to determine if there is any evidence to support the practice. Although there are few publications, one recent trial attempted to compare length of hospital stay among patients who had daily drain irrigation and those who did not. A statistically significant difference was not found. Obviously purulent material should have a patent passage for drainage; but we do not believe that frequent irrigation of drains is the primary factor in patient outcome.[45]

SHOULD TRACHEOSTOMY BE A ROUTINE PROCEDURE IN PATIENTS WITH DEEP NECK SPACE INFECTIONS?

The management of the airway of patients with deep neck space infection is one of the most challenging and potentially dangerous aspects of their treatment. Infection often causes peripharyngeal edema, thus increasing the potential for airway obstruction. If infection also involves the masticatory spaces, trismus may restrict oral access to the airway. Therefore, a plan to secure the airway should precede induction of general anesthesia. It is important that the surgeon is available during induction to facilitate a surgical airway in the event of failed intubation.[46–49]

Direct laryngoscopy is the simplest option, but is feasible only if oral access is possible. Direct laryngoscopy is usually performed following induction, thus this is typically reserved for less severe infections and there is a high degree of confidence that it will be possible to freely ventilate the patient. The advent of modern airway control techniques has dramatically decreased the need for introduction of surgical airways.[48] Video laryngoscopy is a relatively recent technique that permits intubation of more challenging airways. With the aid of video laryngoscopy, it is possible to orally intubate a person with a limited mouth opening or anatomic variation. However, as with a direct laryngoscopy, there should be reasonable assurance that the infection will not obstruct the airway and compromise ventilation.[46]

Awake nasal fiberoptic intubation is a technique reserved for patients with severe deep neck space infection with profound trismus and great concern that the airway will not remain patent following induction. This procedure is performed with a combination of local anesthesia and sedation while the patient sits in an upward position to maintain the airway. Although an excellent option, it is technique-sensitive and effective only when performed by an experienced clinician.[46]

Although video-assisted intubation techniques allow the clinician to safely secure most challenging airways, there is research to suggest that in the case of severe infections, early tracheostomy may offer a therapeutic and resource utilization advantage. Severe head and neck infections often require prolonged intubation due to airway edema; early tracheostomy may facilitate a more rapid transfer of the patient out of a critical care setting, thus potentially decreasing duration of hospitalization intensive care unit–related complications, and health care expenditure.[49]

SUMMARY

We believe that the literature strongly supports guiding surgical decision-making with a combination of clinical evaluation and imaging. It is our view that contrast-enhanced CT is the most practical imaging modality for severe oral and maxillofacial infections; however, ultrasound also can be used in select circumstances. Surgical drainage should focus on areas of defined collections, whereas cellulitis and less severe infections often can be treated medically using appropriately selected antibiotics.

REFERENCES

1. Miller WD, Furst IM, Sandor GK, et al. A prospective, blinded comparison of clinical examination and computed tomography in deep neck infections. Laryngoscope 1999;109(11):1873–9.
2. Vural C, Gungor A, Comerci S. Accuracy of computerized tomography in deep neck infections in the pediatric population. Am J Otolaryngol 2003;24(3): 143–8.
3. Chuang SY, Lin HT, Wen YS, et al. Pitfalls of CT for deep neck abscess imaging assessment: a retrospective review of 162 cases. B-ENT 2013; 9(1):45–52.
4. Kalmovich LM, Gavriel H, Eviatar E, et al. Accuracy of ultrasonography versus computed tomography scan in detecting parapharyngeal abscess in children. Pediatr Emerg Care 2012;28(8):780–2.
5. Lin RH, Huang CC, Tsou YA, et al. Correlation between imaging characteristics and microbiology in patients with deep neck infections: a retrospective review of one hundred sixty-one cases. Surg Infect (Larchmt) 2014;15(6):794–9.
6. Wang B, Gao BL, Xu GP, et al. Images of deep neck space infection and the clinical significance. Acta Radiol 2014;55(8):945–51.
7. Wippold FJ 2nd. Head and neck imaging: the role of CT and MRI. J Magn Reson Imaging 2007;25(3): 453–65.
8. Deshpande SS, Thakur MH, Dholam K, et al. Osteoradionecrosis of the mandible: through a radiologist's eyes. Clin Radiol 2015;70(2):197–205.
9. Woo J. A short history of the development of ultrasound in obstetrics and gynecology. Available at: http://www.ob-ultrasound.net/history1.html. Accessed January 10, 2017.
10. Nogan S, Jandali D, Cipolla M, et al. The use of ultrasound imaging in evaluation of peritonsillar infections. Laryngoscope 2015;125(11):2604–7.

11. Fordham MT, Rock AN, Bandarkar A, et al. Transcervical ultrasonography in the diagnosis of pediatric peritonsillar abscess. Laryngoscope 2015;125(12): 2799–804.

12. Pandey PK, Umarani M, Kotrashetti S, et al. Evaluation of ultrasonography as a diagnostic tool in maxillofacial space infections. J Oral Maxillofac Res 2012; 2(4):e4.

13. Blair AB, Booth R, Baugh R. A unifying theory of tonsillitis, intratonsillar abscess and peritonsillar abscess. Am J Otolaryngol 2015;36(4):517–20.

14. Shah A, Ahmed I, Hassan S, et al. Evaluation of ultrasonography as a diagnostic tool in the management of head and neck facial space infections: a clinical study. Natl J Maxillofac Surg 2015;6(1):55–61.

15. Nisha VA, J P, N S, et al. The role of colour Doppler ultrasonography in the diagnosis of fascial space infections—a cross sectional study. J Clin Diagn Res 2013;7(5):962–7.

16. Davis GG. Acute septic infection of the throat and neck; Ludwig's angina. Ann Surg 1906;44(2): 175–92.

17. Hought RT, Fitzgerald BE, Latta JE, et al. Ludwig's angina: report of two cases and review of the literature from 1945 to January 1979. J Oral Surg 1980; 38(11):849–55.

18. Lawrence R, Bateman N. Controversies in the management of deep neck space infection in children: an evidence-based review. Clin Otolaryngol 2017; 42(1):156–63.

19. Hirasawa K, Tsukahara K, Motohashi R, et al. Deep neck cellulitis: limitations of conservative treatment with antibiotics. Acta Otolaryngol 2017;137(1):86–9.

20. Plaza Mayor G, Martinez-San Millan J, Martinez-Vidal A. Is conservative treatment of deep neck space infections appropriate? Head Neck 2001; 23(2):126–33.

21. Bakir S, Tanriverdi MH, Gun R, et al. Deep neck space infections: a retrospective review of 173 cases. Am J Otolaryngol 2012;33(1):56–63.

22. Wang LF, Kuo WR, Tsai SM, et al. Characterizations of life-threatening deep cervical space infections: a review of one hundred ninety-six cases. Am J Otolaryngol 2003;24(2):111–7.

23. Gervais DA, Brown SD, Connolly SA, et al. Percutaneous imaging-guided abdominal and pelvic abscess drainage in children. Radiographics 2004; 24(3):737–54.

24. Levitt MR, Vaidya SS, Su DK, et al. The "triple-overlay" technique for percutaneous diagnosis and treatment of lesions of the head and neck: combined three-dimensional guidance with magnetic resonance imaging, cone-beam computed tomography, and fluoroscopy. World Neurosurg 2013;79(3–4): 509–14.

25. Cable BB, Brenner P, Bauman NM, et al. Image-guided surgical drainage of medial parapharyngeal abscesses in children: a novel adjuvant to a difficult approach. Ann Otol Rhinol Laryngol 2004;113(2): 115–20.

26. Delides A, Manoli E, Papadopoulos M, et al. Ultrasound-guided transoral drainage of a paediatric parapharyngeal abscess. J Laryngol Otol 2014; 128(12):1120–2.

27. Fating NS, Saikrishna D, Vijay Kumar GS, et al. Detection of bacterial flora in orofacial space infections and their antibiotic sensitivity profile. J Maxillofac Oral Surg 2014;13(4):525–32.

28. Stefanopoulos PK, Kolokotronis AE. The clinical significance of anaerobic bacteria in acute orofacial odontogenic infections. Oral Surg Oral Med Oral Pathol Oral Radiol Endod 2004;98(4):398–408.

29. Brook I. Microbiology and management of peritonsillar, retropharyngeal, and parapharyngeal abscesses. J Oral Maxillofac Surg 2004;62(12):1545–50.

30. Rega AJ, Aziz SR, Ziccardi VB. Microbiology and antibiotic sensitivities of head and neck space infections of odontogenic origin. J Oral Maxillofac Surg 2006;64(9):1377–80.

31. Singh KP, Morris A, Lang SD, et al. Clinically significant Streptococcus anginosus (Streptococcus milleri) infections: a review of 186 cases. N Z Med J 1988;101(859):813–6.

32. Terzic A, Scolozzi P. Deep neck space abscesses of dental origin: the impact of streptococcus group milleri. Eur Arch Otorhinolaryngol 2014;271(10): 2771–4.

33. Law ST, Kong Li MK. Is there any difference in pyogenic liver abscess caused by Streptococcus milleri and Klebsiella spp? Retrospective analysis over a 10-year period in a regional hospital. J Microbiol Immunol Infect 2013;46(1):11–8.

34. Giuliano S, Rubini G, Conte A, et al. Streptococcus anginosus group disseminated infection: case report and review of literature. Infez Med 2012; 20(3):145–54.

35. Foxton CR, Kapila S, Kong J, et al. Streptococcus milleri head and neck abscesses: a case series. Ear Nose Throat J 2012;91(6):246–54.

36. Desai SC, Moradzadeh A, Branham G. Anatomical evidence of microbial biofilms in an alloplastic nasal implant. Aesthetic Plast Surg 2013;37(2):468–71.

37. Mercuri LG. Microbial biofilms: a potential source for alloplastic device failure. J Oral Maxillofac Surg 2006;64(8):1303–9.

38. Vadyvaloo V, Otto M. Molecular genetics of Staphylococcus epidermidis biofilms on indwelling medical devices. Int J Artif Organs 2005;28(11):1069–78.

39. Kong KF, Vuong C, Otto M. Staphylococcus quorum sensing in biofilm formation and infection. Int J Med Microbiol 2006;296(2–3):133–9.

40. Vuong C, Gerke C, Somerville GA, et al. Quorum-sensing control of biofilm factors in Staphylococcus epidermidis. J Infect Dis 2003;188(5):706–18.

41. Wolford LM, Rodrigues DB, McPhillips A. Management of the infected temporomandibular joint total joint prosthesis. J Oral Maxillofac Surg 2010; 68(11):2810–23.

42. Romano CL, Toscano M, Romano D, et al. Antibiofilm agents and implant-related infections in orthopaedics: where are we? J Chemother 2013;25(2):67–80.

43. Lee YJ, Jeong YM, Lee HS, et al. The efficacy of corticosteroids in the treatment of peritonsillar abscess: a meta-analysis. Clin Exp Otorhinolaryngol 2016; 9(2):89–97.

44. Pelaz AC, Allende AV, Llorente Pendas JL, et al. Conservative treatment of retropharyngeal and parapharyngeal abscess in children. J Craniofac Surg 2009;20(4):1178–81.

45. Bouloux GF, Wallace J, Xue W. Irrigating drains in severe odontogenic infection does not improve outcome. J Oral Maxillofac Surg 2012;70(9):e39. oral abstract.

46. Cho SY, Woo JH, Kim YJ, et al. Airway management in patients with deep neck infections: A retrospective analysis. Medicine (Baltimore) 2016;95(27): e4125.

47. Karkos PD, Leong SC, Beer H, et al. Challenging airways in deep neck space infections. Am J Otolaryngol 2007;28(6):415–8.

48. Wolfe MM, Davis JW, Parks SN. Is surgical airway necessary for airway management in deep neck infections and ludwig angina? J Crit Care 2011;26(1): 11–4.

49. Potter JK, Herford AS, Ellis E 3rd. Tracheotomy versus endotracheal intubation for airway management in deep neck space infections. J Oral Maxillofac Surg 2002;60(4):349–54.

Controversies in Oral and Maxillofacial Pathology

Zachary S. Peacock, DMD, MD

KEYWORDS

- Keratocystic odontogenic tumor • Giant cell lesion • Ameloblastoma • Unicystic ameloblastoma
- Odontogenic keratocyst • Giant cell granuloma • Benign jaw tumor

KEY POINTS

- Benign aggressive neoplasms of the maxillofacial region, such as the keratocystic odontogenic tumor, giant cell lesion, and ameloblastoma, remain controversial in etiology and treatment.
- Inconsistency in terminology, classification, and treatment protocols contributes to the lack of consensus in ideal treatment.
- The identification of the genetic profile of these neoplasms is making directed medical treatment possible.

INTRODUCTION

Several benign pathologic entities that are commonly encountered by the oral and maxillofacial surgeon remain controversial. From etiology to treatment, little consensus exists in the literature regarding benign lesions such as the keratocystic odontogenic tumor, giant cell lesion, and ameloblastoma.

Despite being seen in everyday practice, benign maxillofacial tumors are underrepresented in the literature. The lesions are rare in the general population and do not represent "public health problems," like cancer or diabetes. The gold standard in the management of these lesions remains a resection with negative margins given the tendency for recurrence. Other less-invasive treatments have been reported, but success rates do not approach marginal or segmental resections. As we enter the genomic era, it is hoped that many of the controversies outlined herein will be solved with directed medical therapy.

Controversies in the diagnosis and management of the benign aggressive lesions are reviewed here with an update on future directions in management.

KERATOCYSTIC ODONTOGENIC TUMOR

Despite being reclassified and named by the World Health Organization (WHO) as a tumor (keratocystic odontogenic tumor [KCOT]) from a cyst (odontogenic keratocyst), this entity remains a mystery.[1] The etiology is thought to be from the residual dental lamina, similar to a primordial cyst,[2] but has also reported to originate from overlying gingiva/mucosa growing into the jaw.[3] The reclassification did not provide much clarity in etiology of the KCOT,[4] but putative molecular markers have been reported.[5,6] Adding to the confusion, clinicians and researchers alike still commonly refer to the lesion as its longstanding moniker "odontogenic keratocyst." despite being over a decade after the WHO report.[7]

Many aspects of the lesion's behavior and molecular makeup supported the concept of the KCOT as a true neoplasm. The lesion has a high recurrence rate after enucleation and can behave aggressively.[8–13] Although most occur within 5 years of treatment, reports exist of recurrences after more than 10 years.[3,14] Mitotic figures are often identified in the cyst wall above the basal layer and the lesion has been associated with

Department of Oral and Maxillofacial Surgery, Massachusetts General Hospital, Harvard School of Dental Medicine, Warren 1201, 55 Fruit Street, Boston, MA 02114, USA
E-mail address: zpeacock@partners.org

Oral Maxillofacial Surg Clin N Am 29 (2017) 475–486
http://dx.doi.org/10.1016/j.coms.2017.06.005
1042-3699/17/© 2017 Elsevier Inc. All rights reserved.

mutations in the Sonic hedgehog pathway (in isolated lesions in addition to those associated with nevoid basal cell carcinoma syndrome).[14–17]

Management

Management of the KCOT varies immensely, resulting in significant heterogeneity of outcomes studies in the literature. Resection with negative margins has been reported to have recurrence rates approaching 0%.[18–21] Given the benign nature of the disease and morbidity of en bloc resection, less-invasive treatment options have been extensively reported. Resection is still used for cases of extensive disease, aggressive behavior, or exceptional circumstances.[22,23]

Enucleation alone has been problematic. On a macro level, the thin, friable lining, multilocularity, and tendency to be intimately associated with tooth roots makes access difficult and often results in piecemeal removal.[24] The lesion also has the tendency to form "daughter cysts" beyond the main osseous wound not visible to the surgeon after enucleation. On a microscopic level, any remaining neoplastic cells within a daughter cyst or in the overlying mucosa can lead to recurrence.[3]

For the preceding reasons, it is generally agreed on that if treatment is less than en bloc resection, adjunctive measures to enucleation are necessary to avoid recurrence. The type of adjunctive treatment varies immensely in the literature between and even within institutions. The options for adjunctive treatment to enucleation include but are not limited to physical destruction via peripheral ostectomy, cryotherapy, or chemical treatment with Carnoy solution.[25] Another technique used for large lesions is decompression by maintaining an opening from the lesion to the oral cavity. This technique can be carried out via marsupialization or stenting with a drain,[22,26,27] which results in a smaller lesion amenable to enucleation/adjunctive treatment or as definitive treatment.[26,28]

Performing a peripheral ostectomy after enucleation is thought to eliminate remaining neoplastic cells or daughter cysts beyond the lesion's osseous cavity. This technique uses mechanical removal of additional bone (1–2 mm in depth) from the osseous cavity after visible lesion removal. It is typically performed with a carbide bur (round or pineapple shaped). To ensure consistent and complete bone removal, methylene blue can be applied to the cavity. Bone is then removed until the dye is gone.[29] It remains unclear what actually happens to daughter cysts or residual tumor cells in bone when a bur is used. Are cells driven farther into the bone, seeded into

soft tissue, or mechanically destroyed? Regardless, this technique has been shown to decrease recurrence.[30]

Enucleation with adjunctive cryotherapy has recurrence rates comparable to other adjunctive treatments.[31] Liquid nitrogen has been used to freeze the residual osseous cavity, resulting in cell death to a depth of 1.5 mm.[32] The disadvantages are the need to carefully protect the surrounding soft tissue and teeth to avoid tissue necrosis. The liquid nitrogen must be dispensed through a metal cannula, so accessing all areas of the lesion while protecting soft tissue can be challenging (**Fig. 1**). In addition, the mandible is significantly weakened and fractures have been reported particularly with thin residual bone.[33] For this reason, it may be prudent to place autogenous bone graft for defects at risk of fracture, limit the patient's diet, or even place into maxillomandibular fixation. Exposure of the inferior alveolar nerve in a osseous cavity after removal is more amenable to cryotherapy. Use of a surgical drill in an around the nerve for ostectomy is challenging. Cryotherapy applied to exposed nerve has been shown to result in paresthesia, but with reasonable recovery of sensation.[34]

Chemical treatment of the osseous cavity after enucleation has been popular, but current use is contentious. Carnoy solution (absolute alcohol, chloroform, ferric chloride, glacial acetic acid) has been extensively reported to reduce recurrence rate over enucleation alone.[35,36] Chloroform has been classified as a carcinogen and banned as a therapeutic agent. Despite this, chloroform has remained in common use among oral and

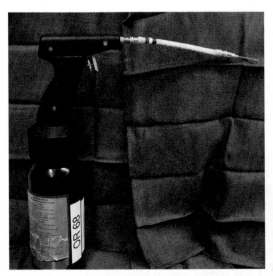

Fig. 1. Liquid nitrogen canister with metal cannula extension.

maxillofacial surgeons.[37] Some have continued to use "modified Carnoy" solution not containing chloroform, but recent studies have shown, however, that chloroform may be the necessary ingredient for success of Carnoy solution. Dashow and colleagues[38] reported that the use of Carnoy solution containing chloroform after enucleation resulted in a 10% recurrence rate compared with 35% with those treated with modified Carnoy solution. Given the liability of using a banned substance, it appears that alternatives should be used rather than a chemical fixative for adjunctive treatment of KCOTs.

Enucleation of larger lesions (>3 cm) with or without the previously described adjunctive treatment remains difficult. Larger lesions are difficult to access and the surrounding bone is thin or perforated, limiting the ability to perform additional ostectomy or cryotherapy. For these reasons, decompression has been used to lessen the size of the lesion. Cystic lesions are thought to enlarge at least in part due to osmosis, with increased fluid shift into the lumen following increased concentration of cell debris or keratin.[39,40] Therefore, opening the lesion to the mouth allows disruption of this concentration gradient and gradual shrinkage of the lesion. Decompression can be achieved by marsupialization, which involves suturing the lining of the cyst to the oral mucosa or placing a physical conduit through an opening into the lesion. Marsupialization is difficult due to the friable nature of the tumor, as mentioned previously, and the tendency of the opening to close. Decompression using a drain of some sort has been extensively reported and is often more reliable than marsupialization[25] (**Fig. 2**).

Decompression using a drain has been reported as a definitive technique, whereas the lesion shrinks to the point that it is not visible radiographically.[28] After initial enthusiasm, the recurrence rate became unacceptably high and it has been recommended that residual cystectomy and adjunctive treatment of the smaller lesion be performed after decompression to significantly decrease recurrence.[29]

In addition to physical shrinkage of the lesions, there have been reports of a change in the histology of the lining of the cystic tumor after long-term decompression. The lining changes from thin and friable to a thicker inflamed lining similar to oral mucosa.[26,28,41,42] It has been suggested that this is a metaplasia, and loss of cytokeratin-10 expression occurs in up to 64% of lesions and may lower recurrence rate.[42] Regardless of any molecular change, the thicker inflamed membrane is easier to enucleate when performing residual cystectomy (**Fig. 3**).

An additional issue is the status of mucosa overlying the lesion. A leading theory of the tissue of origin of KCOT is the epithelial remnants of the dental lamina that develops from the mucosa over the alveolar ridge.[43] An additional theory is that overlying mucosa also has a role in the formation of a KCOT through subsequent invagination well after the dental lamina has ceased functioning.[43] This concept is supported by histologic studies showing epithelial islands and microcysts present within or outside of the lining of KCOTs in both primary and recurrent tumors.[3] Also, recurrences have been reported within bone grafts after resection of KCOTs, presumably from recurrent lesions in the mucosa and penetrating into the grafted bone.[3] Last, excision of overlying mucosa, particularly in nondentate areas and where cortical perforation exists, has been used by several investigators to decrease recurrence.[3,43,44] A recent systematic review recommended that excision of the overlying mucosa should be performed in addition to enucleation and adjuvant treatment for KCOTs of the retromolar trigone, posterior maxilla, and those with cortical perforations.[45] Tissue surrounding the decompression conduit also should be removed during residual cystectomy.

Future Directions

Targeted treatment seems to be possible given the elucidation of several mutations in the KCOT. Several alterations in the sonic hedgehog pathway have been reported in both syndromic and non-syndromic KCOTs. Mutations of the *PTCH1* gene that produces the patched tumor suppressor protein has been the most common mutation in KCOTs associated with the nevoid basal cell carcinoma syndrome (NBCCS).[15] Other reports show *PTCH1* as well as mutations in the gene (*SMO*) coding for the Smoothened protein that activates

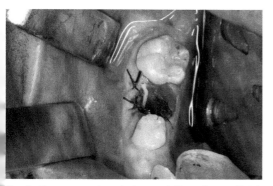

Fig. 2. Decompression drain consisting of a pediatric endotracheal tube flared at the end and secured along the alveolar ridge.

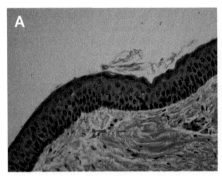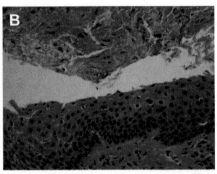

Fig. 3. (*A*) KCOT appearance at the time of incisional biopsy and placement of drain for decompression showing the characteristic wavy parakeratotic cyst lining (6–8 cells thick) with palisading basal layer. (*B*) After 12 months of decompression, the lining is a thick squamous lining without characteristic features of a KCOT. Hematoxylin-eosin, original magnification ×400.

sonic hedgehog (*SHH*) signaling.[17,46,47] Up to 84% of sporadic KCOTs may have mutations in the this pathway.[17] It is likely that other mutations not yet identified exist in the sporadic KCOTs not found to have these known mutations.

Drugs that target the sonic hedgehog pathway may be a treatment that can lessen or eliminate the need for surgical intervention. Vismodegib (Genentech, South San Francisco, CA, USA) has shown to be effective in decreasing the size of KCOTs in those with NBCCS.[48–50] Recently 5-fluorouracil, an antimetabolite that may affect the sonic hedgehog pathway, was shown to be effective as an adjunct after enucleation of KCOTs.[51]

GIANT CELL LESIONS

The giant cell lesion (GCL), a benign osseous neoplasm affecting the maxillofacial skeleton, remains contentious in its origin, relationship to similar lesions found elsewhere, and treatment.

Origin

The biologic origin of the GCL remains undefined. These lesions have been hypothesized to be inflammatory in nature resembling sarcoidosis and response to anti-inflammatory treatment in the form of steroid injections.[52–54] It has been thought of as an endocrine lesion, given the resemblance to the brown tumor of hyperparathyroidism and response to calcitonin.[55–57] Last, it is theorized to be a vascular lesion given the dense vascularity and successful treatment with interferon.[58] The moniker "giant cell lesion" refers to the abundance of multinucleated giant cells, but the neoplastic cell is most likely the mononuclear stromal cells.[59] Stromal cells are thought to recruit and activate the multinucleated giant cells that develop the phenotype of an osteoclast.[60]

Relationship to Giant Cell Lesions in the Axial and Appendicular Skeleton

Significant controversy remains regarding the relationship of maxillofacial GCL (MF GCL) with the giant cell tumor (GCT) that affects the axial and appendicular skeleton (AA GCL).[61–66] The pathogenesis in both locations is thought to involve recruitment of monocytes by stromal cells to form multinucleated giant cells.[60] MF GCLs are more common in female patients and occur in younger patients (1–2 decades) than AA GCLs.[61–63] AA GCLs are more commonly painful than MF GCLs, which are often detected via clinical or radiographic screening.[62]

Multiple reports have proposed that MF and AA GCLs are distinct entities, citing differences in clinical behavior and histologic features.[61,65,67] Other reports postulate that the lesions exist on a continuum of the same disease process.[60,68–71] Comparative studies have generally been limited by inconsistent terminology, and investigators have typically grouped all lesions together not taking into account varying clinical/biologic behavior (ie, aggressiveness).

MF GCLs were first labeled the "giant cell reparative granuloma" by Jaffe in 1953.[67] Reports of spontaneous reparation and resolution are found in the literature,[71–73] but many MF GCLs are destructive and grow rapidly.[74] GCLs have not been shown to be granulomatous lesions resulting from an inciting agent or foreign body. There is a hesitance to refer to MF GCLs as 'giant cell tumors' as reports exist showing AA GCTs metastasizing or undergoing malignant transformation but not for MF GCLs.[75,76] However, retrospective analysis of cases of lung metastases from AA GCLs appear to be separate malignancies that just contain multinucleated giant cells.[77]

When clinical and radiographic features are used to properly classify the lesions, accurate comparisons can be made. MF GCLs are classified as aggressive if they are ≥5 cm, recurrent, or meet 3 of the following 5 criteria: rapid growth, root resorption, tooth displacement, cortical perforation, or thinning.[65] Those that grow slowly and are asymptomatic are considered nonaggressive and less likely to recur after enucleation alone. Similarly, the Enneking classification has been used to classify AA lesions by clinical and radiographic behavior: stage 1 (latent) lesions are static that can heal spontaneously, stage 2 (active) have progressive growth limited by anatomic barriers (ie, cortical bone), and stage 3 are locally destructive of adjacent anatomic barriers.[22,78]

For comparison, the Enneking and the Kaban/Chuong classification systems can be modified to produce a single binary (ie, aggressive or nonaggressive) classification for GCLs in both locations.[69] Using this system, MF and AA GCLs were found to share phenotypic, clinical, and radiographic appearance.[69] In addition, these lesions are histologically similar and cannot be differentiated consistently by masked pathologists.[70]

Subsequent studies have looked at gene expression of GCLs in both locations. These lesions share common genetic expression of MMP9, CTSK, and TC1RG1, which was confirmed by quantifying the protein expression using a tissue microarray.[71] Aggressive lesions in both locations have similar patterns of immune downregulation and may become aggressive by evading immune surveillance.[79] The findings of these studies support the conclusion that they are similar tumors in different locations.

In contrast, recent studies have assessed for mutations in histones, the proteins that package DNA in nucleosomes. One group performed whole genome sequencing and found consistent mutations in histone 3.3 driver variants (H3F3A gene) in the stromal cells of AA GCLs.[80] This group also reported mutations in this gene at different locations in a variety of bone and cartilage tumors.[81] A subsequent study by a different group looking at both aggressive and nonaggressive MF GCLs in the skeleton did not find these specific mutations when sequencing amplified polymerase chain reaction products.[82] Although the studies support that these are different lesions, the studies were not methodologically equivalent. The role histones play in the pathogenesis of these lesions is not clear, despite histone mutations being found in a variety of bone and cartilage tumors, as well as pediatric brain tumors.[83–85] Further studies are needed on the genetics of these neoplasms.

Overall, it seems that enough similarities exist between MF and AA GCLs (particularly between aggressive lesions) to say they exist on a continuous spectrum of disease. Combining them may hasten the development of medical therapy for these historically surgical diseases.

Treatment

MF GCLs are commonly destructive and require operative management. The gold standard for aggressive GCLs remains segmental or marginal resection with negative margins. Contemporarily, this is used sparingly, given the benign nature of the tumor and viable alternatives. No consensus exists regarding the ideal treatment due to the varying clinical behavior and unclear biologic origin. After clinical and radiographic criteria are applied on diagnosis, no biomarker exists to predict behavior. This hampers timely treatment of intermediate lesions (ie, aggressive appearing, but not meeting criteria) in particular.[86]

As in studies comparing MF and AA GCLs, treatment comparisons of MF GCLS have been limited by inconsistent behavior stratification. Many reports assess multiple or varying protocols between and among patients and do not describe tumors uniformly.[87]

Nonaggressive GCLs generally respond to enucleation and curettage alone with few recurrences. Associated teeth and the inferior alveolar nerve can be spared. In contrast, aggressive GCLs are less amenable to enucleation and curettage (eg, due to size) and have a high recurrence rate.[65,74]

Rapid growth and a prominent vascular component have led to the hypothesis that aggressive GCLs are the bone counterparts to the infantile hemangioma.[58] As such, an anti-angiogenic agent, interferon (IFN) alpha-2a, has been used as an adjuvant for aggressive lesions. The protocol in use consists of curettage sparing involved structures, such as teeth and the inferior alveolar nerve, followed by subcutaneous IFN alpha-2a (3 million units/m^2) until the osseous cavity has filled with bone (usually 10–12 months). In a recent study assessing its use in a tightly defined protocol over 20 years, only 6 (13.3%) of 45 patients had progression of disease or recurrence.[88] The main disadvantage of this treatment regimen is the associated side effects of IFN. Fever and flulike symptoms can occur 24 to 48 hours after the initial dose, but only 7 (15.5%) of 45 patients had side effects requiring cessation of therapy before complete bone fill.[88]

As GCLs have a close resemblance to the brown tumor of hyperparathyroidism, adjuvant calcitonin has been reported as both adjuvant and primary treatment of MF GCLs.[55–57] Subcutaneous calcitonin has been reported to be successful for both nonaggressive and aggressive GCLs.[56] The primary disadvantage seems to be the delay in treatment response to calcitonin that can be prohibitive in rapidly growing GCLs.

The hypothesis that MF GCLs are inflammatory in nature has led to the use of intralesional steroid injections. This technique as primary treatment has been shown to have varying success rates.[52–54] Injections are difficult in multilocular or large lesions, but seem to be most effective for small, unilocular nonaggressive lesions.

Future Directions

The binary classification system is helpful for lesions that are obviously aggressive or nonaggressive. Those that are intermediate in behavior are more challenging. Without a reliable biomarker, it is not possible to predict those lesions that are likely to recur with enucleation or grow rapidly with destruction.

Markers of vascularity, such as CD34 and CD31, have been shown to have greater staining intensity in aggressive lesions in immunohistochemical studies.[86,89,90]

Recently, the antibody to nuclear kappa-B receptor (RANK-L) has had some success in both axial-appendicular and maxillofacial GCLs without operative intervention.[91,92] This is based on the prominent role of the pathway in osteoclast-mediated bone resorption. Denosumab is not currently recommended for the skeletally immature, which represents a large portion of MF GCLs. Additional studies are needed to determine the role of denosumab in the management of MF GCLs.

AMELOBLASTOMA

The ameloblastoma represents one of the most controversial lesions managed by oral and maxillofacial surgeons. Despite it being a benign entity, its unmitigated growth and tendency to recur requires operative management similar to that of malignancies (ie, segmental or marginal resection with ≥1-cm margins). Purported successful attempts to lessen the morbidity with "conservative" treatment are found commonly in the literature. Recurrence rates for solid ameloblastoma treated by resection varies from 8% to 17%.[93–95] When treated by treatment less than resection (eg, enucleation), much higher rates are reported (20%–90%).[93–96]

Despite the difference in outcomes, many investigators report on and suggest alternatives to resection with negative margins.[97–100] The most common advocacy for "conservative" management is the classification of ameloblastoma as a "benign" process. Although histologically benign, its behavior is unlike other benign entities encountered in the maxillofacial region. It is highly destructive with boundless growth that can lead to airway compromise, rare metastases, and even death.[101–103] The ameloblastoma has been reported to recur decades after original treatment,[104–106] so one must question the rates of "cure" seen in many reports of "conservative treatment" with more limited follow-up.

Another limitation in the existing literature is the inconsistent reporting of the morphologic or histologic subtype in outcomes studies. The solid/multicystic type is the most common followed by the unicystic and peripheral. The various histologic patterns of the solid/multicystic ameloblastoma have not been shown definitively to affect recurrence rate (eg, desmoplastic, granular cell, follicular, acanthomatous). As compared with the solid/multicystic tumor, the unicystic ameloblastoma (UA) does appear to exhibit different behavior.

Unicystic Ameloblastoma

The existence and proper treatment of the UA has itself been a contentious topic in the literature. The report by Robinson and Martinez[107] of 20 cystic lesions with ameloblastic epithelium (1977) established the UA as a distinct entity from the solid/multicystic ameloblastoma. Before this, Cahn[108] reported that ameloblasts were found in the lining of a dentigerous cyst and described the potential of these cysts to form ameloblastomas. Robinson and Martinez[107] documented 4 configurations of ameloblastic epithelium within the wall of 20 cysts: (1) luminal with ameloblastic epithelium limited to the cyst wall, (2) intramural with growth away from the lumen without extension of the ameloblastic epithelium into the connective tissue, (3) mural with ameloblastic epithelium extending into the connective tissue beneath the cyst wall, and (4) intraluminal with ameloblastic epithelium protruding into the cyst lumen. They reported a recurrence rate of 15% after enucleation, which was far less than solid/multicystic amelobastomas.[107]

Studies since then also have supported that UA appears to be more amenable to less-invasive treatments (eg, enucleation) than the solid/multicystic variety with most reports of recurrence rates less than 21%.[107,109–111] In a systematic review of UA, resection had an average recurrence rate of 3.6%, enucleation with Carnoy solution was 16.0%, and enucleation alone was 30.5%.[112] A recent study reported a 70.5% rate of recurrence after enucleation alone.[113]

Although UA is a commonly known entity, there has been inconsistency in the way the term is applied. Its use has been extended to clinical or radiographic appearance rather than only histologic appearance. Solid ameloblastomas with a prominent cystic component or a unilocular appearance on radiographs have been labeled UA by surgeons, pathologists, or radiologists.[114] The broadening of the definition of UA makes comparison of outcome studies difficult. In addition, the characterization of the epithelial configuration, which affects recurrence, is not always included in existing studies. In a study of only intraluminal UAs, the recurrence rate was 10.7% with enucleation.[115] With mural involvement, the recurrence rates have been much higher and investigators have recommended peripheral ostectomy or resection.[108,116,117]

When faced with a diagnosis of UA, it is clear that the entire cyst wall should be evaluated histologically. This is contrary to the typical practice of most pathology services, in which 1 to 2 portions of the submitted specimen are sectioned and assessed.[114,118–120] If the entire cystic lining is not assessed, mural UA could be missed and recurrence is likely. Similarly, if an incisional biopsy is performed, one may proceed with enucleation if only luminal/intraluminal UA is encountered.[118] Other areas may have mural involvement or even a solid component (**Fig. 4**). For these reasons, it is not recommended to make a diagnosis of UA on incisional biopsy alone and one should proceed with complete histopathologic evaluation of enucleated UAs (ie, excisional biopsy if lesion size allows). If mural involvement is present, resection with negative margins is indicated.[113]

Intraoperative Assessment of Margins

Other aspects of the contemporary treatment of ameloblastoma remain unproven yet common in practice. Histologic studies have suggested that true margins of ameloblastoma extend 4.5 mm (2–8 mm) beyond the radiographic border of the tumor.[116,121] Therefore, most resections are planned for ≥1 cm based on a preoperative computed tomography (CT) scan to achieve negative final histologic margins. To confirm negative margins of a resection, most surgeons obtain frozen sections from the cancellous margin of the residual mandible and/or obtain a 2-dimensional ex vivo radiograph of the specimen.[122,123] Although regularly used, these methods have not been well studied and may not be beneficial.

De Silva and colleagues[124] performed a systematic review of studies assessing imaging and frozen sections to determine margin status in maxillofacial pathology. The investigators concluded that there was only level 4 and 5 evidence supporting use of specimen radiographs and frozen sections. A recent study assessed the utility of frozen sections and intraoperative radiographs to obtain negative margins and prevent recurrence of mandibular ameloblastomas.[125] No difference was found in recurrence rate between subjects who had 1 or more of these modalities used versus no intraoperative assessment. This study was limited by the lack of tumor detected

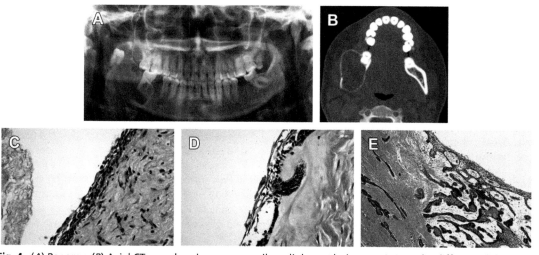

Fig. 4. (*A*) Panorex. (*B*) Axial CT scan showing an expansile radiolucent lesion was UA on the differential diagnosis by the radiologist, given its unilocular appearance. (*C, D*) Incisional biopsy revealed a cystic lesion with ameloblastic epithelium in the lining consistent with UA (hematoxylin-eosin, original magnification ×400). (*E*) Given the size, location, and aggressive behavior, segmental resection was carried out revealing components of the cystic wall that contained solid-type ameloblastoma (hematoxylin-eosin, original magnification ×100).

on any frozen section and soft tissue margins were not included. Furthermore, comparisons of the radiographic margin on the ex vivo radiograph to final histologic margins showed reliability only when the radiographic margin was ≥5 mm. That is, when the radiographic margin was ≥5 mm from visible lesion, then one can reasonably expect the histologic margin to be negative (≥5 mm). Radiographic margins less than 5 mm had far more variability on histologic analysis. Overall, it seems the intraoperative assessments do not add significantly to the management of ameloblastoma when adequate oncologic margins are planned based on a maxillofacial CT scan.

Future Directions

As in the other lesions, the current controversies in treatment may be resolved with molecular diagnosis and treatment. Until recently, the molecular pathogenesis of the ameloblastoma had been largely unknown.[126] Kurppa and colleagues[127] studied primary cell lines of ameloblastoma and found that epidermal growth factor receptor antagonists blocked cell proliferation in 1 of 2 cell lines. Studying downstream mutations, they discovered a mutation in the oncogene BRAF (V600E) within the MAP-kinase pathway. Activating mutations of BRAF, a serine-threonine kinase, results in cell proliferation, survival, and subsequent neoplastic transformation. Mutations in this gene have been reported in melanoma, colorectal carcinoma, and hairy cell leukemia, among other neoplasms.[128–130] They then confirmed that 63% of ameloblastoma samples had BRAF V600E mutations.[127] Within several months, a second group reported BRAF mutations in 46% of ameloblastoma samples and found additional mutations within Smoothened (SMO) of the sonic hedgehog pathway.[131] They determined that BRAF mutations were found commonly in mandibular lesions, whereas SMO mutations were found in maxillary lesions. This second group reported that a cell line harboring the BRAF mutation was sensitive to the clinically available BRAF inhibitor vemurafenib. A third group reported the largest series to date (84 ameloblastomas) and found that 88% had mutations in this MAP-kinase pathway with most of these in BRAF (62%).[132] It seems that detecting these mutations within an ameloblastoma may eventually allow for personalized treatment using known inhibitors and available inhibitors.[133–135]

SUMMARY

The ideal management of several maxillofacial neoplasms remains under question. The KCOT,

GCL, and ameloblastoma can all behave aggressively with a tendency to recur despite their benign histologic appearance. Given the need for potentially morbid treatment to obtain "cure" and prevent recurrence, multiple less-invasive treatments have been reported with widely varying results. As the molecular and genomic pathogenesis of these lesions are better understood, directed treatments could lessen the contention in management.

REFERENCES

1. Philipsen HP. Pathology and genetics of head and neck tumours. In: Barnes L, Eveson JW, Reichart P, et al, editors. World Health Organization classification of tumours. Lyon (France): IARC; 2005. p. 306–7.
2. Partridge M, Towers JF. The primordial cyst (odontogenic keratocyst): its tumour-like characteristics and behaviour. Br J Oral Maxillofac Surg 1987; 25(4):271–9.
3. Stoelinga PJ. Long-term follow-up on keratocysts treated according to a defined protocol. Int J Oral Maxillofac Surg 2001;30(1):14–25.
4. Reichart PA, Philipsen HP, Sciubba JJ. The new classification of head and neck tumours (WHO)—any changes? Oral Oncol 2006;42(8):757–8.
5. Shear M. The aggressive nature of the odontogenic keratocyst: is it a benign cystic neoplasm? Part 3. Immunocytochemistry of cytokeratin and other epithelial cell markers. Oral Oncol 2002;38(5): 407–15.
6. August M, Faquin WC, Troulis M, et al. Differentiation of odontogenic keratocysts from nonkeratinizing cysts by use of fine-needle aspiration biopsy and cytokeratin-10 staining. J Oral Maxillofac Surg 2000;58(9):935–40.
7. Bhargava D, Deshpande A, Pogrel MA. Keratocystic odontogenic tumour (KCOT)—a cyst to a tumour. Oral Maxillofac Surg 2012;16(2):163–70.
8. Shear M. The aggressive nature of the odontogenic keratocyst: is it a benign cystic neoplasm? Part 1. Clinical and early experimental evidence of aggressive behaviour. Oral Oncol 2002;38(3):219–26.
9. Shear M. The aggressive nature of the odontogenic keratocyst: is it a benign cystic neoplasm? Part 2. Proliferation and genetic studies. Oral Oncol 2002;38(4):323–31.
10. Vedtofte P, Praetorius F. Recurrence of the odontogenic keratocyst in relation to clinical and histological features. A 20-year follow-up study of 72 patients. Int J Oral Surg 1979;8(6):412–20.
11. Brannon RB. The odontogenic keratocyst. A clinicopathologic study of 312 cases. Part I. Clinical features. Oral Surg Oral Med Oral Pathol 1976; 42(1):54–72.

12. Rud J, Pindborg JJ. Odontogenic keratocysts: a follow-up study of 21 cases. J Oral Surg 1969; 27(5):323–30.

13. Oikarinen VJ. Keratocyst recurrences at intervals of more than 10 years: case reports. Br J Oral Maxillofac Surg 1990;28(1):47–9.

14. Madras J, Lapointe H. Keratocystic odontogenic tumour: reclassification of the odontogenic keratocyst from cyst to tumour. J Can Dent Assoc 2008; 74(2):165.

15. Barreto DC, Gomez RS, Bale AE, et al. PTCH gene mutations in odontogenic keratocysts. J Dent Res 2000;79(6):1418–22.

16. Shimada Y, Katsube K, Kabasawa Y, et al. Integrated genotypic analysis of hedgehog-related genes identifies subgroups of keratocystic odontogenic tumor with distinct clinicopathological features. PLoS One 2013;8(8):e70995.

17. Qu J, Yu F, Hong Y, et al. Underestimated PTCH1 mutation rate in sporadic keratocystic odontogenic tumors. Oral Oncol 2015;51(1):40–5.

18. Bataineh AB, al Qudah M. Treatment of mandibular odontogenic keratocysts. Oral Surg Oral Med Oral Pathol Oral Radiol Endod 1998;86(1):42–7.

19. el-Hajj G, Anneroth G. Odontogenic keratocysts—a retrospective clinical and histologic study. Int J Oral Maxillofac Surg 1996;25(2):124–9.

20. Chuong R, Donoff RB, Guralnick W. The odontogenic keratocyst. J Oral Maxillofac Surg 1982; 40(12):797–802.

21. Irvine GH, Bowerman JE. Mandibular keratocysts: surgical management. Br J Oral Maxillofac Surg 1985;23(3):204–9.

22. Kolokythas A, Fernandes RP, Pazoki A, et al. Odontogenic keratocyst: to decompress or not to decompress? A comparative study of decompression and enucleation versus resection/peripheral ostectomy. J Oral Maxillofac Surg 2007;65(4):640–4.

23. Warburton G, Shihabi A, Ord RA. Keratocystic odontogenic tumor (KCOT/OKC)-clinical guidelines for resection. J Maxillofac Oral Surg 2015; 14(3):558–64.

24. Forssell K, Forssell H, Kahnberg KE. Recurrence of keratocysts. A long-term follow-up study. Int J Oral Maxillofac Surg 1988;17(1):25–8.

25. Pogrel MA. The keratocystic odontogenic tumor. Oral Maxillofacial Surg Clin N Am 2013;25(1): 21–30.

26. Marker P, Brøndum N, Clausen PP, et al. Treatment of large odontogenic keratocysts by decompression and later cystectomy: a long-term follow-up and a histologic study of 23 cases. Oral Surg Oral Med Oral Pathol Oral Radiol Endod 1996; 82(2):122–31.

27. Nakamura N, Mitsuyasu T, Mitsuyasu Y, et al. Marsupialization for odontogenic keratocysts: long-term follow-up analysis of the effects and changes in growth characteristics. Oral Surg Oral Med Oral Pathol Oral Radiol Endod 2002;94(5):543–53.

28. Pogrel MA, Jordan RC. Marsupialization as a definitive treatment for the odontogenic keratocyst. J Oral Maxillofac Surg 2004;62(6):651–5 [discussion: 655–6]. [Erratum appears in J Oral Maxillofac Surg 2007;65(2):362–3].

29. Pogrel MA. The keratocystic odontogenic tumour (KCOT)—an odyssey. Int J Oral Maxillofac Surg 2015;44(12):1565–8.

30. Sharif FNj, Oliver R, Sweet C, et al. Interventions for the treatment of keratocystic odontogenic tumours (KCOT, odontogenic keratocysts (OKC)). Cochrane Database Syst Rev 2010;(9):CD008464.

31. Schmidt BL, Pogrel MA. The use of enucleation and liquid nitrogen cryotherapy in the management of odontogenic keratocysts. J Oral Maxillofac Surg 2001;59(7):720–5.

32. Pogrel MA, Regezi JA, Fong B, et al. Effects of liquid nitrogen cryotherapy and bone grafting on artificial bone defects in minipigs: a preliminary study. Int J Oral Maxillofac Surg 2002;31(3): 296–302.

33. Fisher AD, Williams DF, Bradley PF. The effect of cryosurgery on the strength of bone. Br J Oral Surg 1978;15(3):215–22.

34. Schmidt BL, Pogrel MA. Neurosensory changes after liquid nitrogen cryotherapy. J Oral Maxillofac Surg 2004;62(10):1183–7.

35. Blanas N, Freund B, Schwartz M, et al. Systematic review of the treatment and prognosis of the odontogenic keratocyst. Oral Surg Oral Med Oral Pathol Oral Radiol Endod 2000;90(5):553–8.

36. Johnson NR, Batstone MD, Savage NW. Management and recurrence of keratocystic odontogenic tumor: a systematic review. Oral Surg Oral Med Oral Pathol Oral Radiol 2013;116(4):e271–6.

37. Ecker J, Horst RT, Koslovsky D. Current role of Carnoy's solution in treating keratocystic odontogenic tumors. J Oral Maxillofac Surg 2016;74(2):278–82.

38. Dashow JE, McHugh JB, Braun TM, et al. Significantly decreased recurrence rates in keratocystic odontogenic tumor with simple enucleation and curettage using Carnoy's versus modified Carnoy's solution. J Oral Maxillofac Surg 2015;73(11):2132–5.

39. Toller PA. Protein substances in odontogenic cyst fluids. Br Dent J 1970;128(7):317–22.

40. Toller PA. The osmolality of fluids from cysts of the jaws. Br Dent J 1970;129(6):275–8.

41. Brøndum N, Jensen VJ. Recurrence of keratocysts and decompression treatment. A long-term follow-up of forty-four cases. Oral Surg Oral Med Oral Pathol 1991;72(3):265–9.

42. August M, Faquin WC, Troulis MJ, et al. Dedifferentiation of odontogenic keratocyst epithelium after cyst decompression. J Oral Maxillofac Surg 2003; 61(6):678–83.

43. Stoelinga PJ. Excision of the overlying, attached mucosa, in conjunction with cyst enucleation and treatment of the bony defect with Carnoy solution. Oral Maxillofac Surg Clin North Am 2003;15(3): 407–14.

44. Stoelinga PJ. The treatment of odontogenic keratocysts by excision of the overlying, attached mucosa, enucleation, and treatment of the bony defect with Carnoy solution. J Oral Maxillofac Surg 2005;63(11):1662–6.

45. Al-Moraissi EA, Pogrel MA, Ellis E 3rd. Does the excision of overlying oral mucosa reduce the recurrence rate in the treatment of the keratocystic odontogenic tumor? A systematic review and meta-analysis. J Oral Maxillofac Surg 2016;74(10):1974–82.

46. Sun LS, Li XF, Li TJ. PTCH1 and SMO gene alterations in keratocystic odontogenic tumors. J Dent Res 2008;87(6):575–9.

47. Rui Z, Li-Ying P, Jia-Fei Q, et al. Smoothened gene alterations in keratocystic odontogenic tumors. Head Face Med 2014;10:36.

48. Goldberg LH, Landau JM, Moody MN, et al. Resolution of odontogenic keratocysts of the jaw in basal cell nevus syndrome with GDC-0449. Arch Dermatol 2011;147(7):839–41.

49. Ally MS, Tang JY, Joseph T, et al. The use of vismodegib to shrink keratocystic odontogenic tumors in patients with basal cell nevus syndrome. JAMA Dermatol 2014;150(5):542–5.

50. Booms P, Harth M, Sader R, et al. Vismodegib hedgehog-signaling inhibition and treatment of basal cell carcinomas as well as keratocystic odontogenic tumors in Gorlin syndrome. Ann Maxillofac Surg 2015;5(1):14–9.

51. Ledderhof NJ, Caminiti MF, Bradley G, et al. Topical 5-fluorouracil is a novel targeted therapy for the keratocystic odontogenic tumor. J Oral Maxillofac Surg 2017;75(3):514–24.

52. Terry B, Jacoway J. Management of central giant cell lesions: an alternative to surgical therapy. Oral Maxillofac Surg Clin North Am 1994;6:579.

53. Carlos R, Sedano HO. Intralesional corticosteroids as an alternative treatment for central giant cell granuloma. Oral Surg Oral Med Oral Pathol Oral Radiol Endod 2002;93:161.

54. Nogueira RL, Teixeira RC, Cavalcante RB, et al. Intralesional injection of triamcinolone hexacetonide as an alternative treatment for central giant-cell granuloma in 21 cases. Int J Oral Maxillofac Surg 2010;39:1204.

55. Harris M. Central giant cell granulomas of the jaws regress with calcitonin therapy. Br J Oral Maxillofac Surg 1993;31:89.

56. Pogrel MA. Calcitonin therapy for central giant cell granuloma. J Oral Maxillofac Surg 2003;61:649.

57. de Lange J, van den Akker HP, Veldhuijzen van Zanten GO, et al. Calcitonin therapy in central giant cell granuloma of the jaw: a randomized double-blind placebo controlled study. Int J Oral Maxillofac Surg 2006;35:791.

58. Kaban LB, Mulliken JB, Ezekowitz RA, et al. Antiangiogenic therapy of a recurrent giant cell tumor of the mandible with interferon alfa-2a. Pediatrics 1999;103:1145.

59. Itonaga I, Hussein I, Kudo O, et al. Cellular mechanisms of osteoclast formation and lacunar resorption in giant cell granuloma of the jaw. J Oral Pathol Med 2003;32:224.

60. Flanagan AM, Nui B, Tinkler SM, et al. The multinucleate cells in giant cell granulomas of the jaw are osteoclasts. Cancer 1988;62:1139.

61. Austin LT Jr, Dahlin DC, Royer RQ. Giant-cell reparative granuloma and related conditions affecting the jawbones. Oral Surg Oral Med Oral Pathol 1959;12:1285.

62. Auclair PL, Cuenin P, Kratochvil FJ, et al. A clinical and histomorphologic comparison of the central giant cell granuloma and the giant cell tumor. Oral Surg Oral Med Oral Pathol 1988;66:197.

63. Waldron CA, Shafer WG. The central giant cell reparative granuloma of the jaws: an analysis of 38 cases. Am J Clin Pathol 1966;45:437.

64. Kauzman A, Li SQ, Bradley G, et al. Central giant cell granuloma of the jaws: assessment of cell cycle proteins. J Oral Pathol Med 2004;33:170.

65. Chuong R, Kaban LB, Kozakewich H, et al. Central giant cell lesions of the jaws: a clinicopathologic study. J Oral Maxillofac Surg 1986;44:708.

66. Murphey MD, Nomikos GC, Flemming DJ, et al. From the archives of AFIP. Imaging of giant cell tumor and giant cell reparative granuloma of bone: radiologic-pathologic correlation. Radiographics 2001;21:1283.

67. Jaffe HL. Giant-cell reparative granuloma, traumatic bone cyst, and fibrous (fibro-osseous) dysplasia of the jawbones. Oral Surg Oral Med Oral Pathol 1953;6:159.

68. Wang C, Song Y, Peng B, et al. Expression of c-Src and comparison of cytologic features in cherubism, central giant cell granuloma and giant cell tumors. Oncol Rep 2006;15:589.

69. Resnick CM, Margolis J, Susarla SM, et al. Maxillofacial and axial/appendicular giant cell lesions: unique tumors or variants of the same disease? A comparison of phenotypic, clinical, and radiographic characteristics. J Oral Maxillofac Surg 2010;68:130.

70. Peacock ZS, Resnick CM, Susarla SM, et al. Do histologic criteria predict biologic behavior of giant cell lesions? J Oral Maxillofac Surg 2012;70:2573.

71. Peacock ZS, Schwab JH, Faquin WC, et al. Genetic analysis of giant cell lesions of the maxillofacial and axial/appendicular skeletons. J Oral Maxillofac Surg 2017;75(2):298–308.

72. Bernier JL, Cahn LR. The peripheral giant cell reparative granuloma. J Am Dent Assoc 1954;49: 141.

73. Worth HM. Principles and practice or oral radiology interpretation. Chicago: Chicago Year Book Medical Publishers; 1963. p. 498–505.

74. Ficarra G, Kaban LB, Hansen LS. Central giant cell lesions of the mandible and maxilla: a clinicopathologic and cytometric study. Oral Surg Oral Med Oral Pathol 1987;64:44.

75. Bertoni F, Present D, Sudanese A, et al. Giant-cell tumor of bone with pulmonary metastases. Six case reports and a review of the literature. Clin Orthop Relat Res 1988;237:275.

76. Siebenrock KA, Unni KK, Rock MG. Giant-cell tumour of bone metastasising to the lungs. A long-term follow-up. J Bone Joint Surg Br 1998; 80:43.

77. Rock MG, Pritchard DJ, Unni KK. Metastases from histologically benign giant-cell tumor of bone. J Bone Joint Surg 1984;66:269.

78. Enneking WF. A system of staging musculoskeletal neoplasms. Clin Orthop Relat Res 1986;204:9.

79. Al-Sukaini A, Hornicek FJ, Peacock ZS, et al. Immune surveillance plays a role in locally aggressive giant cell lesions of bone. Clin Orthop Relat Res 2016.

80. Behjati S, Tarpey PS, Presneau N, et al. Distinct H3F3A and H3F3B driver mutations define chondroblastoma and giant cell tumor of bone. Nat Genet 2013;45:1479.

81. Presneau N, Baumhoer D, Behjati S, et al. Diagnostic value of H3F3A mutations in giant cell tumour of bone compared to osteoclast-rich mimics. J Pathol Clin Res 2015;1:113.

82. Gomes CC, Diniz MG, Amaral FR, et al. The highly prevalent H3F3A mutation in giant cell tumours of bone is not shared by sporadic central giant cell lesion of the jaws. Oral Surg Oral Med Oral Pathol Oral Radiol 2014; 118:583.

83. Lewis PW, Müller MM, Koletsky MS, et al. Inhibition of PRC2 activity by a gain-of-function H3 mutation found in pediatric glioblastoma. Science 2013; 340:857–61.

84. Chan KM, Fang D, Gan H, et al. The histone H3.3K27M mutation in pediatric glioma reprograms H3K27 methylation and gene expression. Genes Dev 2013;27:985–90.

85. Bjerke L, Mackay A, Nandhabalan M, et al. Histone H3.3 mutations drive pediatric glioblastoma through upregulation of MYCN. Cancer Discov 2013;3(5):512–9.

86. Dewsnup NC, Susarla SM, Abulikemu M, et al. Immunohistochemical evaluation of giant cell tumors of the jaws using CD34 density analysis. J Oral Maxillofac Surg 2008;66:928.

87. Schreuder WH, van den Berg H, Westermann AM, et al. Pharmacological and surgical therapy for the central giant cell granuloma: a long-term retrospective cohort study. J Craniomaxillofac Surg 2017;45(2):232–43.

88. Schreuder WH, Peacock ZS, Ebb D, et al. Adjuvant antiangiogenic treatment for aggressive giant cell lesions of the jaw: a 20-year experience at Massachusetts General Hospital. J Oral Maxillofac Surg 2017;75(1):105–18.

89. Susarla SM, August M, Dewsnup N, et al. CD34 staining density predicts giant cell tumor clinical behavior. J Oral Maxillofac Surg 2009;67(5):951–6.

90. Peacock ZS, Jordan RC, Schmidt BL. Giant cell lesions of the jaws: does the level of vascularity and angiogenesis correlate with behavior? J Oral Maxillofac Surg 2012;70(8):1860–6.

91. Chawla S, Henshaw R, Seeger L, et al. Safety and efficacy of denosumab for adults and skeletally mature adolescents with giant cell tumour of bone: interim analysis of an open-label, parallel-group, phase 2 study. Lancet Oncol 2013;14:901.

92. Schreuder WH, Coumou AW, Kessler PA, et al. Alternative pharmacologic therapy for aggressive central giant cell granuloma: denosumab. J Oral Maxillofac Surg 2014;72:1301.

93. Antonoglou GN, Sandor GK. Recurrence rates of intraosseous ameloblastomas of the jaws: a systematic review of conservative versus aggressive treatment approaches and meta-analysis of nonrandomized studies. J Craniomaxillofac Surg 2015;43:149.

94. Almeida RA, Andrade ES, Barbalho JC, et al. Recurrence rate following treatment for primary multicystic ameloblastoma: systematic review and meta-analysis. Int J Oral Maxillofac Surg 2016;45:359.

95. Reichart PA, Philipsen HP, Sonner S. Ameloblastoma: biological profile of 3677 cases. Eur J Cancer B Oral Oncol 1995;31B:86.

96. Sehdev MK, Huvos AG, Strong EW, et al. Ameloblastoma of maxilla and mandible. Cancer 1974; 33:324.

97. Vedtofte P, Hjorting-Hansen E, Jensen BN, et al. Conservative surgical treatment of mandibular ameloblastomas. Int J Oral Surg 1978;7(3):156–61.

98. Huffman GG, Thatcher JW. Ameloblastoma—the conservative surgical approach to treatment: report of four cases. J Oral Surg 1974;32(11): 850–4.

99. Pogrel MA. The use of liquid nitrogen cryotherapy in the management of locally aggressive bone lesions. J Oral Maxillofac Surg 1993;51(3):269–73.

100. Sachs SA. Surgical excision with peripheral ostectomy: a definitive, yet conservative, approach to the surgical management of ameloblastoma. J Oral Maxillofac Surg 2006;64(3):476–83.

101. Mehlisch DR, Dahlin DC, Masson JK. Ameloblastoma: a clinicopathologic report. J Oral Surg 1972;30(1):9–22.

102. Nastri AL, Wiesenfeld D, Radden BG, et al. Maxillary ameloblastoma: a retrospective study of 13 cases. Br J Oral Maxillofac Surg 1995;33(1):28–32.

103. Oka K, Fukui M, Yamashita M, et al. Mandibular ameloblastoma with intracranial extension and distant metastasis. Clin Neurol Neurosurg 1986;88(4):303–9.

104. Hayward JR. Recurrent ameloblastoma 30 years after surgical treatment. J Oral Surg 1973;31(5):368–70.

105. Daramola JO, Ajagbe HA, Oluwasanmi JO. Recurrent ameloblastoma of the jaws—a review of 22 cases. Plast Reconstr Surg 1980;65(5):577–9.

106. Adekeye EO, Lavery KM. Recurrent ameloblastoma of the maxillo-facial region. Clinical features and treatment. J Maxillofac Surg 1986;14(3):153–7.

107. Robinson L, Martinez MG. Unicystic ameloblastoma: a prognostically distinct entity. Cancer 1977;40(5):2278–85.

108. Cahn LR. The dentigerous cyst is a potential adamantinoma. Dent Cosmo 1933;75:889.

109. Leider AS, Eversole LR, Barkin ME. Cystic ameloblastoma. A clinicopathologic analysis. Oral Surg Oral Med Oral Pathol 1985;60:624.

110. Li TJ, Wu YT, Yu SF, et al. Unicystic ameloblastoma: a clinicopathologic study of 33 Chinese patients. Am J Surg Pathol 2000;24:1385.

111. Wang JT. Unicystic ameloblastoma: a clinicopathological appraisal. Taiwan Yi Xue Hui Za Zhi 1985; 84:1363.

112. Lau SL, Samman N. Recurrence related to treatment modalities of unicystic ameloblastoma: a systematic review. Int J Oral Maxillofac Surg 2006;35:681.

113. Chouinard AF, Peacock ZS, Faquin WC, et al. Unicystic ameloblastoma revisited: comparison of Massachusetts General Hospital Outcomes with original Robinson and Martinez report. J Oral Maxillofac Surg 2017. [Epub ahead of print].

114. Kessler HP. Intraosseous ameloblastoma. Oral Maxillofac Surg Clin North Am 2004;16:309.

115. Gardner DG, Corio RL. Plexiform unicystic ameloblastoma, a variant of ameloblastoma with a low-recurrence rate after enucleation. Cancer 1984; 53:1730.

116. Gardner DG, Pecak AMJ. The treatment of ameloblastoma based on pathologic and anatomic principles. Cancer 1980;46:2514.

117. Feinberg SE, Steinberg B. Surgical management of ameloblastoma. Current status of the literature. Oral Surg Oral Med Oral Pathol Oral Radiol Endod 1996;81:383.

118. Guthrie D, Peacock ZS, Sadow P, et al. Preoperative incisional and intraoperative frozen section biopsy techniques have comparable accuracy in the diagnosis of benign intraosseous jaw pathology. J Oral Maxillofac Surg 2012;70:2566.

119. Gardner DG. Some current concepts on the pathology of ameloblastomas. Oral Surg Oral Med Oral Pathol Oral Radiol Endod 1996;82:660.

120. Philipsen HP, Reichart PA. Unicystic ameloblastoma. A review of 193 cases from the literature. Oral Oncol 1998;34:317.

121. Black CC, Addante RR, Mohila CA. Intraosseous ameloblastoma. Oral Surg Oral Med Oral Pathol Oral Radiol Endod 2010;110:585.

122. Carlson ER, Marx RE. The ameloblastoma: primary, curative surgical management. J Oral Maxillofac Surg 2006;64:484.

123. Ghandhi D, Ayoub AF, Pogrel MA, et al. Ameloblastoma: a surgeon's dilemma. J Oral Maxillofac Surg 2006;64:1010.

124. De Silva ID, Rozen WM, Ramakrishnan A, et al. Achieving adequate margins in ameloblastoma resection: the role for intra-operative specimen imaging. Clinical report and systematic review. PLos One 2012;7:e47897.

125. Peacock ZS, Ji YD, Faquin WC. What is important for confirming negative margins when resecting mandibular ameloblastomas? J Oral Maxillofac Surg 2017;75(6):1185–90.

126. Gomes CC, Duarte AP, Diniz MG, et al. Review article: current concepts of ameloblastoma pathogenesis. J Oral Pathol Med 2010;39(8):585–91.

127. Kurppa KJ, Catón J, Morgan PR, et al. High frequency of BRAF V600E mutations in ameloblastoma. J Pathol 2014;232(5):492–8.

128. Salama AK, Flaherty KT. BRAF in melanoma: current strategies and future directions. Clin Cancer Res 2013;19(16):4326–34.

129. Gong J, Cho M, Fakih M. RAS and BRAF in metastatic colorectal cancer management. J Gastrointest Oncol 2016;7(5):687–704.

130. Kreitman RJ. Hairy cell leukemia—new genes, new targets. Curr Hematol Malig Rep 2013;8(3):184–95.

131. Sweeney RT, McClary AC, Myers BR, et al. Identification of recurrent SMO and BRAF mutations in ameloblastomas. Nat Genet 2014;46(7):722–5.

132. Brown NA, Rolland D, McHugh JB, et al. Activating FGFR2-RAS-BRAF mutations in ameloblastoma. Clin Cancer Res 2014;20(21):5517–26.

133. Kaye FJ, Ivey AM, Drane WE, et al. Clinical and radiographic response with combined BRAF-targeted therapy in stage 4 ameloblastoma. J Natl Cancer Inst 2014;107(1):378.

134. Faden DL, Algazi A. Durable treatment of ameloblastoma with single agent BRAFi Re: clinical and radiographic response with combined BRAF-targeted therapy in stage 4 ameloblastoma. J Natl Cancer Inst 2016;109(1) [pii:djw190].

135. Tan S, Pollack JR, Kaplan MJ, et al. BRAF inhibitor therapy of primary ameloblastoma. Oral Surg Oral Med Oral Pathol Oral Radiol 2016;122(4): 518–9.

Controversies in Oral and Maxillofacial Oncology

Jacob G. Yetzer, DDS, MD[a,b]

KEYWORDS

- Oral and maxillofacial • Oncology • Controversy • Cancer

KEY POINTS

- Imaging studies are essential components of tumor diagnosis, staging, assessing tumor response to neoadjuvant and adjuvant therapies, and postoperative surveillance on completion of definitive treatment.
- Contrast-enhanced computed tomography (CT), MRI, ultrasonography, and ^{18}F-fluorodeoxyglucose PET/CT represent the most commonly used imaging modalities in the diagnosis and management of head and neck malignancies.
- Historically, the treatment of early stage (T1/T2) clinically node negative (cN0) oral cavity squamous cell carcinoma has remained a controversial topic in oncologic head and neck surgery.
- Approximately 3% of all head and neck tumors arise within the parotid gland and most often within the superficial lobe, lateral to the facial nerve; among these neoplasms about 80% are benign entities and most are pleomorphic adenoma.
- Although submandibular gland transplant is not an undertaking intended for every patient with dry eyes, in those failing multiple other treatment modalities and facing ongoing pain and loss of vision, microvascular transplant of the gland does remain a viable option.

INTRODUCTION

The world of oral and maxillofacial surgery is full of controversy spanning a broad range of topics. Nowhere is this truer than the area of oncology. Incomplete or insufficient evidence and conflicting opinions often leave surgeons in a state of indecision. It may not be possible at any given time to come to clear consensus, but well-educated surgeons are at least capable of recognizing and evaluating the merits of each side of the controversy and making a decision based on their experience. This article selects 4 controversial topics: imaging modalities in head and neck cancer, sentinel lymph node biopsy (SNB) for oral squamous cell carcinoma, surgical management of parotid masses, and autologous salivary gland transplant for severe dry eye. Differing views regarding each of these topics are discussed with regard to the best supporting evidence.

IMAGING MODALITIES IN HEAD AND NECK SQUAMOUS CELL CARCINOMA

The use of various imaging modalities plays a critical role in the management of head and neck malignancies. Imaging studies are essential components of tumor diagnosis, staging, assessing tumor response to neoadjuvant and adjuvant therapies, and postoperative surveillance on completion of definitive treatment. Contrast-enhanced computed tomography (CT), MRI, ultrasonography (US), and ^{18}F-fluorodeoxyglucose PET/CT represent the most commonly used imaging modalities in the diagnosis and management of head and neck malignancies.[1] Each of these different imaging studies is used to varying degrees depending on the type of malignancy, as well as the anatomic location of the tumor within the head and neck. It remains incumbent on maxillofacial surgeons to understand how and when to use these various imaging modalities

[a] Private Practice, Head and Neck Surgery, Nebraska Oral and Facial Surgery, 2600 S. 56th Street, Suite A, Lincoln, NE 68506, USA; [b] Assistant Professor, Department of Surgery, Creighton University School of Medicine, 2500 California Plaza, Omaha, NE 68178, USA
E-mail address: jakeyetzer@gmail.com

Oral Maxillofacial Surg Clin N Am 29 (2017) 487–501
http://dx.doi.org/10.1016/j.coms.2017.07.004
1042-3699/17/© 2017 Elsevier Inc. All rights reserved.

during the various phases of treatment of head and neck cancer.

Imaging Guidelines

Although there are aspects of imaging for head and neck squamous cell carcinoma (HNSCC) that remain well accepted among surgeons, there continues to be variability among providers in terms of how and when various imaging studies are used. International bodies, such as the European Head and Neck Society/European Society of Medical Oncology/European Society for Radiotherapy & Oncology (EHNS-ESMO-ESTRO) and National Comprehensive Cancer Network (NCCN), have established guidelines for how different imaging studies should be used during the various phases of HNSCC treatment.[2,3] However, each of the guidelines is not entirely rigid, nor do they comprehensively agree with one another in terms of which imaging modality should be selected and for what purpose.[1] There continues to be inherent allowances built into the recommendations from both NCCN and EHNS-ESMO-ESTRO that allow individualized selection of various imaging modalities to be made by providers. At present, there is no universally accepted algorithm for selection of diagnostic, staging, or surveillance imaging as it pertains to HNSCC. Nevertheless, it remains important for surgeons to maintain an understanding of the various imaging modalities at their disposal in order to ensure that patients with HNSCC are being managed and surveilled appropriately within the generally accepted standards of care.

Staging

According to the most recently updated NCCN guidelines (version 1.2016) the appropriate clinical staging of HNSCC should be composed of a complete head and neck examination (including mirror and fiberoptic endoscopy when indicated), a diagnostic biopsy, a contrast-enhanced CT scan of the head and neck and/or MRI with contrast to assess the primary tumor and regional nodal basins, chest imaging as clinically indicated, and consideration of PET/CT for advanced stage (III–IV) disease.[2] The rationale for the inclusion of PET/CT for advanced stage disease is the potential for diagnostically upstaging patients if distant metastatic disease is identified, because this would alter the overall management strategy.[4] The NCCN guidelines do not make explicit recommendations on the specific type of chest imaging that should be pursued. Thus the potential imaging modalities implemented for chest interrogation (chest radiograph, chest CT, or PET/CT) are left at the discretion of the provider.

The European guidelines (EHNS-ESMO-ESTRO) are similar to those of the NCCN as they pertain to clinical staging of HNSCC; however, there are subtle differences in the recommendations. The European guidelines also recommend that routine staging be based on physical examination, diagnostic biopsy, chest radiograph, head and neck endoscopy, and a head and neck CT scan and/or MRI.[3] The European guidelines state that contrast-enhanced MRI of the head and neck is the preferred imaging modality for every head and neck tumor subsite with the exception of laryngeal and hypopharyngeal cancers.[3] The European guidelines also specifically recommend chest CT as a method for ruling out distant metastatic disease and/or second lung primaries; however, they do not delineate specific clinical scenarios in which this should be explicitly used rather than chest radiograph.[3] In addition, the European stance on the use of PET/CT for routine HNSCC staging remains more equivocal, citing PET/CT's lower specificity and higher sensitivity for detecting metastatic disease, but that, for the purposes of HNSCC staging, PET/CT is still currently under investigation.[1,3]

The primary differences between the NCCN and European guidelines as they pertain to diagnostic staging of HNSCC primarily come down to the role of PET/CT, minor variation in the preferred imaging modality (CT vs MRI) for staging, and subtle differences in the recommendations on chest interrogation. Clearly, with as high as 90% of the distant metastatic disease of HNSCC occurring within the lungs,[5–8] it remains of critical importance to use some form of interrogative imaging of the chest. Distant metastases isolated to other organ systems such as the liver and bone are exceedingly rare in the absence of a concomitant pulmonary malignancy,[7] and this highlights why some clinicians think that full-body imaging in the form of PET/CT is unwarranted in the routine work-up of HNSCC. Even in the current oncologic paradigm, chest radiograph continues to remain a favored method of lung screening among surgeons treating HNSCC[9] owing to its wide availability, low cost, ease of interpretation, and low radiation dose. Although some studies have suggested that chest radiography is becoming an outdated imaging method for HNSCC,[10–12] there remains inadequate evidence to currently recommend a specific chest imaging modality as a standard of care in assessing the lung fields for the presence of distant metastases.

Although the European guidelines have suggested that contrast-enhanced MRI is the preferred imaging modality of HNSCC staging, the NCCN guidelines consider CT and MRI to be interchangeable, with no stipulation on superiority of one method to the other. Before the year 2000, contrast-enhanced CT was widely considered to be the gold standard for detection of malignant cervical lymph nodes in HNSCC[2,13]; however, further advances in MR technology have subsequently improved the diagnostic accuracy of MRI in the detection of regional nodal disease.[14,15] Compared with CT, MRI carries the advantages of higher soft tissue contrast resolution, lack of iodine-based contrast agents, and higher sensitivity for identifying perineural invasion.[16] However, MRI is also associated with lower patient tolerance owing to the time required for image acquisition, contraindication in the presence of pacemakers, greater sensitivity to motion artifact, and higher overall cost compared with CT. In contrast, CT is generally well tolerated secondary to its rapid acquisition time, it is readily available at most centers, and it has reduced cost compared with MRI. However, CT is more susceptible to beam hardening and streaking artifact in the presence of metal materials such as dental amalgam and dental implants, which can obscure visualization of certain primary tumor subsites and some areas of the upper neck.[17]

The diagnostic criteria used for CT and MRI in the assessment of metastatic regional lymph nodes in HNSCC predominantly relies on nodal size, nodal architecture, and the presence of nodal necrosis.[15] Typically the reported pathologic size criterion for metastatic lymph nodes in HNSCC is a maximum nodal axis diameter of greater than or equal to 10 mm.[15,17,18] Emerging evidence has suggested potential utility in using differing pathologic size criteria for different levels of the neck as a method of reducing misdiagnosis of small (<10 mm) metastatic lymph nodes[15,17–19]; however, differing pathologic size criteria based on neck level is not universally used. Nodal necrosis continues to remain a virtually pathognomonic feature of metastatic cervical lymph nodes in HNSCC and the presence of necrosis is critically important to assess for on imaging of regional nodal basins for staging purposes. Nodal necrosis is known to occur even in nodes with very small tumor deposits and it has been reported to occur in up to 35% of metastatic nodes with less than 10 mm greatest axial diameter.[18] Identification of nodal necrosis in subcentimeter lymph nodes remains a challenge with contrast-enhanced CT images owing to the similarity of necrotic areas (water density) to those of normal lymphatic hilar structures (water to fat density).[15] MRI is more sensitive in distinguishing between nodal necrosis and normal hilar structures on both T1-weighted images and on fat-suppressed T2-weighted images.[15] These distinctive features on MRI contribute to the slightly improved performance of MRI in distinguishing between small metastatic lymph nodes and reactive lymph nodes in HNSCC.[15,17] However, emerging evidence has recently suggested that combined protocols using contrast-enhanced CT with PET/CT may be the most sensitive method of identifying metastatic regional lymph nodes in HNSCC,[1,20] but these protocols require further corroboration with future studies.

Ultimately, the primary question of CT versus MRI in HNSCC staging generally comes down to cases in which regional disease is subclinical and ambiguous, rather than cases in which cervical adenopathy is grossly obvious from a clinical and radiographic standpoint. Of primary concern is the inadequate clinical staging of individuals who harbor occult nodal metastasis at the time of their initial diagnosis, but in whom preoperative imaging suggests a lack of regional disease. This naturally harkens back to the age-old question of how to adequately treat the clinically node negative (cN0) neck. However, with more recent evidence suggesting survival benefits conferred through elective neck dissection[21] as well as the potentially increasing role of SNB in the management of cN0 disease,[22–26] the question of staging equivalence between MRI and CT may ultimately be rendered a moot point. Nevertheless, based on the currently available evidence, providers can remain confident in selecting either modality for staging purposes, with the selection of either method largely depending on the local availability, the specific anatomic subsite of the primary tumor, and overall patient characteristics.

Assessment of Response to Treatment/Surveillance

Recurrence rates following curative-intent therapy for HNSCC are reported to range from approximately 10% to 48% depending on tumor subsite and initial stage at primary diagnosis.[27,28] Accordingly, approximately 75% to 90% of HNSCC recurrences occur within the first 2 to 3 years following definitive oncologic treatment,[29–31] which underscores the importance of close regular follow-up for tumor surveillance. The purpose of surveillance is 2-fold, with the primary objective to detect locoregional and/or distant metastasis as quickly as possible but also, secondarily, to detect second primary malignancies outside the head and neck region.[10] The NCCN guidelines recommend an explicit surveillance regimen with deescalating frequency of clinical and radiographic evaluations over an initial 5-year time frame.[2] Specifically, the NCCN recommends that surveillance examinations occur every 1 to 3 months during year 1, every 2 to 6 months in year 2, every 4 to 8 months in years 3 to 5, and an annual surveillance visit greater after 5 years from the definitive treatment.[2] The NCCN also recommends that baseline posttreatment imaging of the primary and tumor site and the neck should be obtained within 6 months of definitive therapy and that additional reimaging should be pursued based on worrisome clinical examination findings and for routine assessment of clinically inaccessible anatomic areas.[2] The surveillance recommendations from the European guidelines are much less explicit in terms of the cadence of patient follow-up examinations; however, the guidelines do recommend assessment of treatment response with either CT scan or MRI depending on the initial curative-intent procedure rendered.[3] The European guidelines reference the utility of PET/CT in assessing the treatment response of HNSCC primaries that are treated either with definitive radiation therapy or definitive concomitant chemoradiation therapy, because functional imaging can aid in decision making regarding the utility of a posttreatment neck dissection for residual regional disease.[1,3] In addition, the European guidelines specifically recommend that a chest radiograph be obtained on an annual basis to assess for distant metastases and/or new lung primaries,[3] whereas the NCCN guidelines only recommend regular surveillance chest imaging for patients with prior smoking history as a routine screening method for lung cancer.[2]

Although the NCCN and European guidelines both recommend CT or MRI as the favored strategies for assessing treatment response on completion of curative-intent therapy, there are certain drawbacks to the use of each of these modalities in the posttreatment time frame. Surgery and adjuvant therapies have the potential to cause fibrosis and scarring both within the primary tumor bed and within the regional nodal basins of the neck. Fibrosis and postsurgical changes greatly limit the capabilities of cross-sectional imaging modalities such as CT and MRI to distinguish between residual or recurrent tumor and surrounding fibrotic tissue.[1] In contrast, functional imaging strategies such as PET/CT are not limited by the presence of posttreatment fibrosis and can thus identify residual or recurrent disease with a high degree of precision, enabling prompt introduction of salvage treatment strategies[1] (**Figs. 1** and **2**). However, the diagnostic performance of functional imaging such as PET/CT depends on the time elapsed between completion of therapy and the time of image acquisition. Procuring functional imaging too early in the posttreatment window invariably leads to a falsely positive study from the increased metabolic activity and unresolved tissue inflammation within the tissue beds. Accordingly, it is recommended that PET/CT should not be obtained until 3 months have elapsed from the completion of curative-intent therapy in order to improve accuracy and precision in detecting recurrent locoregional disease.[32,33]

In spite of the limitations mentioned earlier, cross-sectional imaging studies, including CT and MRI, remain the mainstay surveillance modalities used for HNSCC in the posttreatment window. Although no consensus exists in the preferred

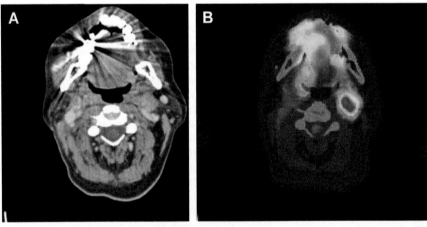

Fig. 1. A 61-year-old man with history of metachronous squamous cell carcinomas of the oral cavity previously treated with surgical resection, microvascular reconstruction, and adjuvant radiation therapy. (*A*) Postoperative contrast-enhanced CT scan of head and neck showing mildly enhancing nodular swelling in level II of the left neck. (*B*) PET/CT scan showing intense fluorodeoxyglucose (FDG) avidity in the previously identified level II mass, suggestive of recurrent regional metastatic disease. Fine-needle aspirate biopsy confirmed presence of regionally recurrent squamous cell carcinoma.

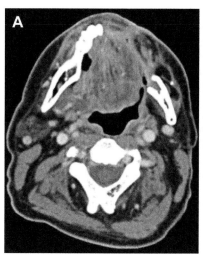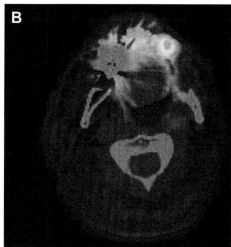

Fig. 2. A 60-year-old man with history of multiply recurrent squamous cell carcinomas of the oral cavity previously treated with multiple surgical resections, locoregional flaps, microvascular reconstruction, and adjuvant radiation therapy. (*A*) Postoperative contrast-enhanced CT scan of head and neck showing mildly enhancing nodular soft tissue thickening involving the previous radial forearm free flap reconstruction of the left buccal mucosa. Imaging was thought to be inconclusive for postoperative changes versus recurrent disease. (*B*) Subsequent PET/CT scan showing intense FDG avidity in anterior margin of left buccal mucosal reconstruction site. Incisional biopsy ultimately confirmed presence of locally recurrent squamous cell carcinoma.

method or frequency of surveillance imaging, anatomic subsites that are easily evaluated by physical and/or fiberoptic examination (ie, oral cavity or larynx) likely do not require routine surveillance imaging in the absence of clinical findings in otherwise asymptomatic patients.[10] When interval surveillance imaging is pursued, consideration should be given to maintaining consistency with the initial posttreatment baseline study as a means of easing the radiologic interpretation through equivalent study comparison. Equivocal clinical examination and indeterminate cross-sectional imaging findings should prompt the provider to pursue additional diagnostic modalities such as PET/CT or possibly neck ultrasonography with subsequent fine-needle aspiration, particularly in light of the potentially grave prognostic implications of a delayed or missed diagnosis of recurrent disease.

Ultimately, the present lack of consensus relative to posttreatment imaging strategies underscores the importance of the provider's duty in maintaining both a high level of suspicion for residual or recurrent disease and a frequent follow-up schedule to evaluate patients treated for HNSCC. Although it remains possible that future investigations may eventually provide adequate evidence to support a unified surveillance strategy, this is not presently a reality for practicing head and neck oncologic surgeons in the current time frame. Accordingly, providers must remain aware of the imaging studies that are actively available to them in their day-to-day practice and they must ensure that they are using these imaging modalities appropriately within the presently defined standards of care.

SENTINEL LYMPH NODE BIOPSY IN ORAL CAVITY SQUAMOUS CELL CARCINOMA

Historically, the treatment of early stage (T1/T2) cN0 oral cavity squamous cell carcinoma (OSCC) has remained a controversial topic in oncologic head and neck surgery. The management of the cN0 neck has typically been encompassed by 1 of 2 distinct approaches for early stage disease: elective neck dissection at the time of primary tumor resection or watchful waiting with subsequent therapeutic neck dissection at the time of regional recurrence. With the presence of occult nodal metastasis reaching as high as 30% in early stage cN0 OSCC coupled with the important prognostic implications held by the pathologic status of the cervical lymph nodes in terms of locoregional recurrence rates and overall survival,[34] elective neck dissection has largely become the standard treatment methodology. Controversy surrounding the practice of elective neck dissection in the management of early stage OSCC has also been greatly diminished by the recent publication of a randomized controlled trial identifying improved overall survival and higher rates of disease-free survival among patients undergoing elective neck dissection compared with individuals randomized to watchful waiting and therapeutic neck dissection for regional recurrence.[21] Nevertheless, routine use of elective neck dissection inherently leads to an overtreatment of 70% to 80% of patients with early stage OSCC who do not harbor occult nodal metastases at the time of their initial diagnosis.[35] Compared with a watchful waiting strategy, elective neck dissection is also associated with higher initial health care costs and increased surgical morbidity, including potential risk of injury to the marginal mandibular branch of the facial nerve, chronic pain, decreased shoulder strength, limited neck mobility, and poor cosmetic outcomes.

With an increasing body of evidence supporting the need for interrogation of the cervical lymph node basins as an integral component of the management of early stage OSCC, the use of SNB has emerged as a less invasive alternative staging modality for cN0 disease.[36–39] The technique of SNB for OSCC involves the preoperative mapping of sentinel lymph nodes via injection of a radiotracer (m-99 technetium)–labeled colloid solution, administered at 4 to 6 injection sites circumferentially within the healthy mucosa surrounding the primary tumor from 2 to 24 hours before surgery. Conventional dynamic planar lymphoscintigraphy and/or single-photon emission CT (SPECT) with CT is then used for preoperative image-guided localization of sentinel nodes. Intraoperative identification of the sentinel lymph nodes is facilitated by the use of handheld gamma probes, which are used to distinguish sentinel nodes from background radioactivity (**Fig. 3**). Patients with positive SNB results then typically undergo therapeutic neck dissection in a delayed fashion if traditional serial sectioning with hematoxylin and eosin is performed or, more rarely, in an immediate fashion if fresh frozen section analysis is used.[23]

SNB is commonly used for staging of cutaneous melanoma and breast cancer; however, it has not attained universal acceptance for staging of OSCC. The premise of SNB application to OSCC staging remains well founded in that the stereotypical lymphatic drainage patterns have previously been well delineated by multiple large-scale studies.[11,40] However, within the current oncologic paradigm, elective neck dissection continues to remain the gold standard staging procedure for OSCC and the routine use of SNB for staging and treatment of the cN0 neck remains largely relegated to a limited number of institutions across the world. Nevertheless, SNB for early stage OSCC remains an attractive alternative given its potential to detect subclinical nodal metastases while concomitantly reducing the risk of morbidity incurred from traditional staging elective neck dissection.

Although SNB has been increasing in popularity in specific centers around the world, there remains a limited amount of data relative to the outcomes and accuracy of SNB for early stage OSCC. An increasing number of published studies have provided evidence that SNB can be effectively used for OSCC nodal staging and that it is capable of reliable detection of occult cervical metastasis.[23,24,26,37,41,42] However, the adoption of SNB into standard-of-care pathways for OSCC has largely been hampered by several concerns relative to the technique's accuracy, institutional learning curve, false-negative rates, and anatomic subsite–specific reliability, as well as apprehensions about its overall impact on recurrence rates, disease-free survival, and overall survival.

Largely a historical concern at present, the accuracy of SNB in identifying sentinel nodes for OSCC has now been well established by numerous feasibility and validation studies over the past 2 decades.[23,26,42–46] Detection rates of sentinel lymph nodes is reported to range from 90% to 100%,[23,26,42–46] leaving little concern as to the reliability of applying this technique to the lymphatic drainage pattern of OSCC. However, institutional learning curves remain a viable impediment to the universal acceptance of SNB for OSCC staging.[37] This impediment is further compounded by interinstitutional variability in the availability and sensitivity of the fresh frozen section techniques that are required for performing single-stage therapeutic neck dissection at the time of positive SNB results. In contrast, patients undergoing SNB staging that is based on permanent section inherently require a secondary procedure during which a delayed therapeutic neck dissection is performed for the positive SNB disorder. The need to potentially stage therapeutic neck dissection until after primary tumor resection introduces the need for an additional surgical procedure and additional general anesthetic, both of which can be undesirable from the surgeon's and patient's perspective.

False-negative rates for SNB for OSCC are reported to range from 3% to 14%.[22,23,26,37] By comparison, the false-negative rates for SNB reported from large-scale meta-analyses on malignant melanoma staging range from 12.5% to 20%[47,48] and the currently accepted false-negative rate of SNB for breast cancer staging is 7%.[49] Although false-negative rates for OSCC SNB are reported to be comparable with those of malignant melanoma and breast cancer, it is likely that further reduction in the false-negative rate will be required before the widespread use of SNB for OSCC staging becomes universally accepted, particularly in light of the recent evidence supporting potential survival benefit conferred by elective neck dissection in the management of early stage OSCC.[21] Primary

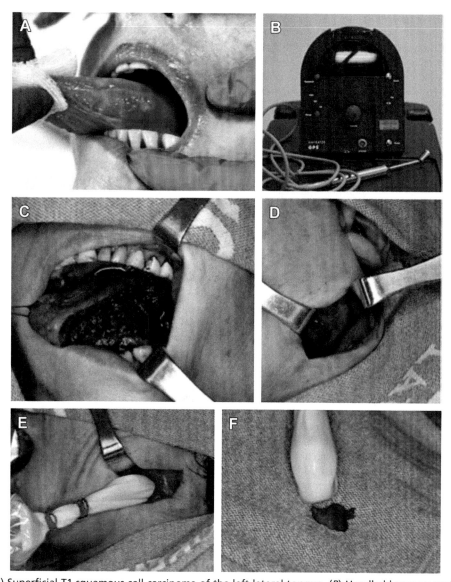

Fig. 3. (*A*) Superficial T1 squamous cell carcinoma of the left lateral tongue. (*B*) Handheld gamma probe setup. (*C*) Resection of primary tumor before sentinel lymph node localization to minimize radiation shine-through. (*D*) Surgical access for SNB. (*E*) Gamma probe guidance for identification of sentinel lymph node. (*F*) Ex-vivo confirmation of gamma signal from surgically removed sentinel lymph node. (*Courtesy* of Dr Allen C. Cheng, DDS, MD, Portland, OR, with permission; and Dr Felix Sim, BDS, MBBS, FRACDS (OMS), Portland, OR, with permission.)

tumor subsite has been suggested as a potential factor influencing the false-negative rate with SNB for OSCC. Floor-of-mouth tumors have been implicated in causing shine-through that obscures the signal from sentinel nodes leading to difficulty in sentinel node identification.[22,39,50] However, this phenomenon has not been universally shown across all studies[23,26] and the relationship between primary tumor subsite and accuracy of SNB for OSCC requires additional clarification through future investigations. Some investigators have advocated for targeted sentinel lymph node basin

dissection as a failsafe method for reducing the impact of false-negative results from SNB alone.[22,25] This technique involves elective dissection of the corresponding lymph node basins from which the negative sentinel lymph nodes are identified. This method relies on the premise that nonsentinel lymph nodes potentially harboring occult metastatic disease are likely to be contained within the same neck level as the identified sentinel nodes that are ultimately found negative for metastatic deposits.[22,25] This hybridized technique allows for a targeted interrogation of at-risk lymph node basins while simultaneously reducing the morbidity that would be incurred by a traditional multilevel staging elective neck dissection. However, this technique has only recently been investigated by a limited number of validation studies[22,25] and the ongoing utility of this technique as an OSCC staging method requires further validation.

A small but increasing number of studies have reported comparable regional control rates for SNB compared with elective neck dissection as a staging and treatment modality for OSCC. Regional control rates for SNB are reported to range from 2% to 15%,[23,26,37,39,51] whereas the calculated regional control rate for elective neck dissection in early stage cN0 OSCC was 18% in a recently published systematic review.[52] Although the regional control rates for SNB are based on much smaller patient cohorts than the data obtained from studies evaluating traditional elective neck dissection, the low rates of regional recurrence with SNB argue against prior concerns that SNB would potentially predispose toward regional failures through inadvertent seeding of the neck with metastatic deposits during sentinel node identification and dissection. In spite of these findings, the prognostic value of SNB remains controversial. Emerging evidence suggests that patients with positive SNB results tend to show poor regional control rates, reduced disease-specific survival, and lower overall survival compared with those with negative SNB.[22,26,37,51,53] However, there remains a paucity of data on survival outcomes for SNB in OSCC because many of the recently published studies evaluating SNB are validation studies that are without robust survival analyses or long-term follow-up intervals. Ultimately, the further delineation of the prognostic significance of SNB in the management and staging of early stage OSCC will require future investigation with large multi-institutional prospective trials.

In spite of the limited number of centers currently performing SNB for early stage cN0 OSCC, there are a multitude of advantages to the technique that are likely to contribute to its increasing use in the future, particularly if it continues to show equivalent oncologic safety relative to traditional staging elective neck dissection. The most obvious advantage of SNB is its minimally invasive nature and its potential for reducing the morbidity incurred by traditional elective neck dissection. The efficacy of SNB in reducing surgical complications and morbidity is not simply theoretic, because several recently published studies have corroborated reduced morbidity following SNB compared with elective neck dissection.[54–56] SNB also carries the advantage of being able to identify aberrant lymphatic drainage patterns that would otherwise be inadequately addressed by reflex ipsilateral neck dissection for unilateral tumors. This advantage is highlighted by findings of a recently published study wherein an unexpected contralateral lymphatic drainage was identified in 12% (49 of 369) of patients with a unilateral primary OSCC tumor.[23] In 7 of these 49 patients with unexpected contralateral lymphatic drainage patterns, the contralateral sentinel node was positive for occult metastasis, which would have been missed by a conventional treatment consisting of ipsilateral elective neck dissection.[23] SNB also has the potential to target specific areas of the neck for pathologic interrogation among patients with midline primary tumors who would otherwise be prescribed bilateral neck dissection under current standard of practice patterns. Targeting limited areas of the neck would not only have the added benefit of limiting the invasiveness of surgery but also greatly reduce the length of hospital stay and, in turn, reduce the cost of health care delivery. Limiting dissection of the neck can also aid in the subsequent performance of salvage surgery if this is ultimately required by disease progression. Preserving undissected levels of the neck allows for preservation of vascular targets for subsequent microvascular reconstructions that might otherwise not be possible in the salvage setting. This preservation in turn has the potential to postpone the earlier need for regional flaps owing to vessel depletion in the neck and thus potentially allows for greater reconstructive options during the treatment course of recurrent OSCC.

Ultimately, SNB is not currently recommended as the standard staging procedure for early stage OSCC. However, there is an increasing body of evidence suggesting equivalent oncologic safety in its use for early stage cN0 disease. Accordingly, the 2014 update of the NCCN guidelines for head and neck cancer has included the option of using SNB for the identification of occult cervical metastasis in T1 to T2, N0 oral cavity cancer.[57] However, the NCCN guidelines stipulate that SNB should only be used in medical centers with specific expertise in the technique.[57] With the long-term follow-up results of large-scale prospective trials such as the Sentinel European Node Trial (SENT) less than a half a decade away, it remains likely that SNB will continue to play an increasing role in the management of early stage cN0 disease for OSCC.

MANAGEMENT OF PAROTID MASSES

Management of parotid gland neoplasms is a subject of controversy in oral and maxillofacial surgery. It is a deserving topic of discussion because approximately 3% of all head and neck tumors arise within the parotid gland and most often within the superficial lobe, lateral to the facial nerve. Among these neoplasms about 80% are benign entities and most are pleomorphic adenoma. Because of their high incidence and troublesome potential for recurrence, pleomorphic adenoma has come to play a central role in the discussion of management of parotid masses in general.

Head and neck surgeons have seen a gradual evolution of the management of salivary gland neoplasms. In the nineteenth century, enucleation was advocated. In this procedure, intracapsular shelling out of the tumor was performed. The perceived value of enucleation was avoidance of injury to the facial nerve, which is recognized as the most morbid complication associated with parotid surgery. Enucleation of parotid gland masses remained the preferred approach until the early part of the twentieth century, when it was recognized that the strategy left much to be desired in terms of recurrence.[58] Histologic evaluation of pleomorphic adenoma led to the discovery that the capsule was often incomplete and included pseudopodia, or satellite lesions.[59] These characteristics of pleomorphic adenoma were cited as the cause of residual tumor or tumor spillage and resultant recurrence when using enucleation. Therefore, broader resection with a cuff of parotid parenchyma was advocated. A more comprehensive dissection of the facial nerve was required, from the trunk to the major branches. This procedure is recognized as the superficial parotidectomy.[60,61] Parotidectomy with nerve dissection has become the most common and recognized treatment of salivary gland neoplasms, often regarded as the gold standard for parotid neoplasms.

More recently, a limited resection has been offered as an alternative to superficial parotidectomy and is referred to as extracapsular dissection. Initially described by McGurk and colleagues,[62] it by definition excludes the identification and dissection of the main trunk of the facial nerve, which differentiates this procedure from superficial parotidectomy. Advocates of this technique cite equivalent rates of control and recurrence and the minimization of the complications commonly associated with complete removal of the superficial lobe.

Certain aspects of the management of parotid masses are free of controversy. First, it is well recognized that the most appropriate treatment of nearly all parotid neoplasms is surgical excision. For malignant neoplasms, a sound margin must be achieved whenever anatomically feasible, which

usually necessitates superficial or total parotidectomy with dissection of the facial nerve. With regard to benign neoplasms in general, and pleomorphic adenoma specifically, it is recognized that without complete removal of the tumor there is a high likelihood of recurrence, and can result in multifocal recurrences, which are highly challenging to address secondarily. However, in these cases, an oncologic margin is often not always achieved, nor is it considered mandatory.[63] In addition to the goal of total removal, it is desirable to avoid the common complications most often associated with parotid surgery. These complications include but are not limited to facial nerve injury, Frey syndrome, salivary fistula, and cosmetic deformity. It is because of the desire to limit these complications that extracapsular dissection has been offered as an alternative to traditional superficial parotidectomy.

Supporters of the more limited extracapsular dissection for benign parotid tumors cite evidence that similar rates of recurrence are achieved with a diminished rate of complications compared with parotidectomy. McGurk and colleagues[62] published a large series at a single unit comparing traditional parotidectomy with nerve dissection with more limited extracapsular dissection. This group showed similar rates of recurrence between superficial parotidectomy (1.8%) and extracapsular dissection (1.7%), and revealed significantly lower rates of facial nerve paresis and Frey syndrome, which are two of the most serious complications associated with parotid surgery. In the McGurk and colleagues[62] series, the decision of which procedure to perform was determined intraoperatively. Those tumors undergoing extracapsular dissection were selected based on size (with the upper limit at 4 cm), tumor mobility, and degree of lateral position within the gland. These criteria have been replicated by other investigators, many of whom have reported similar success with the extracapsular dissection technique.[64,65] Additional evidence in support of extracapsular dissection comes in the form of several large meta-analyses showing similar rates of recurrence with lower or similar complication rates in extracapsular dissection groups compared with parotidectomy.[66,67]

Many investigators have found fault with the available evidence for extracapsular dissection and caution against the abandonment of superficial parotidectomy as the primary modality for treatment of benign neoplasms of the parotid. These individuals point out that there are significant shortcomings within most of the larger series and meta-analyses. All available evidence is retrospective and based on intraoperative decision making for determination of extracapsular dissection versus superficial parotidectomy. In addition, the decision-making criteria that are most often applied ensure that the smaller, mobile, laterally located, and most easily dissected tumors are selected for extracapsular dissection.[66] This process potentially introduces strong bias against the parotidectomy approach, which would represent the larger tumors and those more likely to be in close proximity or adherent to the facial nerve. Furthermore, all of the available literature is derived from large-volume centers and written by highly experienced parotid surgeons, thus limiting the value of these findings for small-volume centers or those surgeons less experienced in parotid surgery. In addition, there is a lack of long-term follow-up in the available literature. It is well known that pleomorphic adenoma may recur well beyond 5 years. Series using shorter time frames risk an increased rate of false-negative findings with regard to recurrence rates.

The question of the most appropriate parotid surgery for benign parotid neoplasms benefits from better clinical research, with trials and appropriate comparison groups. At present, oral and maxillofacial surgeons must make a decision based on best available evidence. Like much of modern medicine, a one-size-fits-all approach is unlikely to prove satisfactory. In an era of individualized medicine, clinicians seek to apply the best surgery given the specific patient, tumor, and availability of surgical expertise. For highly experienced surgeons, with the anatomic knowledge and surgical skill required to safely achieve extracapsular dissection, it may be appropriate to use that skill set for smaller, more easily dissected tumors. However, traditional parotidectomy techniques with facial nerve dissection are likely to remain a mainstay in the management of parotid tumors, particularly those larger and less ideally located within the gland. In selecting either surgical approach, clinicians must consider the limits of their own competence and experience and apply this knowledge toward the optimal care of the patient.

AUTOLOGOUS SUBMANDIBULAR GLAND TRANSFER

Because of the great breadth and depth of training oral and maxillofacial surgeons undergo, the specialty has become extremely diverse in its areas of focus, with applications spanning both medicine and dentistry. Even among this diversified group, salivary gland transplant for the purpose of treating severe dry eye continues to be relegated to the outer fringes of the specialty. It is not considered a standard treatment, particularly in disease states in which both the lacrimal and salivary glands are affected, such as graft-versus-host disease. Considerations for a new application of autogenous submandibular gland transplant for refractory dry eye related to graft-versus-host disease are presented here, with an accompanying case presentation.

The modern history of salivary gland transplant for ophthalmologic purposes dates to 1951, when the first Stenson duct transposition was described.[68] This procedure was effective in increasing salivary-tear flow, but the serous character of the parotid duct and the variability of flow rate prohibited its use as a common treatment of dry eye. It was in 1986 that Murube-del-Castillo[69] first described the microvascular transplant of the submandibular gland to the temporal fossa. This procedure was later described successfully in larger numbers[70–73] among other groups. The benefits of submandibular gland transplant were notable across several series for the ability to increase moisture in severe and refractory cases of dry eye. Indications have included patients with zero or near-zero lacrimal flow and corneal injury associated with this deficit and who have failed to improve with more traditional and less invasive therapies. The retrospective series evaluating this procedure have repeatedly shown success in improving patient symptoms as well as clinical metrics of tear production and corneal injury.[71,73,74] Long-term follow-up suggests that these benefits can be maintained over the course in several years.[75]

Submandibular gland autotransplant has risks. Notably, epiphora is present in approximately 50% of the patients undergoing this procedure and is usually associated with warmth, caffeine ingestion, and exercise.[76] Attempts to address this complication have included partial gland transplant, secondary excision, and injection with botulinum toxin.[72,77] Other less frequently occurring complications include venous thrombosis, ischemic necrosis of the gland, or ductal occlusion following transplant. Importantly, most of the series have included as indications a broad array of pathologic causes of dry eye, but have specifically excluded any systemic conditions that may diminish salivary function, such as Sjögren syndrome and graft-versus-host disease.

There is evidence that, although multiple excretory glands may be affected in the setting of graft-versus-host disease, the salivary gland function may be differentially involved compared with the lacrimal glands.[78] In addition, because these patients often face debilitating corneal injury and

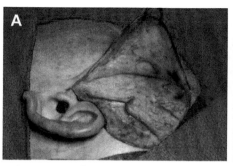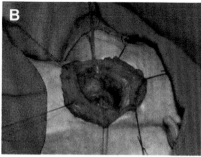

Fig. 4. Operative images of submandibular gland transfer showing recipient site preparation with superficial temporal vessels exposed (*A*) and harvest of the submandibular gland, including the duct and vascular supply (*B*).

potential loss of vision, they are often left with few alternatives for treatment of their dry eye. Because epiphora is a common complaint in patients undergoing submandibular gland transplant, it is possible that a hypofunctioning submandibular gland would provide a more appropriate amount of secretion for eye lubrication. For these reasons, our group reconsidered graft-versus-host disease as a contraindication to submandibular gland transfer.

This article presents a case of submandibular gland transplant for severe and refractory dry eye in the setting of graft-versus-host disease. The patient is a 34-year-old woman with a history of graft-versus-host disease–related severe dry eye following bone marrow transplant for treatment of acute lymphoblastic leukemia. Over the course of 4 years, she underwent several ophthalmologic interventions, including artificial and autologous serum drops, punctual occlusion, and scleral lenses. Despite these interventions, persistent symptoms included chronic eye pain and loss of vision. After an ophthalmologic evaluation, which showed a diminished Schirmer test of 5 mm, rapid tear breakup time, and severe bilateral corneal staining, she was offered evaluation by the authors for potential gland transplant. Important clinical findings included clear and consistent flow from the submandibular duct on bimanual manipulation. Moreover, salivary scintigraphy was performed with a technetium 99m pertechnetate scan. Although the scan did reveal diminished uptake in the bilateral submandibular glands, they were both clearly viable with retained excretory function. Because the left eye was deemed most at risk, the decision was made to proceed with unilateral transfer and revisit the right eye based on clinical outcome and patient desires.

The procedure was performed under general anesthesia and nasotracheal intubation. The ipsilateral submandibular gland transferred to the temporal fossa. The temporal incision was made first and a recipient bed was prepared. The

superficial temporal artery and vein were prepared for anastomosis. A tunnel was made toward the superolateral fornix of the eye and a 3-mm incision was made within the upper eyelid conjunctiva. At this point, the gland and its vascular supply were harvested. An incision was made inferior to the border of the mandible and the submandibular gland was dissected just superficial to the capsule until the facial artery and its branches into the submandibular gland were identified. In addition, the facial vein was identified and careful dissection of its branches supplying the submandibular gland was performed in order to preserve venous drainage. The duct was identified and dissected from proximal to distal up to the floor of mouth. The most distal portion was dissected from a transoral incision. This portion was passed through the neck and the facial artery and facial vein, where it was ligated and divided. The flap was then brought to the temporal fossa and inset with the submandibular gland sutured into the superolateral fornix of the upper eyelid, and vascular anastomosis was performed in the usual manner. Immediate flow was noted, as shown in **Figs. 4** and **5**.

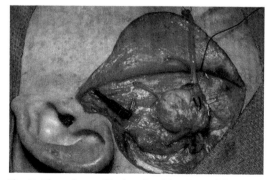

Fig. 5. The submandibular gland is oriented for insetting such that the duct is tunneled to the superolateral fornix of the ipsilateral eye and the arterial and venous supply can be anastomosed to the superficial temporal vessels.

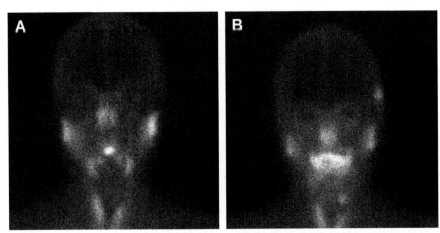

Fig. 6. Preoperative (*A*) and postoperative (*B*) sialoscintigraphy imaging for left submandibular gland transfer to the temporal fossa. Viable gland is shown in left temporal fossa postoperatively.

Postoperatively, the patient immediately showed subjective improvement in dry eye symptoms compared with preoperative findings, as well as compared with the contralateral eye. The patient was discharged on postoperative day 3. She did complain of epiphora at the 1-month follow-up, in which the Schirmer test was 25 mm in the left eye. The right eye remained unchanged. By the 6-month follow-up the epiphora had largely resolved, the patient endorsed improved comfort in the left eye, as well as 12 mm on repeat Schirmer. Postoperative salivary scan showed viable gland within the left temporal fossa, as shown in **Fig. 6**.

Although submandibular gland transplant is not an undertaking intended for every patient with dry eyes, in those failing multiple other treatment modalities and facing ongoing pain and loss of vision, microvascular transplant of the gland remains a viable option. This option should be considered to include those patients having disease entities such as graft-versus-host, which may involve salivary tissue as long as sufficient salivary function is retained. Careful preoperative assessment and discussion with the patient is critical regarding optimal outcome and realistic expectations. Ongoing experience will ultimately determine the value of this procedure.

REFERENCES

1. Evangelista L, Cervino AR, Chondrogiannis S, et al. Comparison between anatomical cross-sectional imaging and 18F-FDG PET/CT in the staging, restaging, treatment response, and long-term surveillance of squamous cell head and neck cancer: a systematic literature overview. Nucl Med Commun 2013;35(2): 123–34.

2. Curtin HD, Ishwaran H, Mancuso AA, et al. Comparison of CT and MR imaging in staging of neck metastases. Radiology 1998;207(1):123–30.

3. Gregoire V, Lefebvre JL, Licitra L, et al, EHNS–ESMO–ESTRO Guidelines Working Group. Squamous cell carcinoma of the head and neck: EHNS-ESMO-ESTRO Clinical Practice Guidelines for diagnosis, treatment and follow-up. Ann Oncol 2010;21(Suppl 5):v184–186.

4. Fleming AJ Jr, Smith SP Jr, Paul CM, et al. Impact of [18F]-2-fluorodeoxyglucose-positron emission tomography/computed tomography on previously untreated head and neck cancer patients. Laryngoscope 2007;117(7):1173–9.

5. de Bree R, Deurloo EE, Snow GB, et al. Screening for distant metastases in patients with head and neck cancer. Laryngoscope 2000;110(3 Pt 1):397–401.

6. Slaughter DP, Southwick HW, Smejkal W. Field cancerization in oral stratified squamous epithelium; clinical implications of multicentric origin. Cancer 1953;6(5):963–8.

7. Spector ME, Chinn SB, Rosko AJ, et al. Diagnostic modalities for distant metastasis in head and neck squamous cell carcinoma: are we changing life expectancy? Laryngoscope 2012;122(7):1507–11.

8. Zbaren P, Lehmann W. Frequency and sites of distant metastases in head and neck squamous cell carcinoma. An analysis of 101 cases at autopsy. Arch Otolaryngol Head Neck Surg 1987;113(7):762–4.

9. Madana J, Morand GB, Barona-Lleo L, et al. A survey on pulmonary screening practices among otolaryngology-head & neck surgeons across Canada in the post treatment surveillance of head and neck squamous cell carcinoma. J Otolaryngol Head Neck Surg 2015;44:5.

10. Digonnet A, Hamoir M, Andry G, et al. Post-therapeutic surveillance strategies in head and neck squamous cell carcinoma. Eur Arch Otorhinolaryngol 2013;270(5):1569–80.

11. Shah JP. Patterns of cervical lymph node metastasis from squamous carcinomas of the upper aerodigestive tract. Am J Surg 1990;160(4):405–9.

12. Warner GC, Cox GJ. Evaluation of chest radiography versus chest computed tomography in screening for pulmonary malignancy in advanced head and neck cancer. J Otolaryngol 2003;32(2):107–9.

13. Chong VF, Fan YF, Khoo JB. MRI features of cervical nodal necrosis in metastatic disease. Clin Radiol 1996;51(2):103–9.

14. King AD, Tse GM, Ahuja AT, et al. Necrosis in metastatic neck nodes: diagnostic accuracy of CT, MR imaging, and US. Radiology 2004;230(3):720–6.

15. Sumi M, Kimura Y, Sumi T, et al. Diagnostic performance of MRI relative to CT for metastatic nodes of head and neck squamous cell carcinomas. J Magn Reson Imaging 2007;26(6):1626–33.

16. Alberico RA, Husain SH, Sirotkin I. Imaging in head and neck oncology. Surg Oncol Clin N Am 2004;13(1):13–35.

17. Kato H, Kanematsu M, Watanabe H, et al. Metastatic retropharyngeal lymph nodes: comparison of CT and MR imaging for diagnostic accuracy. Eur J Radiol 2014;83(7):1157–62.

18. Eida S, Sumi M, Yonetsu K, et al. Combination of helical CT and Doppler sonography in the follow-up of patients with clinical N0 stage neck disease and oral cancer. AJNR Am J Neuroradiol 2003;24(3):312–8.

19. van den Brekel MW, Stel HV, Castelijns JA, et al. Cervical lymph node metastasis: assessment of radiologic criteria. Radiology 1990;177(2):379–84.

20. Rodrigues RS, Bozza FA, Christian PE, et al. Comparison of whole-body PET/CT, dedicated high-resolution head and neck PET/CT, and contrast-enhanced CT in preoperative staging of clinically M0 squamous cell carcinoma of the head and neck. J Nucl Med 2009;50(8):1205–13.

21. D'Cruz AK, Vaish R, Kapre N, et al. Elective versus therapeutic neck dissection in node-negative oral cancer. N Engl J Med 2015;373(6):521–9.

22. Miura K, Hirakawa H, Uemura H, et al. Sentinel node biopsy for oral cancer: a prospective multicenter phase II trial. Auris Nasus Larynx 2016;44(3):319–26.

23. Schilling C, Stoeckli SJ, Haerle SK, et al. Sentinel European Node Trial (SENT): 3-year results of sentinel node biopsy in oral cancer. Eur J Cancer 2015;51(18):2777–84.

24. Thompson CF, St John MA, Lawson G, et al. Diagnostic value of sentinel lymph node biopsy in head and neck cancer: a meta-analysis. Eur Arch Otorhinolaryngol 2013;270(7):2115–22.

25. Antonio JK, Santini S, Politi D, et al. Sentinel lymph node biopsy in squamous cell carcinoma of the head and neck: 10 years of experience. Acta Otorhinolaryngol Ital 2012;32(1):18–25.

26. Broglie MA, Haile SR, Stoeckli SJ. Long-term experience in sentinel node biopsy for early oral and oropharyngeal squamous cell carcinoma. Ann Surg Oncol 2011;18(10):2732–8.

27. Cooney TR, Poulsen MG. Is routine follow-up useful after combined-modality therapy for advanced head and neck cancer? Arch Otolaryngol Head Neck Surg 1999;125(4):379–82.

28. Virgo KS, Paniello RC, Johnson FE. Costs of posttreatment surveillance for patients with upper aerodigestive tract cancer. Arch Otolaryngol Head Neck Surg 1998;124(5):564–72.

29. Boysen M, Lovdal O, Tausjo J, et al. The value of follow-up in patients treated for squamous cell carcinoma of the head and neck. Eur J Cancer 1992;28(2–3):426–30.

30. de Visscher AV, Manni JJ. Routine long-term follow-up in patients treated with curative intent for squamous cell carcinoma of the larynx, pharynx, and oral cavity. Does it make sense? Arch Otolaryngol Head Neck Surg 1994;120(9):934–9.

31. Wensing BM, Merkx MA, Krabbe PF, et al. Oral squamous cell carcinoma and a clinically negative neck: the value of follow-up. Head Neck 2011;33(10):1400–5.

32. Isles MG, McConkey C, Mehanna HM. A systematic review and meta-analysis of the role of positron emission tomography in the follow up of head and neck squamous cell carcinoma following radiotherapy or chemoradiotherapy. Clin Otolaryngol 2008;33(3):210–22.

33. Porceddu SV, Jarmolowski E, Hicks RJ, et al. Utility of positron emission tomography for the detection of disease in residual neck nodes after (chemo) radiotherapy in head and neck cancer. Head Neck 2005;27(3):175–81.

34. Layland MK, Sessions DG, Lenox J. The influence of lymph node metastasis in the treatment of squamous cell carcinoma of the oral cavity, oropharynx, larynx, and hypopharynx: N0 versus N+. Laryngoscope 2005;115(4):629–39.

35. Werner JA, Dunne AA, Ramaswamy A, et al. The sentinel node concept in head and neck cancer: solution for the controversies in the N0 neck? Head Neck 2004;26(7):603–11.

36. Alex JC, Krag DN. The gamma-probe-guided resection of radiolabeled primary lymph nodes. Surg Oncol Clin N Am 1996;5(1):33–41.

37. Alkureishi LW, Ross GL, Shoaib T, et al. Sentinel node biopsy in head and neck squamous cell cancer: 5-year follow-up of a European multicenter trial. Ann Surg Oncol 2010;17(9):2459–64.

38. Rigual N, Douglas W, Lamonica D, et al. Sentinel lymph node biopsy: a rational approach for staging T2N0 oral cancer. Laryngoscope 2005;115(12):2217–20.

39. Ross GL, Soutar DS, MacDonald DG, et al. Improved staging of cervical metastases in clinically

node-negative patients with head and neck squamous cell carcinoma. Ann Surg Oncol 2004;11(2): 213–8.

40. Lindberg R. Distribution of cervical lymph node metastases from squamous cell carcinoma of the upper respiratory and digestive tracts. Cancer 1972;29(6): 1446–9.

41. Goerkem M, Braun J, Stoeckli SJ. Evaluation of clinical and histomorphological parameters as potential predictors of occult metastases in sentinel lymph nodes of early squamous cell carcinoma of the oral cavity. Ann Surg Oncol 2010;17(2):527–35.

42. Civantos FJ, Zitsch RP, Schuller DE, et al. Sentinel lymph node biopsy accurately stages the regional lymph nodes for T1-T2 oral squamous cell carcinomas: results of a prospective multi-institutional trial. J Clin Oncol 2010;28(8):1395–400.

43. Haerle SK, Hany TF, Strobel K, et al. Is there an additional value of SPECT/CT over planar lymphoscintigraphy for sentinel node mapping in oral/oropharyngeal squamous cell carcinoma? Ann Surg Oncol 2009; 16(11):3118–24.

44. Khafif A, Schneebaum S, Fliss DM, et al. Lymphoscintigraphy for sentinel node mapping using a hybrid single photon emission CT (SPECT)/CT system in oral cavity squamous cell carcinoma. Head Neck 2006;28(10):874–9.

45. Kontio R, Leivo I, Leppanen E, et al. Sentinel lymph node biopsy in oral cavity squamous cell carcinoma without clinically evident metastasis. Head Neck 2004;26(1):16–21.

46. Stoeckli SJ, Steinert H, Pfaltz M, et al. Sentinel lymph node evaluation in squamous cell carcinoma of the head and neck. Otolaryngol Head Neck Surg 2001;125(3):221–6.

47. Valsecchi ME, Silbermins D, de Rosa N, et al. Lymphatic mapping and sentinel lymph node biopsy in patients with melanoma: a meta-analysis. J Clin Oncol 2011;29(11):1479–87.

48. Morton DL, Thompson JF, Cochran AJ, et al. Final trial report of sentinel-node biopsy versus nodal observation in melanoma. N Engl J Med 2014; 370(7):599–609.

49. Pesek S, Ashikaga T, Krag LE, et al. The false-negative rate of sentinel node biopsy in patients with breast cancer: a meta-analysis. World J Surg 2012;36(9):2239–51.

50. Borbon-Arce M, Brouwer OR, van den Berg NS, et al. An innovative multimodality approach for sentinel node mapping and biopsy in head and neck malignancies. Rev Esp Med Nucl Imagen Mol 2014;33(5):274–9.

51. Kovacs AF, Stefenelli U, Seitz O, et al. Positive sentinel lymph nodes are a negative prognostic factor for survival in T1-2 oral/oropharyngeal cancer-a long-term study on 103 patients. Ann Surg Oncol 2009;16(2):233–9.

52. Brown JS, Shaw RJ, Bekiroglu F, et al. Systematic review of the current evidence in the use of postoperative radiotherapy for oral squamous cell carcinoma. Br J Oral Maxillofac Surg 2012;50(6):481–9.

53. Terada A, Hasegawa Y, Yatabe Y, et al. Follow-up after intraoperative sentinel node biopsy of N0 neck oral cancer patients. Eur Arch Otorhinolaryngol 2011;268(3):429–35.

54. Schiefke F, Akdemir M, Weber A, et al. Function, postoperative morbidity, and quality of life after cervical sentinel node biopsy and after selective neck dissection. Head Neck 2009;31(4):503–12.

55. Murer K, Huber GF, Haile SR, et al. Comparison of morbidity between sentinel node biopsy and elective neck dissection for treatment of the n0 neck in patients with oral squamous cell carcinoma. Head Neck 2011;33(9):1260–4.

56. Hernando J, Villarreal P, Alvarez-Marcos F, et al. Comparison of related complications: sentinel node biopsy versus elective neck dissection. Int J Oral Maxillofac Surg 2014;43(11):1307–12.

57. National Comprehensive Cancer Network. Head and neck cancers (version 2.2016). Available at: https://www.nccn.org/professionals/physician_gls/pdf/head-and-neck.pdf. Accessed January 1, 2017.

58. McFarland J. The mysterious mixed tumors of the salivary glands. Surg Gynecol Obstet 1943;76:23.

59. Zbären P, Stauffer E. Pleomorphic adenoma of the parotid gland: histopathologic analysis of the capsular characteristics of 218 tumors. Head Neck 2007;29(8):751–7.

60. Patey DH, Thackray A. The treatment of parotid tumours in the light of a pathological study of parotidectomy material. Br J Surg 1958;45(193):477–87.

61. Bailey H. Parotidectomy: indications and results. Br Med J 1947;1(4499):404.

62. McGurk M, Renehan A, Gleave E, et al. Clinical significance of the tumour capsule in the treatment of parotid pleomorphic adenomas. Br J Surg 1996; 83(12):1747–9.

63. Donovan DT, Conley JJ. Capsular significance in parotid tumor surgery: reality and myths of lateral lobectomy. Laryngoscope 1984;94(3):324–9.

64. Iro H, Zenk J, Koch M, et al. Follow-up of parotid pleomorphic adenomas treated by extracapsular dissection. Head Neck 2013;35(6):788–93.

65. Zhang S, Ma D, Guo C, et al. Conservation of salivary secretion and facial nerve function in partial superficial parotidectomy. Int J Oral Maxillofac Surg 2013;42(7):868–73.

66. Xie S, Wang K, Xu H, et al. PRISMA—extracapsular dissection versus superficial parotidectomy in treatment of benign parotid tumors: evidence from 3194 patients. Medicine 2015;94(34):e1237.

67. Albergotti WG, Nguyen SA, Zenk J, et al. Extracapsular dissection for benign parotid tumors: a meta-analysis. Laryngoscope 2012;122(9):1954–60.

68. Bennett JE, Bailey AL. A surgical approach to total xerophthalmia: transplantation of the parotid duct to the inferior cul-de-sac. AMA Arch Ophthalmol 1957;58(3):367–71.

69. Murube-del-Castillo J. Transplantation of salivary gland to the lacrimal basin. Scand J Rheumatol Suppl 1985;61:264–7.

70. Geerling G, Sieg P, Bastian G-O, et al. Transplantation of the autologous submandibular gland for most severe cases of keratoconjunctivitis sicca. Ophthalmology 1998;105(2):327–35.

71. Paniello RC. Submandibular gland transfer for severe xerophthalmia. Laryngoscope 2007;117(1): 40–4.

72. Qin J, Zhang L, Cai ZG, et al. Microvascular autologous transplantation of partial submandibular gland for severe keratoconjunctivitis sicca. Br J Ophthalmol 2013;97(9):1123–8.

73. Yu G-Y, Zhu Z-H, Mao C, et al. Microvascular autologous submandibular gland transfer in severe cases of keratoconjunctivitis sicca. Int J Oral Maxillofac Surg 2004;33(3):235–9.

74. Sieg P, Geerling G, Kosmehl H, et al. Microvascular submandibular gland transfer for severe cases of keratoconjunctivitis sicca. Plast Reconstr Surg 2000;106(3):554–60.

75. Jacobsen H-C, Hakim SG, Lauer I, et al. Long-term results of autologous submandibular gland transfer for the surgical treatment of severe keratoconjunctivitis sicca. J Craniomaxillofac Surg 2008; 36(4):227–33.

76. Geerling G, Sieg P. Transplantation of the major salivary glands. Dev Ophthalmol 2008;41:255–68. Karger Publishers.

77. Keegan DJ, Geerling G, Lee JP, et al. Botulinum toxin treatment for hyperlacrimation secondary to aberrant regenerated seventh nerve palsy or salivary gland transplantation. Br J Ophthalmol 2002; 86(1):43–6.

78. Imanguli MM, Atkinson JC, Mitchell SA, et al. Salivary gland involvement in chronic graft-versus-host disease: prevalence, clinical significance, and recommendations for evaluation. Biol Blood Marrow Transplant 2010;16(10):1362–9.

Controversies in Obstructive Sleep Apnea Surgery

Carolyn C. Dicus Brookes, DMD, MD[a],*,
Scott B. Boyd, DDS, PhD[b]

KEYWORDS

- Obstructive sleep apnea • Upper airway obstruction • Continuous positive airway pressure
- Polysomnography • Maxillomandibular advancement (MMA) • Surgical management/treatment

KEY POINTS

- Obstructive sleep apnea (OSA) is a common chronic disease characterized by repetitive pharyngeal collapse during sleep.
- Untreated OSA results in sleep fragmentation, which leads to excessive daytime somnolence. Untreated OSA is associated with decreased quality of life, increased risk of cardiovascular disease and all-cause mortality, and impaired cognitive function.
- Continuous positive airway pressure (CPAP) is first line therapy for OSA, but is not always tolerated. Alternative treatments are reviewed.
- Dynamic assessment of the airway in the OSA patient allows targeted intervention and plays a crucial role in surgical planning.
- Maxillomandibular advancement (MMA) is the most successful surgical intervention for OSA aside from tracheostomy; outcomes have been equated to those with CPAP.
- Multiple controversies and unresolved questions surrounding OSA remain and are explored in this article.

Obstructive sleep apnea (OSA) is a common chronic disease characterized by repetitive pharyngeal collapse during sleep. The estimated prevalence of OSA in middle-aged adults is between 20% and 25%,[1,2] and the overall prevalence of moderate to severe OSA is estimated to be 6.7% to 10.0%.[2,3]

Untreated OSA results in sleep fragmentation, which decreases time in deep sleep and leads to excessive daytime somnolence. Hypoxia and hypercarbia occur, and sympathetic activation increases.[4–6] Decreased vigilance, motor coordination, and executive functioning may result.[7] Depression[8] and decreased quality of life[9] may be seen. Untreated OSA has also been linked to hypertension,[1,10–12] arrhythmias,[10,12] congestive heart failure,[12] and increased risk of cardiovascular events,[13] as well as type 2 diabetes mellitus.[14,15] Stroke and all-cause mortality are associated with untreated OSA; risk seems to increase with OSA severity.[16] Because of the significant impact of untreated moderate to severe OSA, there is no question that treatment is indicated.

DIAGNOSIS

OSA is diagnosed based on polysomnography (PSG). This multimodal analysis reports several

The authors have no disclosures.
[a] Division of Oral and Maxillofacial Surgery, Froedtert & the Medical College of Wisconsin, CFAC 5th Floor, 9200 W Wisconsin Avenue, Milwaukee, WI 53226, USA; [b] Vanderbilt University School of Medicine, 1161 21st Avenue S, Nashville, TN 37232, USA
* Corresponding author.
E-mail address: cbrookes@mcw.edu

Oral Maxillofacial Surg Clin N Am 29 (2017) 503–513
http://dx.doi.org/10.1016/j.coms.2017.07.005

metrics, among which are the apnea hypopnea index (AHI), respiratory disturbance index (RDI), nadir oxygen saturation, and percentage of time spent with oxygen saturation below specified thresholds. Severity of OSA is based on the AHI or RDI (mild OSA: 5–15 events per hour, moderate OSA: >15–30 events per hour, severe OSA: >30 events per hour), although other metrics must be considered during patient assessment. Per the American Association of Sleep Medicine, streamlined, more convenient and cost-effective home studies may be used in patients with a high pretest probability of moderate to severe OSA without certain comorbidities.[17] Additional components of the diagnostic evaluation are discussed later in this article.

NONOPERATIVE TREATMENT OF OBSTRUCTIVE SLEEP APNEA

Continuous positive airway pressure (CPAP) is the first-line treatment for OSA; it works by splinting the upper airway open to improve patency during sleep. When used appropriately and regularly, CPAP is highly effective for most patients. CPAP virtually eliminates OSA[18] and improves quality of life and sleepiness.[5,19,20] Unfortunately, nonadherence rates (with adherence defined as CPAP use for 4 or more hours nightly) of 46% to 83% have been reported.[21] Multiple mask designs and alternative positive airway pressure (PAP) delivery modes (eg auto-PAP) are available, and should be explored to help improve adherence. Intranasal steroids and nasal surgery may also improve PAP tolerance. The surgical provider should help encourage PAP use if possible. Nonetheless, treatment alternatives are necessary for patients who refuse or cannot tolerate CPAP.

Oral appliances (OAs) improve the upper airway by modifying the position of the tongue and associated upper airway structures. Custom, titratable, tooth-borne appliances designed to advance the mandible are the preferred OA.[22] OAs reduce AHI and improve nadir SpO2, although to a lesser degree than CPAP.[22] They improve sleepiness, control of hypertension, and quality of life.[22] Adherence to OAs appears to be similar to or slightly higher than adherence to CPAP.[23] OAs tend to work better for nonobese patients with skeletofacial deformities,[24] and patients must have reasonable protrusive range of motion to derive benefit from OAs. Monitoring for dental and skeletal changes is requisite.[22,25]

Additional nonoperative management strategies include positional aids if AHI is worse in the supine position,[5] sleep hygiene (including avoidance of alcohol, caffeine, and screen time before bed),[5]

and weight loss. A 10% weight loss has been linked to a 26% reduction in AHI[26]; however, OSA can recur even in the absence of weight gain, so follow-up is crucial.[27] Bariatric surgery may be used to help facilitate weight loss, and has also been linked to a decrease in AHI.[28]

Sleepiness that is unresponsive to OSA therapy may be managed by modafinil as long as other causes of daytime somnolence have been ruled out.[5]

SURGICAL TREATMENT OF OBSTRUCTIVE SLEEP APNEA

Many surgical approaches to adult OSA have been described. The more common are briefly reviewed.

Tracheostomy bypasses the upper airway and is thus nearly universally successful in managing OSA. However, the significant morbidity associated with tracheostomy limits its application in the OSA population.[29]

Bariatric surgery, as mentioned previously, is a surgical option in patients with morbid obesity.

Tonsillectomy with adenoidectomy is the first-line surgical therapy for children with OSA without craniofacial anomalies.

Nasal surgery may play a role in OSA management by improving nasal airflow. Particularly for those with moderate to severe sleep apnea, isolated nasal surgery is unlikely to lead to resolution of OSA. However, it may increase CPAP use in some patients.[30]

Multiple palatal procedures have been described; the most common is uvulopalatopharyngoplasty (UPPP), which involves removal of the tonsils, uvula, and posterior velum. Multiple variations of UPPP have been described. One meta-analysis reported a mean reduction in AHI of 33% to a mean postoperative AHI of 29.8[31]; however, UPPP does not reliably result in AHI normalization and is thus not recommended by the American Academy of Sleep Medicine (AASM) as a sole procedure for treating moderate to severe OSA.[32] A recent meta-analysis evaluated predictors for successful UPPP and found that only Friedman stage I (large tonsils and relatively normal palatal position) predicted surgical success; Friedman stage III and low hyoid position were negative predictors.[33]

Myriad tongue base procedures, robotic or conventional, have been described and may involve partial glossectomy or various ablative techniques to volumetrically reduce the tongue. Reported surgical success varies from 20% to 83%.[34]

Genioglossal advancement (GA) involves advancement of the genial tubercles, and may be accompanied by hyoid suspension. In conjunction with other therapies addressing palatal obstruction (or for those with isolated collapse at the retrolingual level) these interventions may be helpful. Multilevel surgery may be performed concomitantly or in a staged fashion. The AASM acknowledges multilevel surgery as an acceptable option for patients with multisite obstruction, but notes that the quality of evidence is low.[32] Reported surgical success rates for GA with or without hyoid suspension in conjunction with palatal surgery vary widely from 22% to 78%[34]; success rates seem to drop in the long term (65.2% vs 78.3% in one series).[35] Many procedures may be involved in multilevel surgical treatment of OSA, and less invasive combination procedures such as nasal surgery, palatal stiffening (eg, with implants) and radiofrequency ablation of the tongue have been reported on with a short-term success rate of 47.5%. The success rate in this series was higher for those with a body mass index (BMI) less than 30 kg/m^2.[36] A recent meta-analysis of radiofrequency ablation (RFA) for OSA found that most data were on management of mild-moderate OSA. Multilevel RFA showed an overall 41% reduction in RDI.[37]

Hypoglossal nerve stimulators are a relatively new addition to the array of surgical options for treatment of OSA, and were approved by the Food and Drug Administration for treatment of moderate to severe OSA in 2014. Postoperative titration is required. A multicenter trial reported surgical success in 74% at 3 years, although not all recipients used the device nightly[38]; another study reported 55% surgical success at 1 year postimplantation.[39] The device seems to improve symptoms and quality of life.[38,39] Hypoglossal nerve stimulation seems to be more successful when AHI is less than 50 in patients with a lower BMI and an anteroposterior pattern of palatal collapse.[40,41]

Maxillomandibular advancement (MMA) is the most successful surgical intervention for OSA aside from tracheostomy. MMA has been equated to CPAP in terms of outcomes. This procedure involves advancement of both jaws and addresses airway obstruction at multiple levels; airway collapsibility decreases due to advancement of its skeletal framework.[42] Its high success rate is likely because most patients with moderate-severe OSA exhibit multilevel obstruction.[43,44] Because of its high success rate and increased utilization, many of the controversies addressed in the remainder of this article focus on questions surrounding MMA.

Additional controversies with broader applications that are explored include evaluation of the airway and definition of successful treatment.

WHAT IMAGING/AIRWAY ASSESSMENT MODALITIES SHOULD BE USED ALONE OR IN COMBINATION FOR DIAGNOSIS, TREATMENT PLANNING, AND OUTCOMES ASSESSMENT?

Assessing the level of upper airway obstruction is a critical component of evaluation and surgical treatment planning for the patient with OSA, and has classically been done using awake nasopharyngoscopy. Additional imaging has been used to characterize the airway, to guide treatment planning, and to help assess outcomes.

WHAT IS THE ROLE OF LATERAL CEPHALOGRAMS?

Lateral cephalometric radiographs are readily obtained with low radiation, and may be used for preoperative planning before MMA. Attempts have been made to use them to predict levels of obstruction and anticipated treatment response to non-CPAP OSA therapies. However, lateral cephalograms have several important limitations when used for airway assessment.

A 2-dimensional image is inherently suboptimal for evaluation of a 3-dimensional structure, and lateral cephalograms for airway assessment are no exception. Clinically significant airway narrowing can be missed on a 2-dimensional view, which only demonstrates narrowing in the sagittal plane. Interestingly, lateral pharyngeal wall collapse has been linked to more severe sleep apnea than retropalatal and retrolingual collapse as assessed with dynamic MRI, and this change would not be noted on a lateral cephalogram.[45,46]

Airway measurements change throughout the respiratory cycle, so any measurements should be taken at a standardized point in the cycle. Even with every effort made to expose an image at a consistent point, though, different films could easily be taken at slightly different phases in the cycle. This could skew results when comparing measurements. Differences in head position at the time of imaging can also influence measurements.[47,48] Many individuals with OSA assume a head-up posture; it is important to obtain radiographs in a neutral head position.

Additionally, because lateral cephalograms are typically taken with the patient upright and awake, they do not characterize the asleep (or even supine) airway. The concept of supine cephalograms has been explored, but they are technically more challenging to obtain, which negates one of the main advantages of this imaging modality. Further, supine cephalometry still may not represent sleeping anatomy: An awake patient likely stents the airway when supine, and this may be more pronounced in the patient with OSA.[49]

Overall literature on the utility of lateral cephalograms in predicting treatment response to OAs, UPPP, multilevel surgery, or MMA is conflicting, with some studies showing no predictive value of various parameters, whereas others have linked specific measurements to success rates after various interventions. A recent review describes these studies nicely.[50] The role of cephalometry may continue to evolve; currently lateral cephalometric radiographs serve as an adjunctive airway assessment tool but cannot supplant direct airway assessment with endoscopy.

WHAT DOES 3-DIMENSIONAL CONE-BEAM COMPUTED TOMOGRAPHY AIRWAY ASSESSMENT ADD?

Three-dimensional airway assessment using cone-beam computed tomography (CBCT) has been used, and the addition of the third dimension offers an advantage over traditional plain films. When a CBCT is obtained as part of treatment planning for MMA, any data gleaned from the CBCT is available at no additional cost or potential harm to the patient. Although CT also can be used (and has the advantage of better soft tissue imaging), the additional radiation is difficult to justify. MRI is another option, but is used less frequently. Visually striking airway depictions make this modality particularly appealing in publications and to patients.

Multiple 3-D studies describe volumetric airway changes after MMA. These include increases in airway volume, minimal cross-sectional area, and both anteroposterior and lateral dimensions. Decreased airway length also has been shown,[51–54] as has anterosuperior movement of the hyoid.[55] Computational fluid dynamics can be used to assess theoretical airway flow and resistance, and this has been proposed as a method to predict surgical outcomes.[56–58] Increased airway volume after MMA has been linked to decrease in RDI and AHI,[51,55] although the magnitude of movement and changes in AHI are unlikely to fully correlate even with additional data because the dynamic nature of the airway is simply not accounted for when using this modality.

Despite increased data available on 3-D airway morphology before and after MMA and with use of OAs, there are limitations. As with lateral cephalometry, studies have reported data obtained in both the upright and supine positions. Measurements are similarly based on static images of the dynamic airway in awake patients, and respiratory phase and patient position may influence them.

Different anatomic boundaries may be used to define the airway; the impact of this is likely minimal, but still poses a challenge when comparing studies. The optimal interval from surgery to reassessment has not been defined, and the impact of time on results remains to be characterized. Perhaps most importantly, little is known about which parameters predict success with certain treatment modalities.

The primary roles of both lateral cephalograms and CBCTs remain characterization of baseline skeletal morphology and of postoperative skeletal changes. Three-dimensional airway analysis is likely to continue to be used primarily because it can be obtained from imaging taken for preoperative planning. It may contribute to our understanding of the airway in OSA and of the gross airway changes that result from various treatments, but it remains limited by its static nature, the challenges associated with precisely timing the image with respiratory cycle, and its exposure during the awake state.

WHAT ROLE DOES DYNAMIC UPPER AIRWAY IMAGING PLAY?

Dynamically assessing the level of upper airway obstruction in the patients with OSA allows targeted intervention and plays a crucial role in selecting a surgical procedure by allowing a description of the site, degree, and pattern of obstruction. It is also critical to rule out pathologic sources of obstruction, such as an obstructive tumor.

Awake nasopharyngoscopy with the Müller maneuver, or inspiration against closed nasal and oral airways, is used to assess level and degree of airway obstruction. Obstruction is scored by the observer but can be recorded for later review. Obstruction of more than 75% is typically considered severe and suggests the need for surgical correction at that site. The most significant limitation to this technique is that it is performed while the patient is awake.

Dynamic sleep MRI[45,59] and drug-induced sleep CT[44] have been used to characterize the airway in OSA. Advantages include the dynamic nature, the ability to evaluate the airway in a multiplane fashion, and the fact that these are obtained in the sleeping state or a simulated sleep state. One study explored airway differences between BMI-matched subjects with mild and severe OSA using sleep MRI; all subjects had retropalatal collapse, and all subjects with severe OSA had lateral pharyngeal wall collapse (vs <7% of those with mild OSA).[59] Lateral pharyngeal wall collapse as assessed by drug-induced sleep endoscopy has previously been correlated with hypoxemia in

OSA.[60] This is one example of the type of information that may be derived from studies using these modalities. Although currently used in the research setting, these approaches may help further our understanding of levels of obstruction and impact of various treatments.

Drug-induced sleep endoscopy (DISE) has been introduced as an alternative to conventional endoscopy with the goal of more accurately representing patterns of collapse during the sleeping state. The introduction of DISE brings us closer to understanding the dynamic airway during sleep, but still has some shortcomings. The optimal anesthetic agent for DISE that most closely emulates the sleeping state has not been established,[61] and the results of DISE seem to vary based on agent used; for instance, propofol seems to lead to more airway obstruction and oxygen desaturations than does dexmedetomidine.[62] It seems that awake endoscopy and DISE detect retropalatal collapse equally well, but DISE may identify retrolingual collapse more often.[63] A systematic review reported that performing DISE after awake endoscopy changed the surgical plan in slightly more than 50% of cases, typically due to detection of additional hypopharyngeal or laryngeal obstruction. It is unclear, though, whether DISE improves surgical outcomes, and there is concern that DISE may lead to unnecessary surgical interventions.[61] More and more data are emerging about patterns of collapse on DISE that predict success with various surgical interventions and on DISE findings in treatment failures.

Accomplishing 3-D airway assessment while accurately reproducing the sleeping state has the potential to impact sleep apnea surgery significantly.

WHAT MEDICAL CONDITIONS PRECLUDE TREATMENT WITH MAXILLOMANDIBULAR ADVANCEMENT?

No definitive guidelines outline medical conditions that preclude MMA. As with any surgical procedure, the perioperative risk to the patient must be weighed against potential benefits, including risk reduction for sequelae of untreated OSA and improvement in quality of life. When in doubt, collaboration with the patient's medical team is paramount to guide decision making and, for the MMA candidate, to medically optimize the patient preoperatively.

First a decision must be made about whether the patient has sufficient reserve to tolerate a major procedure. Second, consideration must be given to medical comorbidities that could impact MMA in particular. For instance, severe osteoporosis could impact stability. Conditions with compromised wound healing, such as chronic immunosuppression or poorly controlled diabetes should be taken into account. Diabetes-associated microvascular and macrovascular disease could compromise blood supply, leading to loss of teeth, gingiva, or bone. Significant peripheral vascular disease, vasoactive drug use (eg, cocaine), or ongoing tobacco use can cause similar issues. Delay procedures could be considered in select cases to mitigate this risk. Conditions or medications that increase bleeding risk also merit consideration and, if surgery is pursued, require involvement of the appropriate specialists to guide management.

Uncontrolled hypertension should be optimized preoperatively. Baseline hypertension limits the safety of deliberate intraoperative hypotension, and can thus contribute to increased blood loss. This should be discussed with the patient and the anesthesia care team before surgery.

Uncontrolled or severe psychiatric disease may impact the patient's ability to adhere to postoperative guidelines and to integrate a new facial appearance. Preoperative discussion with the managing psychiatrist is crucial to ensure that management of psychiatric conditions is optimized and social support systems are in place. Careful consideration must be given to the use of steroids in this population.

There is no universally accepted age cutoff for candidacy for MMA, and general physical condition is more important than chronologic age. Age-related changes in sleep architecture should be incorporated into PSG interpretation. An additional consideration is that an older patient will likely enjoy the benefits of treatment for a shorter period, which may impact the risk-to-benefit ratio. For some patients, alternative treatments must be explored to minimize surgical risk.

SHOULD MAXILLOMANDIBULAR ADVANCEMENT CANDIDATES BE OFFERED OTHER SURGICAL OPTIONS FIRST?

Initially a staged approach was recommended for surgical management of OSA. Phase I procedures included UPPP with or without adjunctive procedures, such as GA with or without hyoid myotomy, and phase II surgery involved MMA.[64] In theory this approach minimized morbidity while maximizing opportunity for successful outcomes. However, a recent comparative study confirmed that MMA alone is more effective than UPPP alone and reported that a traditional staged approach is no more effective than MMA alone.[65] Though UPPP is less morbid, its unpredictable success rate for those with moderate to severe OSA may make

MMA as a primary treatment quite reasonable provided a patient can tolerate the larger procedure. Potential benefits of this approach over staged surgery for those who fail the latter include decreased total treatment time and earlier effective management of disease, a more favorable cost-to-benefit ratio, and reduced anesthetic and surgical risks.

Severe lateral pharyngeal collapse and laryngeal collapse on DISE have been linked to treatment failures in patients who received targeted interventions with multilevel surgery (most often palato-pharyngoplasty and a base of tongue procedure); this cohort did not include patients who underwent MMA.[63] MMA, in contrast, has been shown to improve lateral pharyngeal wall collapsibility on DISE, and this change was correlated with surgical success.[46] Particularly for those with lateral pharyngeal collapse, strong consideration should be given to MMA as first-line therapy.

WHAT ARE THE INDICATIONS FOR ORTHODONTICS BEFORE MAXILLOMANDIBULAR ADVANCEMENT?

An absolute indication for preoperative orthodontics is patient desire to address a preexisting malocclusion in the absence of severe disease necessitating more urgent therapy. When a malocclusion is present that is not bothersome to the patient or when orthodontic therapy is not financially feasible, a discussion of potential benefits of definitive treatment of the malocclusion must take place. For instance, if a patient has a class II malocclusion or maxillary transverse hypoplasia, the patient should understand that orthodontic decompensation will allow further advancement of the mandible or widening of the maxilla, both of which may improve results. With baseline poor intercuspation, orthodontic treatment to improve dental relationships may enhance stability. However, it must be borne in mind that the goal of MMA is to treat a serious medical condition and to drop the associated risks; because of this, MMA without orthodontics may be pursued even if this yields a less optimal occlusal result.

The delay in MMA caused by orthodontic decompensation also must be considered, and patients should be strongly encouraged to adhere to nonsurgical treatment modalities and to strive for weight loss (if indicated) while awaiting skeletal sleep surgery. In some cases, early surgery (either before orthodontics entirely or before complete decompensation) may be performed, although this involves some guesswork on the final optimal jaw position.

When correction of a significant transverse deficiency is planned, surgically assisted rapid maxillary expansion (and/or surgical mandibular expansion) should be considered. A recent systematic review reported that maxillary expansion with or without mandibular expansion decreases AHI and improves nadir oxygen saturation.[66] The location of the transverse deficiency and stability will factor into selection of a surgical maxillary expansion versus a multipiece osteotomy.

IS THERE A ROLE FOR PREOPERATIVE SPEECH/SWALLOW ASSESSMENT BEFORE MAXILLOMANDIBULAR ADVANCEMENT?

No guidelines exist regarding preoperative speech assessment before MMA. Although regurgitation and hypernasal speech appear to be rare after MMA, improved ability to predict which patients might develop postoperative velopharyngeal insufficiency or swallowing dysfunction would be quite valuable. One systematic review noted that velopharyngeal insufficiency was reported only in patients who had undergone UPPP before MMA.[67] Patients with a history of palatal surgery should be counseled about the risk of velopharyngeal dysfunction. Consideration also could be given to preoperative speech/swallow assessment for those at high risk of postoperative dysfunction, such as individuals who have undergone previous palatal surgery.

WHAT IS THE IDEAL MAGNITUDE OF ADVANCEMENT IN MAXILLOMANDIBULAR ADVANCEMENT?

Scant data are available about the magnitude of advancement in MMA required to maximally benefit the patient with OSA. One frequently cited study suggests that mandibular advancement should be at least 10 mm.[68] However, a subsequent systematic review reported no association between degree of mandibular advancement and surgical success; data were analyzed at the study level and the patient level.[67] Study-level as well as univariate and multivariate patient-level analyses showed a higher surgical success rate with larger maxillary advancement (mean 9.9 vs 8.4 mm). The odds ratio for surgical success was 1.97 per 1 mm maxillary advancement based on multivariate analysis.[67] A recent small cohort study (n = 43 subjects) underwent smaller advancements (mean 5.2 mm in maxilla and 8.3 mm in mandible) with reported surgical success rate of 100% and surgical cure rate of 50% in the subset of patients with AHI data (n = 12).[69] These data suggest that the amount of advancement required to achieve surgical success remains poorly understood. Dynamic airway assessment may help improve our understanding of the optimal magnitude of advancement, and will ideally allow us to tailor this to each patient's needs.

WHAT ROLE DO ESTHETICS PLAY IN TREATMENT PLANNING FOR MAXILLOMANDIBULAR ADVANCEMENT? WHAT ARE SOME ALTERNATIVES TO CONVENTIONAL MAXILLOMANDIBULAR ADVANCEMENT?

Given the lack of literature supporting a specific magnitude of advancement, it seems prudent to factor in patient esthetics when planning the degree of advancement. This is particularly true in situations in which the patient is likely to develop an abnormal appearance after 1 cm of advancement and has less severe disease. Modifications to a straightforward maxillomandibular advancement also have been described and these or other variations can be applied to individual patients. Direct comparisons of outcomes with these different techniques are lacking.

Counterclockwise rotation of the maxillomandibular complex has been touted as a method to maximize mandibular advancement while minimizing the cosmetic impact of the surgery in the nasomaxillary region,[70] and may be appropriate for select patients. A recent meta-analysis demonstrated that both traditional and counterclockwise rotation result in a significant AHI reduction, but reported that there are insufficient data to determine superiority of either operation.[71]

A recently published alternative aimed at improving esthetic outcomes in the Asian face describes bimaxillary osteotomies coupled with anterior segmental maxillary setback; the result is advancement of the posterior maxilla with minimal effect on incisor position.[72]

Addition of a genioplasty can be esthetically beneficial, and should be offered if indicated. The potential airway benefits of genial tubercle advancement are discussed in the next section.

In the absence of strong literature support for one technique over another, careful discussion of the patient's goals and a detailed esthetic assessment should factor into decisions about the magnitude and direction of maxillomandibular movement as well as any additional modifications.

IS CONCOMITANT GENIAL TUBERCLE ADVANCEMENT OR NASAL SURGERY INDICATED DURING MAXILLOMANDIBULAR ADVANCEMENT?

In theory, genial tubercle advancement (either independently or as part of a genioplasty) may yield greater overall airway improvement. At present, though, there are few data to support the benefit of a genioplasty or genial tubercle advancement along with MMA on sleep parameters; this may be due to limited case numbers or a relatively small contribution of the genioplasty to AHI reduction. One review included 72 subjects who had undergone MMA with genioplasty as clinically indicated; there was no difference in AHI reduction or improvement in nadir oxygen saturation between those who had a genioplasty and those who did not.[65] A recent meta-analysis also showed that genial tubercle advancement in addition to MMA did not impact PSG outcomes.[73]

Concomitant nasal surgery may be considered to improve nasal airflow during MMA in select patients, although case selection is currently guided only by clinical judgment.

IS BONE GRAFTING DURING MAXILLOMANDIBULAR ADVANCEMENT BENEFICIAL?

Although some surgeons routinely graft during MMA, many do not. Good stability has been demonstrated with and without bone grafting.[68,74,75] If there are large lateral wall defects, autogenous or allogeneic grafts may be helpful. Grafting also may be helpful when treating the patient with an edentulous maxilla. Stepped osteotomies are advocated by some to ensure plates at the zygomaticomaxillary buttress are in thick bone while protecting the nasolacrimal apparatus medially.

HOW DO WE DEFINE TREATMENT SUCCESS?

Surgical success is classically defined as a 50% or greater reduction in AHI to less than 20 events per hour.[76] Surgical cure is defined as a reduction in AHI to less than 5 events per hour. Nadir oxygen saturation and percentage of time spent at a saturation below a threshold are among other metrics that merit consideration when evaluating polysomnographic changes. No consensus exists regarding optimal timing of the postsurgical PSG, although they are often obtained 3 to 6 months postoperatively to allow full surgical recovery and normalization of sleep patterns. Because OSA is a chronic, life-long disease, a long-term, durable treatment response is critical, and more information is needed about long-term outcomes.

The recently introduced effective AHI considers the time during which therapy is not used.[77] This is important when comparing interventions. For instance, MMA and CPAP result in similar AHI reductions.[78] However, CPAP and hypoglossal nerve stimulators may not be used for the entire sleep period, whereas MMA yields reduction in AHI during every hour of sleep. Taking this into account is crucial for outcome comparison.

Resolution of sleepiness, improvement in quality of life, and positive changes in cardiovascular health are also critical outcomes, and their incorporation into sleep medicine practices has been recommended by the AASM.[79] Sleepiness is most often assessed subjectively with the Epworth Sleepiness Scale.[5,80,81] Multiple quality-of-life questionnaires are also available; the Functional Outcomes of Sleep Questionnaire is an easily self-administered 30-question disease-specific quality-of-life assessment. It assesses several domains, including activity level, vigilance, intimacy/sexual relations, general productivity, and social outcomes.[82] Blood pressure and BMI are also important to follow, and are easily obtained.

WHAT ARE THE PREDICTORS OF SUCCESS OR FAILURE OF MAXILLOMANDIBULAR ADVANCEMENT IN TREATMENT OF OBSTRUCTIVE SLEEP APNEA?

One systematic review and meta-analysis of post-MMA outcomes concluded that, in addition to a larger maxillary advancement, a lower preoperative BMI was linked to an increased likelihood of surgical success.[67] Another meta-analysis of 45 studies including more than 500 subjects found that younger age and less severe preoperative OSA (as indicated by lower AHI and higher nadir SpO2) were associated with surgical cure. However, those with more severe preoperative OSA had a larger improvement in nadir SpO2 and a greater reduction in AHI than did those with a lower baseline AHI.[73] Although the surgical success and cure rates of MMA are quite high, we have much to learn about reasons for treatment failure.

SUMMARY

Although much is known about OSA, unanswered questions remain. Our understanding of the optimal airway evaluation in surgical candidates should continue to grow, as will our knowledge about predictors of successful treatment through various modalities. The inclusion of multiple outcome metrics in future case series in a more standardized fashion will also deepen our understanding of the impact of surgical treatment on individuals with significant OSA, particularly as reports on long term outcomes increase. Additionally, as reports emerge with larger sample sizes, we will develop a deeper appreciation for the impact of nuances in treatment planning on outcomes after MMA.

Multidisciplinary teams will lay the foundation for exploration of the unanswered questions in this field, and will facilitate delivery of the highest level of care to the CPAP-intolerant OSA population.

REFERENCES

1. Duran J, Esnaola S, Rubio R, et al. Obstructive sleep apnea-hypopnea and related clinical features in a population-based sample of subjects aged 30 to 70 yr. Am J Respir Crit Care Med 2001;163:685.
2. Peppard PE, Young T, Barnet JH, et al. Increased prevalence of sleep-disordered breathing in adults. Am J Epidemiol 2013;177:1006.
3. Young T, Peppard PE, Gottlieb DJ. Epidemiology of obstructive sleep apnea: a population health perspective. Am J Respir Crit Care Med 2002; 165:1217.
4. Eckert DJ, Malhotra A. Pathophysiology of adult obstructive sleep apnea. Proc Am Thorac Soc 2008;5:144.
5. Epstein LJ, Kristo D, Strollo PJ Jr, et al. Clinical guideline for the evaluation, management and long-term care of obstructive sleep apnea in adults. J Clin Sleep Med 2009;5:263.
6. Somers VK, White DP, Amin R, et al. Sleep apnea and cardiovascular disease: an American Heart Association/American College of Cardiology Foundation Scientific Statement from the American Heart Association Council for High Blood Pressure Research Professional Education Committee, Council on Clinical Cardiology, Stroke Council, and Council On Cardiovascular Nursing. In collaboration with the National Heart, Lung, and Blood Institute National Center on Sleep Disorders Research (National Institutes of Health). Circulation 2008;118:1080.
7. Beebe DW, Groesz L, Wells C, et al. The neuropsychological effects of obstructive sleep apnea: a meta-analysis of norm-referenced and case-controlled data. Sleep 2003;26:298.
8. BaHammam AS, Kendzerska T, Gupta R, et al. Comorbid depression in obstructive sleep apnea: an under-recognized association. Sleep Breath 2016;20:447.
9. Reimer MA, Flemons WW. Quality of life in sleep disorders. Sleep Med Rev 2003;7:335.
10. Golbin JM, Somers VK, Caples SM. Obstructive sleep apnea, cardiovascular disease, and pulmonary hypertension. Proc Am Thorac Soc 2008;5:200.
11. Peppard PE, Young T, Palta M, et al. Prospective study of the association between sleep-disordered breathing and hypertension. N Engl J Med 2000; 342:1378.
12. Phillips B. Sleep-disordered breathing and cardiovascular disease. Sleep Med Rev 2005;9:131.
13. Marin JM, Carrizo SJ, Vicente E, et al. Long-term cardiovascular outcomes in men with obstructive

sleep apnoea-hypopnoea with or without treatment with continuous positive airway pressure: an observational study. Lancet 2005;365:1046.

14. Vgontzas AN, Bixler EO, Chrousos GP. Sleep apnea is a manifestation of the metabolic syndrome. Sleep Med Rev 2005;9:211.

15. Wang X, Bi Y, Zhang Q, et al. Obstructive sleep apnoea and the risk of type 2 diabetes: a meta-analysis of prospective cohort studies. Respirology 2013;18:140.

16. Yaggi HK, Concato J, Kernan WN, et al. Obstructive sleep apnea as a risk factor for stroke and death. N Engl J Med 2005;353:2034–41.

17. Collop NA, Anderson WM, Boehlecke B, et al. Clinical guidelines for the use of unattended portable monitors in the diagnosis of obstructive sleep apnea in adult patients. Portable Monitoring Task Force of the American Academy of Sleep Medicine. J Clin Sleep Med 2007;3:737.

18. Giles TL, Lasserson TJ, Smith BH, et al. Continuous positive airways pressure for obstructive sleep apnoea in adults. Cochrane Database Syst Rev 2006;(3):CD001106.

19. Antic NA, Catcheside P, Buchan C, et al. The effect of CPAP in normalizing daytime sleepiness, quality of life, and neurocognitive function in patients with moderate to severe OSA. Sleep 2011;34:111.

20. Gordon P, Sanders MH. Sleep. 7: positive airway pressure therapy for obstructive sleep apnoea/hypopnoea syndrome. Thorax 2005;60:68.

21. Weaver TE, Grunstein RR. Adherence to continuous positive airway pressure therapy: the challenge to effective treatment. Proc Am Thorac Soc 2008;5:173.

22. Ramar K, Dort LC, Katz SG, et al. Clinical practice guideline for the treatment of obstructive sleep apnea and snoring with oral appliance therapy: an update for 2015. J Clin Sleep Med 2015;11:773.

23. Li W, Xiao L, Hu J. The comparison of CPAP and oral appliances in treatment of patients with OSA: a systematic review and meta-analysis. Respir Care 2013;58:1184.

24. Sutherland K, Vanderveken OM, Tsuda H, et al. Oral appliance treatment for obstructive sleep apnea: an update. J Clin Sleep Med 2014;10:215.

25. Goldberg R. Treatment of obstructive sleep apnea, other than with continuous positive airway pressure. Curr Opin Pulm Med 2000;6:496.

26. Peppard PE, Young T, Palta M, et al. Longitudinal study of moderate weight change and sleep-disordered breathing. JAMA 2000;284:3015.

27. Pillar G, Peled R, Lavie P. Recurrence of sleep apnea without concomitant weight increase 7.5 years after weight reduction surgery. Chest 1994;106:1702.

28. Ashrafian H, Toma T, Rowland SP, et al. Bariatric surgery or non-surgical weight loss for obstructive sleep apnoea? A systematic review and comparison of meta-analyses. Obes Surg 2015;25:1239.

29. Camacho M, Certal V, Brietzke SE, et al. Tracheostomy as treatment for adult obstructive sleep apnea: a systematic review and meta-analysis. Laryngoscope 2014;124:803.

30. Camacho M, Riaz M, Capasso R, et al. The effect of nasal surgery on continuous positive airway pressure device use and therapeutic treatment pressures: a systematic review and meta-analysis. Sleep 2015;38:279.

31. Caples SM, Rowley JA, Prinsell JR, et al. Surgical modifications of the upper airway for obstructive sleep apnea in adults: a systematic review and meta-analysis. Sleep 2010;33:1396.

32. Aurora RN, Casey KR, Kristo D, et al. Practice parameters for the surgical modifications of the upper airway for obstructive sleep apnea in adults. Sleep 2010;33:1408.

33. Choi JH, Cho SH, Kim SN, et al. Predicting outcomes after uvulopalatopharyngoplasty for adult obstructive sleep apnea: a meta-analysis. Otolaryngol Head Neck Surg 2016;155:904–13.

34. Kezirian EJ, Goldberg AN. Hypopharyngeal surgery in obstructive sleep apnea: an evidence-based medicine review. Arch Otolaryngol Head Neck Surg 2006;132:206.

35. Neruntarat C. Genioglossus advancement and hyoid myotomy: short-term and long-term results. J Laryngol Otol 2003;117:482.

36. Friedman M, Lin HC, Gurpinar B, et al. Minimally invasive single-stage multilevel treatment for obstructive sleep apnea/hypopnea syndrome. Laryngoscope 1859;117:2007.

37. Baba RY, Mohan A, Metta VV, et al. Temperature controlled radiofrequency ablation at different sites for treatment of obstructive sleep apnea syndrome: a systematic review and meta-analysis. Sleep Breath 2015;19:891.

38. Woodson BT, Soose RJ, Gillespie MB, et al. Three-year outcomes of cranial nerve stimulation for obstructive sleep apnea: the STAR trial. Otolaryngol Head Neck Surg 2016;154:181.

39. Kezirian EJ, Goding GS Jr, Malhotra A, et al. Hypoglossal nerve stimulation improves obstructive sleep apnea: 12-month outcomes. J Sleep Res 2014;23:77.

40. Van de Heyning PH, Badr MS, Baskin JZ, et al. Implanted upper airway stimulation device for obstructive sleep apnea. Laryngoscope 2012;122:1626.

41. Vanderveken OM, Maurer JT, Hohenhorst W, et al. Evaluation of drug-induced sleep endoscopy as a patient selection tool for implanted upper airway stimulation for obstructive sleep apnea. J Clin Sleep Med 2013;9:433.

42. Waite PD, Shettar SM. Maxillomandibular advancement surgery: a cure for sleep apnea syndrome. Oral Maxillofacial Surg Clin N Am 1995;7:327.

43. Kezirian EJ. Nonresponders to pharyngeal surgery for obstructive sleep apnea: insights from

drug-induced sleep endoscopy. Laryngoscope 2011;121:1320.

44. Li HY, Lo YL, Wang CJ, et al. Dynamic drug-induced sleep computed tomography in adults with obstructive sleep apnea. Sci Rep 2016;6:35849.

45. Liu SY, Huon LK, Lo MT, et al. Static craniofacial measurements and dynamic airway collapse patterns associated with severe obstructive sleep apnoea: a sleep MRI study. Clin Otolaryngol 2016; 41:700.

46. Liu SY, Huon LK, Powell NB, et al. Lateral pharyngeal wall tension after maxillomandibular advancement for obstructive sleep apnea is a marker for surgical success: observations from drug-induced sleep endoscopy. J Oral Maxillofac Surg 2015;73:1575.

47. Muto T, Takeda S, Kanazawa M, et al. The effect of head posture on the pharyngeal airway space (PAS). Int J Oral Maxillofac Surg 2002;31:579.

48. Hellsing E. Changes in the pharyngeal airway in relation to extension of the head. Eur J Orthod 1989;11:359.

49. Martin SE, Marshall I, Douglas NJ. The effect of posture on airway caliber with the sleep-apnea/hypopnea syndrome. Am J Respir Crit Care Med 1995;152:721.

50. Denolf PL, Vanderveken OM, Marklund ME, et al. The status of cephalometry in the prediction of non-CPAP treatment outcome in obstructive sleep apnea patients. Sleep Med Rev 2016;27:56.

51. Abramson Z, Susarla SM, Lawler M, et al. Three-dimensional computed tomographic airway analysis of patients with obstructive sleep apnea treated by maxillomandibular advancement. J Oral Maxillofac Surg 2011;69:677.

52. Butterfield KJ, Marks PL, McLean L, et al. Linear and volumetric airway changes after maxillomandibular advancement for obstructive sleep apnea. J Oral Maxillofac Surg 2015;73:1133.

53. Fairburn SC, Waite PD, Vilos G, et al. Three-dimensional changes in upper airways of patients with obstructive sleep apnea following maxillomandibular advancement. J Oral Maxillofac Surg 2007;65:6.

54. Rosario HD, Oliveira GM, Freires IA, et al. Efficiency of bimaxillary advancement surgery in increasing the volume of the upper airways: a systematic review of observational studies and meta-analysis. Eur Arch Otorhinolaryngol 2016;274:587–8.

55. Hsieh YJ, Liao YF, Chen NH, et al. Changes in the calibre of the upper airway and the surrounding structures after maxillomandibular advancement for obstructive sleep apnoea. Br J Oral Maxillofac Surg 2014;52:445.

56. Sittitavornwong S, Waite PD, Shih AM, et al. Computational fluid dynamic analysis of the posterior airway space after maxillomandibular advancement for obstructive sleep apnea syndrome. J Oral Maxillofac Surg 2013;71:1397.

57. Yu CC, Hsiao HD, Lee LC, et al. Computational fluid dynamic study on obstructive sleep apnea syndrome treated with maxillomandibular advancement. J Craniofac Surg 2009;20:426.

58. Yu CC, Hsiao HD, Tseng TI, et al. Computational fluid dynamics study of the inspiratory upper airway and clinical severity of obstructive sleep apnea. J Craniofac Surg 2012;23:401.

59. Huon LK, Liu SY, Shih TT, et al. Dynamic upper airway collapse observed from sleep MRI: BMI-matched severe and mild OSA patients. Eur Arch Otorhinolaryngol 2016;273:4021.

60. Lan MC, Liu SY, Lan MY, et al. Lateral pharyngeal wall collapse associated with hypoxemia in obstructive sleep apnea. Laryngoscope 2015;125:2408.

61. Certal VF, Pratas R, Guimaraes L, et al. Awake examination versus DISE for surgical decision making in patients with OSA: A systematic review. Laryngoscope 2016;126:768.

62. Chang ET, Certal V, Song SA, et al. Dexmedetomidine versus propofol during drug-induced sleep endoscopy and sedation: a systematic review. Sleep Breath 2017. [Epub ahead of print].

63. Soares D, Folbe AJ, Yoo G, et al. Drug-induced sleep endoscopy vs awake Muller's maneuver in the diagnosis of severe upper airway obstruction. Otolaryngol Head Neck Surg 2013;148:151.

64. Riley RW, Powell NB, Guilleminault C. Obstructive sleep apnea syndrome: a surgical protocol for dynamic upper airway reconstruction. J Oral Maxillofac Surg 1993;51:742.

65. Boyd SB, Walters AS, Song Y, et al. Comparative effectiveness of maxillomandibular advancement and uvulopalatopharyngoplasty for the treatment of moderate to severe obstructive sleep apnea. J Oral Maxillofac Surg 2013;71:743.

66. Abdullatif J, Certal V, Zaghi S, et al. Maxillary expansion and maxillomandibular expansion for adult OSA: a systematic review and meta-analysis. J Craniomaxillofac Surg 2016;44:574.

67. Holty JE, Guilleminault C. Maxillomandibular advancement for the treatment of obstructive sleep apnea: a systematic review and meta-analysis. Sleep Med Rev 2010;14:287.

68. Riley RW, Powell NB, Li KK, et al. Surgery and obstructive sleep apnea: long-term clinical outcomes. Otolaryngol Head Neck Surg 2000;122:415.

69. Ubaldo ED, Greenlee GM, Moore J, et al. Cephalometric analysis and long-term outcomes of orthognathic surgical treatment for obstructive sleep apnoea. Int J Oral Maxillofac Surg 2015;44:752.

70. Brevi BC, Toma L, Pau M, et al. Counterclockwise rotation of the occlusal plane in the treatment of obstructive sleep apnea syndrome. J Oral Maxillofac Surg 2011;69:917.

71. Knudsen TB, Laulund AS, Ingerslev J, et al. Improved apnea-hypopnea index and lowest

oxygen saturation after maxillomandibular advancement with or without counterclockwise rotation in patients with obstructive sleep apnea: a meta-analysis. J Oral Maxillofac Surg 2015;73:719.

72. Liao YF, Chiu YT, Lin CH, et al. Modified maxillomandibular advancement for obstructive sleep apnoea: towards a better outcome for Asians. Int J Oral Maxillofac Surg 2015;44:189.

73. Zaghi S, Holty JE, Certal V, et al. Maxillomandibular advancement for treatment of obstructive sleep apnea: a meta-analysis. JAMA Otolaryngol Head Neck Surg 2016;142:58.

74. Lee SH, Kaban LB, Lahey ET. Skeletal stability of patients undergoing maxillomandibular advancement for treatment of obstructive sleep apnea. J Oral Maxillofac Surg 2015;73:694.

75. Louis PJ, Waite PD, Austin RB. Long-term skeletal stability after rigid fixation of Le Fort I osteotomies with advancements. Int J Oral Maxillofac Surg 1993;22:82.

76. Sher AE, Schechtman KB, Piccirillo JF. The efficacy of surgical modifications of the upper airway in adults with obstructive sleep apnea syndrome. Sleep 1996;19:156.

77. Boyd SB, Upender R, Walters AS, et al. Effective Apnea-Hypopnea Index ("Effective AHI"): a new measure of effectiveness for positive airway pressure therapy. Sleep 1961;39:2016.

78. Vicini C, Dallan I, Campanini A, et al. Surgery vs ventilation in adult severe obstructive sleep apnea syndrome. Am J Otolaryngol 2010;31:14.

79. Aurora RN, Collop NA, Jacobowitz O, et al. Quality measures for the care of adult patients with obstructive sleep apnea. J Clin Sleep Med 2015;11:357.

80. Johns MW. A new method for measuring daytime sleepiness: the Epworth sleepiness scale. Sleep 1991;14:540.

81. Johns MW. Reliability and factor analysis of the Epworth Sleepiness Scale. Sleep 1992;15:376.

82. Weaver TE, Laizner AM, Evans LK, et al. An instrument to measure functional status outcomes for disorders of excessive sleepiness. Sleep 1997;20:835.

Controversies in Anesthesia for Oral and Maxillofacial Surgery

 CrossMark

Brett J. King, DDS[a],*, Adam Levine, MD[b,c,d]

KEYWORDS

- Office-based outpatient anesthesia • Anesthesia team model • Autonomy in anesthesia
- Safety in anesthesia • Controversy in anesthesia

KEY POINTS

- The future of self-performed office-based outpatient anesthesia for oral and maxillofacial surgery is at risk.
- Oral and maxillofacial surgeons have a long history of providing safe and effective outpatient office-based anesthesia.
- Changes in Centers for Medicare and Medicaid Services guidelines are affecting the ability to adequately train oral and maxillofacial surgery residents in outpatient anesthesia.

INTRODUCTION

The modern worlds of medicine and dentistry are fraught with a multitude of controversies that present in various forms: from clinical, including diagnostic and therapeutic, to legislative and administrative. This discussion of controversies in anesthesia for oral and maxillofacial surgery will focus predominately on the legislative.

The provision of anesthesia services for office-based oral and maxillofacial surgical procedures has been an integral and inherent facet of the practice of Oral and Maxillofacial Surgery since its inception as a specialty. Oral and maxillofacial surgeons (OMSs) have a long history of providing safe and effective anesthesia in conjunction with a multitude of common procedures performed in the outpatient setting.[1–3] The provision of anesthesia by OMSs, however, has not come without controversy. It is certainly reasonable to recognize that there could be a variety of differing opinions regarding surgical and anesthetic techniques, some of which may seem more "controversial" than others; however, when it comes to the provision of anesthesia care by non–anesthesiologist providers, the "flood gates of controversy" tend to swing wide open. Even if one were to assume that all anesthesia services provided by the OMS were considered safe and within the standard-of-care, the general idea that these services are being provided by these specialists at all still remains somewhat controversial to both the medical community and the public at large. To further complicate the matters, the wide variety in the level of training and experience for the non–anesthesiologist dental

Disclosures: The authors of this article have no commercial or financial conflicts of interest to disclose. Funding for this article was provided by the authors' respective academic departments.
[a] Department of Oral and Maxillofacial Surgery and General Surgery, LSU Health New Orleans, University Medical Center–New Orleans, Children's Hospital of New Orleans, Touro Infirmary, 1100 Florida Avenue, Box 220, New Orleans, LA 70119, USA; [b] Department of Anesthesiology, Perioperative and Pain Medicine, Mount Sinai Health System, Icahn School of Medicine at Mount Sinai, New York, NY 10029, USA; [c] Department of Pharmacological Sciences, Mount Sinai Health System, Icahn School of Medicine at Mount Sinai, New York, NY 10029, USA; [d] Department of Otolaryngology, Mount Sinai Health System, Icahn School of Medicine at Mount Sinai, New York, NY 10029, USA
* Corresponding author.
E-mail address: bking6@lsuhsc.edu

Oral Maxillofacial Surg Clin N Am 29 (2017) 515–523
http://dx.doi.org/10.1016/j.coms.2017.07.006
1042-3699/17/© 2017 Elsevier Inc. All rights reserved.

provider, whether it be an OMS versus another dental specialist or general practitioner, is often not clearly delineated to those outside of the specialty of OMS, and thus, all dentists are often inappropriately considered as a single group.

BACKGROUND

For decades, most practicing OMSs have used "the *anesthesia team model* for the delivery of office-based anesthesia in which the OMS, along with trained anesthesia and surgical assistants, carries out the administration of the anesthetic, monitors the airway, and performs the surgical procedure. This model is unique and different from a medical anesthesiologist's practice in which a dedicated anesthesia provider is responsible for the anesthetic management of the patient."[3] Although a team approach is used, there still remains a single surgeon operator/anesthetist in this model for the delivery of office-based anesthetics (OBA). The single-operator/anesthetist technique has not come without controversy and is often viewed skeptically by practitioners of other medical specialties. The single surgeon operator/anesthetist model, regardless of the team approach used, creates an easy target for outside specialists who provide anesthesia services solely, while a separate physician or dentist provides the surgical treatment. In addition, the background and training of OMS in relation to the providing of anesthesia services could also be viewed with skepticism by outside parties, often because of a general lack of familiarity of the specialty.

In 2012, the Committee on Dental Accreditation (CODA) increased the required length of the dedicated anesthesia rotation for OMS residents from 4 months to 5 months; however, these 5 months do not clearly depict the totality of the experience and training in anesthesia for the OMS during their residency. The OMS resident experience in anesthesia is intended to be a cumulative experience over the minimum of 4 to 6 years of training because it is an integral part of many of the most commonly performed OMS office/clinic-based procedures. Clearly, the training in any particular procedure or technique occurs as an amalgamation of experience over time. The anesthesia training of the OMS resident involves not only pure general anesthesiology training during the formal anesthesia rotation but also the added experience of providing anesthesia for OMS-specific office-based outpatient procedures, often as the sole provider of anesthesia and surgical services, which frequently occurs throughout the complete length of the 4- to 6-year training program.

HISTORICAL CONTROVERSY

The history of anesthesiology is replete with significant contributions from the field of dentistry in general, and oral and maxillofacial surgery in particular. The "discovery" and early history of anesthesiology are inherently linked to the practice of dentistry, with dentists such as Horace Wells and William T. Morton among the first clinicians to demonstrate and publicize anesthetic techniques for surgical procedures. From the time of Wells' demonstration and promotion of nitrous oxide/oxygen anesthesia in 1844 through the 1940s, the paths of dentistry and anesthesiology were intertwined. In the late 1800s, "dentistry was the qualitative and quantitative leader in the provision of anesthesia."[4] The symbiotic relationship of dentistry and anesthesia was clearly evident in the literature of the time. In 1891, from Pittsburgh, Pennsylvania, *The Dental and Surgical Microcosm* proclaimed to be the world's first journal "devoted chiefly to the science of Anaesthesia and Anaesthetics"[5] (**Fig. 1**). There were only a few hundred medical anesthesia providers in the country during this era; however, many dentists administered thousands of anesthetics annually in their own offices.[4] Charles Teeter, DDS, an early innovator of anesthesia equipment and designer of the first nasopharyngeal tubes for clinical use, was elected an early President of the American Society of Anesthesiologists (ASA).[4] In 1909, Teeter published a paper in the *Journal of the American Medical Association* entitled, "13,000 administrations of nitrous oxide with oxygen as an anesthetic."[6] A significant number of cases described in the paper were anesthetics performed for surgeries distant to the oral cavity, and it appears that it was not uncommon at the time for dentists to provide the anesthesia so that physician surgeons could perform general surgical procedures. Even throughout the 1940s, and especially during World War II, it was common that anesthesia for general surgical procedures was performed by dentist anesthetists who were invariably OMS-trained practitioners.[7] Up until this time in history, seemingly the trajectories of practice for the OMS dentist-anesthetist and the physician-anesthetist seemed aligned, and there was a clear acceptance and interchange of information, technologies, and techniques between the 2 fields.

Although the American Board of Oral Surgery and the American Board of Anesthesiology were each formed only a year apart, in 1940 and 1941, respectively, it is evident that medical anesthesiology began to see significant and increased growth of practitioners focused solely on anesthesia from the early 1900s onwards. In 1911,

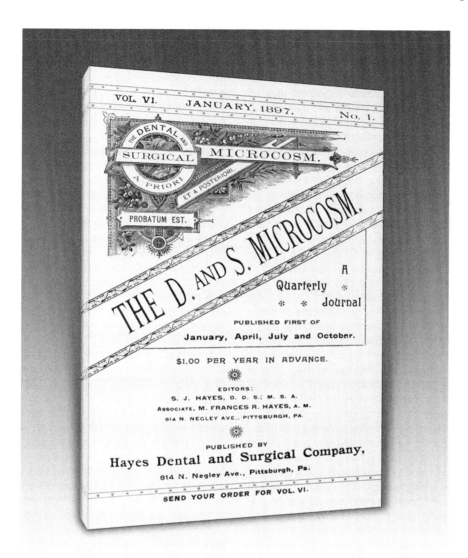

Fig. 1. The Dental and Surgical Microcosm first published in 1891 proclaimed to be the world's first journal "devoted chiefly to the science of Anaesthesia and Anaesthetics." (*Image courtesy of* the Wood Library-Museum of Anesthesiology, Schaumburg, Illinois.)

there were 23 members of the forerunner of the ASA; this increased to 487 members in 1936 and slightly greater than 50,000 in 2012.[5] In comparison, in 2012, the membership of the American Society of Oral and Maxillofacial Surgeons was just over 9000.[8]

The rapid growth of anesthesiology as an independent medical specialty led to the first major "turf war" in the 1950s. In 1951, the ASA rescinded unrestricted membership for dentists, thereby excluding dentist anesthetists and many OMSs members from its ranks.[9] To further stoke the fire of competition and attempt to restrict freedom to practice, the American Medical Association (AMA) has twice, once in the early 1950s and again

in 2009, published documentation that would attempt to directly define or refute the "scope of practice" for OMS, even though oral and maxillofacial surgery is a singularly recognized specialty of dentistry and is thus not under the purview of the AMA.[10,11] This type of controversy, where an attempt has been made by practitioners outside of dentistry to limit a dentist's, and more specifically an OMS's scope of practice, has appeared in multiple forms throughout the years. An easy and convincing argument could seemingly be made to the uninitiated and uninformed simply by mentioning the term "dentist." Most medical professionals and laypeople have a clearly defined definition of what they think a dentist is, and this most frequently correlates with the duties and practice of a general dentist and does not typically correlate with the scope of practice of an OMS. Even more confounding is that multiple studies have shown that there exists a general lack of recognition and understanding of the overall scope of practice of the OMS, which only further confuses both medical professionals and the public at large.[12,13] Even senior dental students have demonstrated a clear lack of understanding of the scope of training and expertise of the OMS.[14] In addition, there are numerous well-known instances in which the lay press will wantonly use the term "dentist," rather than the appropriate designated specialist title, to sensationalize a story in order to make it sound as if "dentists" are practicing well outside their scope of expertise.

A 2004 article addressing cosmetic facial surgery in the New York Times entitled, "A Nip and Tuck With That Crown?," is typical of the problem of negligent omission and general misunderstanding of what an OMS is, how they are trained, and what they practice.[15] Because there is no similar counterpart in medicine to the general dentist, one could, however, make the analogy that it would be inflammatory to write a story that suggests that a family practice physician is routinely performing complex neurosurgical procedures. Most readers and authors would typically understand that their neighborhood "family doctor" is not performing brain surgery, but yet, they are still often willing to imply or accept the concept that their local "family dentist" may be inappropriately performing cosmetic facial surgery, providing general anesthesia, removing cancerous tumors, and so forth...all possibly because of the inherent perception of what a "dentist" is and by the manner in which dentists are frequently portrayed by the mass media. There exists a sometimes subtle, and at other times, outright implication by the mass media and health care/medical community that a "dentist" is somewhat of a second-class citizen when compared with their medical physician colleagues. This type of labeling is unfair to the profession of dentistry as a whole and to the OMS in particular. When one implies that a dentist is not qualified to perform a certain procedure simply because they are a dentist, it is clearly a play on what the general public perceives a dentist to be. Those who persist in arguing that the scope of practice for dentists in general, and for OMS specifically, should be limited do not have a clear understanding of the significant amount of training and expertise that an OMS obtains above and beyond that of training in general dentistry, nor do they have an understanding of how the practice of dentistry and the recognized specialty of oral and maxillofacial surgery are actually defined. The American Dental Association (ADA) official definition of dentistry, which has additionally been adopted by the regulating dental boards of many US states, is as follows:

Dentistry is the evaluation, diagnosis, prevention and/or treatment (nonsurgical, surgical or related procedures) of diseases, disorders and/or conditions of the oral cavity, maxillofacial area and/or the adjacent and associated structures and their impact on the human body; provided by a dentist, within the scope of his/her education, training and experience, in accordance with the ethics of the profession and applicable law.[16]

The ADA official definition of the specialty of oral and maxillofacial surgery reads as follows:

Oral and maxillofacial surgery is the specialty of dentistry which includes the diagnosis, surgical and adjunctive treatment of diseases, injuries and defects involving both the functional and aesthetic aspects of the hard and soft tissues of the oral and maxillofacial region.[17]

Referring to the New York Times "A Nip and Tuck With That Crown," the original article stated: "An oral surgeon...has a D.D.S. or a D.M.D. degree, which is conferred after a 4-year course of study limited to oral health, followed by another 4-year period of study in dental surgery, of which only 18 months are usually spent in surgical rotation."[15] Although the American Association of Oral and Maxillofacial Surgeons (AAOMS) quickly penned a strongly worded rebuttal letter to the editor that factually corrected many of the faults of the original article, the letter was not published in the paper. A simple correction note that was published by the New York Times in an edition 2 weeks after the original article did not present any of the points of fact made by AAOMS regarding scope of practice and training, but rather only stated that OMS "received 30 months of clinical oral and maxillofacial training...not merely 18 months."[15]

The above scenario is demonstrated in this piece as an example to lay the groundwork for a current and increasingly pressing issue for OMSs regarding the ability of the OMS to continue to provide their own anesthesia services. Whether accepted and understood by the lay public and medical physician colleagues or not, OMSs have a clear legislatively accepted mandate from their professional governing societies (ADA, AAOMS) and from their respective state dental and licensing boards to perform a variety of levels of anesthesia, not to mention an impressive longstanding record of safety. Furthermore, AAOMS "Parameters of Care for Anesthesia and Outpatient Facilities" are reviewed and concurred with by the ASA.[3]

CENTERS FOR MEDICARE AND MEDICAID SERVICES CHANGES EVERYTHING

"AAOMS recognized early on that to continue the privilege of administering outpatient anesthesia, three issues had to be addressed: residents needed adequate formal general anesthesia training; the public needed the assurance that oral surgeons were maintaining the highest standard of care; and outpatient general anesthesia had to remain an integral part of our specialty."[8]

In 2010, the Centers for Medicare and Medicaid Services (CMS) issued a memorandum that clarified and added new requirements and interpretive guidelines for anesthesia services in Medicare-certified hospitals that took effect in 2011. The new rules made explicit the requirement "for there to be a single anesthesia service or department responsible for developing policies and procedures for all anesthesia services including sedation and analgesia. This department shall also determine the minimum qualifications for each practitioner permitted to provide anesthesia services of all forms in all locations within the hospital."[18] "Anesthesia services must be under the direction of one individual who is a qualified doctor of medicine (MD) or doctor of osteopathic medicine (DO)."[19] The effective outcome of this rule change in many hospitals was that oral and maxillofacial surgery departments or divisions and/or dental departments lost their autonomy and control over the anesthesia services that they were already providing in their own hospital-based clinics. Many non–anesthesiologist physicians, such as gastroenterologists, provide sedation for their own procedures. However, unlike dental/OMS providers, there is typically no additional state licensing or training documentation required. Anecdotally, in many institutions, the overriding policies that anesthesia departments created to oversee the delivery of anesthesia services as required by CMS ignored the fact that OMS and dental providers are specifically licensed by their state boards to provide various levels of anesthesia depending on their training. As anesthesia departments became the gatekeeper for their institutions and thus gained control and oversight of the anesthetics and sedations performed in clinics previously outside the realm of the anesthesia department, in order to create blanket policies for all sedation, analgesia, and anesthesia, OMS often became "lumped in" with other non–anesthesiologist providers of varying levels of training and often lost significant amounts of autonomy. A frequently noted result of these changes is that hospital-based OMS departments are losing the ability to perform single-provider anesthetist-operator procedures (regardless of the anesthesia team model being in place), losing the ability to use specific anesthesia medications in the clinic (propofol, ketamine, and sevoflurane are commonly reported examples), and occasionally losing the ability to provide anything beyond the level of conscious or moderate sedation. The first author's personal experience at a prior institution demonstrates an extreme of the impractical, and arguably egregious, effects of this type of blanket hospital policy change when an OMS or dental department must follow an outside department's rules: this particular institution has a large, 20+ resident General Practice Residency (GPR) Program in addition to being a rotation site for an affiliated OMS program. The anesthesia and analgesia policy for all locations in this institution's hospital and clinics, crafted by the chair of the Department of Anesthesiology and approved by the hospital administration, disallowed any and all single anesthetist-operator procedures for both residents and attending staff. This policy included the administering of nitrous oxide above the concentration of 30% N_2O. The practical effect of this rule required that the manpower necessary for a patient to be given nitrous oxide–oxygen would be as follows: One GPR or OMS resident to perform the dental or surgical work, one GPR or OMS attending to staff the resident performing the work, a second GPR or OMS resident to deliver and monitor the $N_2O:O_2$, and a second attending staff member to oversee this resident. This formula was also in affect for all sedations in the OMS clinic, each thus requiring at least 2 faculty members in the room at all times because no one faculty member could oversee both the procedure and the sedation/anesthesia. The only anesthesia/analgesia method exempt from this rule at this particular institution was local or topical anesthesia. These rules create a significant and specific problem regarding the training and accreditation of OMS residents in regards to meeting the specific CODA requirements for anesthesia training by essentially doubling the number of cases the residents need to perform.

At the first author's current academic institution, the overriding policy crafted by the Department of Anesthesiology, with little to no input from the Department of Oral and Maxillofacial Surgery, disallows the use of both propofol and ketamine outside the general operating rooms and without a physician anesthesiologist present, thus de facto removing the possibility of providing adequate levels of deep sedation and/or general anesthesia in the OMS outpatient surgi-center.

In fact, the Department's 2 recently acquired anesthesia machines remain in a locked closet unable to be placed into service and used for patient care. The approximately 250-ft² purpose-designed, fully equipped recovery suite is thus currently functioning as a disorganized storage space (**Fig. 2**).

Rules and guidelines similar to the above description have been enacted in hospitals and academic teaching centers throughout the nation as a direct result of the change in CMS policy in 2011. Many hospital-based OMS programs have lost their ability to use the techniques such as the OMS operator-anesthetist model and the use of commonly used medications for sedation anesthesia such as propofol and ketamine in the training of their residents. These changes will inevitably create a long-lasting effect on the specialty of Oral and Maxillofacial Surgery as a whole.

CURRENT INTERPRETIVE GUIDELINES

It is important at this point in the discussion to review the specific guidelines regarding the delivery of anesthesia and analgesia as described by CMS and based on ASA definitions. These guidelines have become widely accepted by governing bodies and hospitals. The ADA has also incorporated the ASA definitions for use in its own published guidelines.

Adapted from Department of Health & Human Services (DHHS) Certification Centers for Medicare & Medicaid Services (CMS), CMS Manual System, Pub. 100-07 State Operations Provider Certification, Transmittals 59 and 74, May 21, 2010 and December 2, 2011:

Anesthesia

"*Anesthesia*" involves the administration of a medication to produce a blunting or loss of: pain perception (analgesia); voluntary and involuntary movements; autonomic function; and memory and/or consciousness, depending on where along the central neuraxial (brain and spinal cord) the medication is delivered. In contrast, "*analgesia*" involves the use of a medication to provide relief of pain through the blocking of pain receptors in the peripheral and/or central nervous system. The patient does not lose consciousness, but does not perceive pain to the extent that may otherwise prevail.

General Anesthesia

General anesthesia is a drug-induced loss of consciousness during which patients are not arousable, even by painful stimulation. The ability to independently maintain ventilatory support is often impaired. Patients often require assistance in maintaining a patent airway, and positive pressure ventilation may be required because of depressed spontaneous ventilation or drug-induced depression of neuromuscular function. Cardiovascular function may be impaired. For example, a patient undergoing major abdominal surgery involving the removal of a portion or all of an organ would require general anesthesia in order to tolerate such an extensive surgical procedure. General anesthesia is used for those procedures when loss of consciousness is required for the safe and effective delivery of surgical services.

Monitored Anesthesia Care

Anesthesia care that includes the monitoring of the patient by a practitioner who is qualified to administer anesthesia as defined by the regulations listed in later discussion (see section, "Who May Administer Anesthesia"). Indications for monitored anesthesia care (MAC) depend on the nature of the procedure, the patient's clinical condition, and/or the potential need to convert to a general or regional anesthetic. Deep sedation/analgesia is included in MAC.

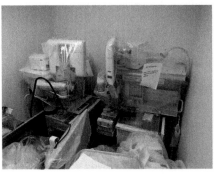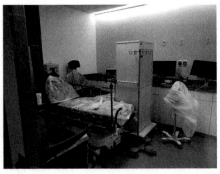

Fig. 2. Fully functional anesthesia machines in the OMS Department at primary author's institution that can not be utilized in the outpatient surgery suites due to the current interpretation of CMS guidelines in the institution. Disused custom-built recovery room space in the same institution.

Deep Sedation/Analgesia

Deep sedation/analgesia is a drug-induced depression of consciousness during which patients cannot be easily aroused but respond purposefully following repeated or painful stimulation. The ability to independently maintain ventilatory function may be impaired. Patients may require assistance in maintaining a patent airway, and spontaneous ventilation may be inadequate. Cardiovascular function is usually maintained. Because of the potential for the inadvertent progression to general anesthesia in certain procedures, it is necessary that the administration of deep sedation/analgesia be delivered or supervised by a practitioner as listed in later discussion (see section, "Who May Administer Anesthesia").

Moderate Sedation/Analgesia ("Conscious Sedation")

Moderate sedation/analgesia ("conscious sedation") is a drug-induced depression of consciousness during which patients respond purposefully to verbal commands, either alone or accompanied by light tactile stimulation. No interventions are required to maintain a patent airway, and spontaneous ventilation is adequate. Cardiovascular function is usually maintained. *CMS, consistent with ASA guidelines, does not define moderate or conscious sedation as anesthesia.*

Minimal Sedation

Minimal sedation is a drug-induced state during which patients respond normally to verbal commands. Although cognitive function and coordination may be impaired, ventilator and cardiovascular functions are unaffected. This is also not anesthesia.

Topical or Local Anesthesia

Topical or local anesthesia is the application or injection of a drug or combination of drugs to stop or prevent a painful sensation to a circumscribed area of the body where a painful procedure is to be performed. There are generally no systemic effects of these medications, which also are not anesthesia, despite the name.

Who May Administer Anesthesia

Topical/local anesthetics, minimal sedation, moderate sedation: The requirements concerning who may administer anesthesia do not apply to the administration of topical or local anesthetics, minimal sedation, or moderate sedation. However, the hospital must have policies and procedures, consistent with State scope of practice law,

governing the provision of these types of anesthesia services. Furthermore, hospitals must assure that all anesthesia services are provided in a safe, well-organized manner by qualified personnel.

General anesthesia, regional anesthesia, and monitored anesthesia, including deep sedation/analgesia, may only be administered by the following:

- A qualified anesthesiologist;
- An MD or DO (other than an anesthesiologist);
- A dentist, oral surgeon, or podiatrist who is qualified to administer anesthesia under State law;
- A certified registered nurse anesthetist (CRNA) who is supervised by the operating practitioner or by an anesthesiologist who is immediately available if needed;
- An anesthesiologist's assistant under the supervision of an anesthesiologist who is immediately available if needed.[19]

Arguably, most OMSs performing office-based anesthesia are practicing at the level of MAC: deep sedation/analgesia or moderate sedation/analgesia, while other hospital-based non–anesthesiologist sedation providers are practicing at or below the level of moderate sedation only. A patient undergoing either technique could easily fluctuate between the 2 because anesthesia exists along a continuum and individual patients will respond differently to different types of medication. There is no clear boundary between anesthesia and analgesia and this is particularly the case with moderate versus deep sedation; however, the organization and staffing required by CMS and AAOMS for the 2 are quite different.

DISCUSSION

Completion of formal residency training in oral and maxillofacial surgery provides the OMS with a pathway to obtain either a state license or a permit for general anesthesia or at the least, deep sedation. Other dental practitioners (except for residency-trained dental anesthesiologists) can likely only obtain sedation permits. Although an OMS may have graduated from an accredited residency program and obtained a state license or permit for anesthesia, this may or may not be reflected in the OMS's ability to obtain hospital privileges for anesthesia and sedation because hospital-based anesthesia departments, rather than licensing or state law, define who can do what under the CMS guidelines. Although these guidelines will rarely have a direct effect on current private practice OMSs who do not provide anesthesia services themselves in a hospital setting, it will overall affect the ability to appropriately train OMS residents in many institutions. Any trend in a decrease in anesthesia training for OMS residents can theoretically lead to a delayed indirect effect for all OMS, whether private practice or institution/hospital based.

OMSs as a specialty have an excellent track record of safety in anesthesia. "The Oral and Maxillofacial Surgery National Insurance Company (OMSNIC) insures approximately 80% of the practicing OMS in the United States...For the 14-year period from 2000 to 2013, OMSNIC estimates that its insured practitioners administered 39,392,008 office-based anesthetics. During this time, there were 113 cases that resulted in patient death or brain injury. This is an occurrence of 1 patient death or brain injury per every 348,602 anesthestic procedures."[1] If OMS residents do not receive adequate training in OBA, including the utilization of all common medications and using the anesthesia team model in which a single OMS is the operator and anesthetist with a team of assistants (as they will likely practice "in the real world"), it can only be expected that the complication rate for OBA will increase over time as these residents enter the private practice community. When a serious anesthetic complication occurs, that is, death, from an otherwise low-risk surgical procedure such as third-molar extractions, the backlash can be swift and powerful. The news media commonly grab hold of these stories when they occur and in today's connected digital and social media environment an otherwise local story will quickly gain national traction and attention.

When an anesthetic complication hits the news cycle or becomes a medico-legal issue, one can be assured that any statements or positions from medical anesthesiologists or the ASA will be actively sought after and highly regarded. In 2010, the ASA House of Delegates approved the "Advisory on Granting Privileges for Deep Sedation to Non-Anesthesiologist Sedation Providers." The semantics and terminology in the advisory are most telling, but not surprising.

"The American Society of Anesthesiologists is vitally interested in the safe administration of all anesthesia services including moderate and deep sedation...It has genuine concern that individuals, however well intentioned, who are not anesthesia professionals may not recognize that sedation and general anesthesia area on a continuum and thus deliver levels of sedation that may, in fact, be general anesthesia without having the training and experience to respond appropriately-...ASA believes that anesthesiologist participation

in all deep sedation is the best means to achieve the safest care, ASA acknowledges, however, that Medicare regulations permit some non-anesthesiologists to administer or supervise the administration of deep sedation. This advisory should not be considered an endorsement, or absolute condemnation, of this practice by ASA but rather to serve as a potential guide to its members who may be called upon by administrators or others to provide input in this process...Unrestricted general anesthesia shall only be administered by anesthesia professionals within their scope of practice..."[20]

The advisory then clearly provides 2 definitions (from ASA advisory):

1.1. Anesthesia Professional: An anesthesiologist, anesthesiologist assistant, or CRNA
1.2. Non–Anesthesiologist *Sedation Practitioner*: A licensed physician (allopathic or osteopathic); or dentist, *oral surgeon*, or podiatrist who is qualified to administer anesthesia under State law: who has not completed postgraduate training in anesthesiology but is specifically trained to administer personally or to supervise the administration of deep sedation.[20]

THE FUTURE

Medical anesthesiologists and the ASA have acknowledged the long history of safety in outpatient OMS anesthesia[3,21]; however, the relatively recent changes to CMS guidelines and the ASA's position on general anesthesia will only make it increasingly difficult to adequately train OMS residents in all levels of anesthesia. Ironically, medical anesthesiology residency training programs have identified that they themselves are lacking in exposure to office-based anesthesia during their own residency training.[21] A 2014 article in the ASA Newsletter titled: "Safe Anesthesia in the Office-Based Surgical Setting" by Shapiro and Osman reiterated the ASA statement regarding anesthesiology providers being the gatekeepers for OBA. They reported that "a recent review of the literature suggested that cosmetic and dental procedures are potentially high-risk interventions in the office setting."[22] In *Paediatric Anaesthesia* in 2013, Lee and colleagues[23] reviewed Lexis-Nexis and a private foundation Web site to study trends in death associated with pediatric dental sedation and general anesthesia. Of the deaths, 56.8% occurred when a general or pediatric dentist was the anesthesia provider. Eight deaths occurred when an OMS was the anesthesia provider, and 7 deaths occurred when an anesthesiologist was the anesthesia provider.[23] Although OMSs and anesthesiologists had practically the same number of deaths in this study, the data ignore the likely fact that a significantly greater number of OBA are performed in this patient population by OMS than by medical anesthesiologists. No number of overall cases or rate was reported.

The OMS approach to office-based anesthesia is unique when compared with the delivery of anesthesia by physician anesthesiologists or other dental providers. The OMS track record of safety for OBA and the anesthesia team model has withstood the test of time. It must be fair to say that OMSs have the most experience as a specialty overall in the performance of outpatient anesthesia for oral and maxillofacial procedures, including concomitant airway management, especially when considering that outpatient OBA is considered a weakness in medical anesthesiology training. It is a matter of particular pride for many OMSs. Recent changes in CMS rules are hampering the ability to appropriately train OMS residents in the tried and true techniques of their specialty, the long-term results of which are yet to fully present themselves. Ideally, the ASA and AAOMS can continue to work together to recognize these important issues and craft unique solutions for the betterment of both specialties, to increase access to care for patients, and to provide the safest and most efficient care possible.

REFERENCES

1. Bennett JD, Kramer KJ, Bosack RC. How safe is deep sedation or general anesthesia while providing dental care? J Am Dent Assoc 2015;146(9):705–8.

2. Perrot DH, Yuen JP, Andreson RV, et al. Office-based ambulatory anesthesia: outcomes of clinical practice of oral and maxillofacial surgery. J Oral Maxillofac Surg 2003;61:983–95.

3. American Association of Oral and Maxillofacial Surgeons White Paper: Office-based anesthesia provided by the oral and maxillofacial surgeon. 2016.

4. Orr DL. The development of anesthesiology in oral and maxillofacial surgery. Oral Maxillofacial Surg Clin N Am 2013;25:341–55.

5. History of Anesthesia. Wood library of anesthesiology. Available at: www.woodlibrarymuseum.org/history-of-anesthesia/. Accessed February 23, 2017.

6. Teeter CK. 13,000 administrations of nitrous oxide with oxygen as an anesthetic. JAMA 1909;53:448–54.

7. Diaz JH. Calling all anesthetists to service in World War II. Anesthesiology 2002;96:776–7.

8. Lew D. A historical overview of the American Association of Oral and Maxillofacial Surgeons. 2013. p. 5–13.

9. American Society of Anesthesiologists Newsletter 1951;5:15.

10. Lynch DF. Are you interested in the definition of oral surgery? Anesth Prog 1957;4:7–8.

11. American Medical Association. AMA scope of practice data series, oral and maxillofacial surgeons. Chicago: American Medical Association; 2009.

12. Hunter MJ, Rubeiz T, Rose L. Recognition of the scope of oral and maxillofacial surgery by the public and healthcare professionals. J Oral Maxillofac Surg 1996;54:1227–32.

13. Rangarajan S, Kaltman S, Rangarajan T, et al. The general public's recognition of oral and maxillofacial surgery. Oral Surg Oral Med Oral Path Oral Rad 2008;506.

14. Guerrero AV, Elo JA, Sun H, et al. What name best represents our specialty? Oral and maxillofacial surgeon versus oral and facial surgeon. J Oral Maxillofac Surg 2017;75:9–20.

15. Kuczynski A. A nip and tuck with that crown? New York Times 2004. Correction May 30, 2004.

16. American Dental Association. Current Policies. 2017;75.

17. American Dental Association. Current Policies. 2017;189.

18. Rosing JR. CMS anesthesia rules are stiffened. OR Manager 2010;26:1–3.

19. Department of Health & Human Services (DHHS) Certification Centers for Medicare & Medicaid Services (CMS), CMS Manual System, Pub. 100–107 State Operations Provider Certification, Transmittals 59 and 74, May 21, 2010 and December 2, 2011.

20. American Society of Anesthesiologists. Advisory on granting privileges for deep sedation to non-anesthesiologist sedation practitioners. Approved by the ASA House of Delegates October 20, 2010.

21. Hausman LM, Levine AI, Rosenblatt MA. A survey evaluating the training of anesthesiology residents in office-based anesthesia. J Clin Anesth 2006;18:499–503.

22. Shapiro FE, Osman BM. Safe anesthesia in the office-based surgical setting. ASA Newsletter 2014;78.

23. Lee HH, Milgrom P, Starks H, et al. Trends in death associated with pediatric dental sedation and general anesthesia. Paediatr Anaesth 2013;23:741–8.

Controversies in Implant Surgery

Tara L. Aghaloo, DDS, MD, PhD*, Martin Mardirosian, DDS, MD, Brando Delgado, BS

KEYWORDS

- Implants • Mini implants • Short implants • Growing patients

KEY POINTS

- Dental implants are a mainstream treatment protocol to replace missing teeth; because they enjoy a high survival and success rate, patients and clinicians continue to increase the demand for more economical, less time consuming, and less complicated surgical procedures.
- These patient and clinician demands have led to shorter length and narrower diameter implants, immediately placed implants into infected sites, and the use of implants in children.
- With all new techniques and procedures, case reports and case series are the first publications to appear in the literature, and there are many favorable reports to justify their use; however, appropriate well-designed, long-term studies are not always available to support clinical practice.
- Because long-term studies are often not available, especially for implants in infected sites, mini implants, and implants in the growing patient, the field continues to evolve.

INTRODUCTION

Implant therapy is an effective and desirable treatment option for fully and partially edentulous patients. With implant survival rates greater than 95% in many studies, and a plethora of long-term data, it is not surprising that the dental profession has truly been transformed by the concept of osseointegration. There are still, however, difficult clinical situations for which a true consensus has not been reached in the literature. Furthermore, many newer protocols, less invasive techniques, and procedures that do not follow conventional implant therapy are often performed in clinical practice without extensive literature support. Therefore, it is important to address some of these controversial topics and review the available publications that may or may not justify altering diagnostic, treatment planning, surgical, and prosthetic principles. Atrophic alveolar bone represents a major obstacle to implant success and ideal implant placement in the mandible and maxilla. Often, extensively atrophic regions of bone require large and complex bone augmentation procedures that require lengthened healing periods, increase the rate of complications, and ultimately increase implant failure. Many implant options have been developed and publicized to circumvent these augmentation procedures to decrease the complexity of treatment and increase patient comfort and potential for implant success. Other points of contention within implant dentistry include the use of implants in growing patients, which has traditionally been avoided entirely; use of mini implants; and the new concept of immediate implant placement in actively infected extraction sockets. These controversial topics are discussed in this article, and evidence in support and in opposition is presented.

SHORT IMPLANTS

Conventional length dental implants have extremely high and predictable survival rates in

Section of Oral and Maxillofacial Surgery, UCLA School of Dentistry, 10833 LeConte Avenue, CHS Rm. 53-076, Los Angeles, CA 90095-1668, USA
* Corresponding author.
E-mail address: taghaloo@dentistry.ucla.edu

Oral Maxillofacial Surg Clin N Am 29 (2017) 525–535
http://dx.doi.org/10.1016/j.coms.2017.07.007
1042-3699/17/© 2017 Elsevier Inc. All rights reserved.

many long-term studies with few complications.[1-3] When faced with a vertically deficient ridge, options available to facilitate successful implant placement include various bone augmentation procedures and placement of a traditional length implant or placement of a short implant. First, defining short implants is important for discussion. Classic short implant length was considered less than 10 mm, but many authors and clinicians consider a short implant as less than or equal to 8 mm or less than or equal to 6 mm.[4-7] Obvious advantages exist for short implants, especially in the posterior maxilla and mandible.[6] Reduced treatment time, less invasive surgery, and decreased morbidity from lack of a bone augmentation procedure, and lower overall cost are major driving forces for the use of short implants.[8] In addition, other potential advantages include easier removal if complications occur, more possible implant sites, and less surgical skill needed for placement.[6] For some patients, particularly with advanced age, decreased healing ability, or complex medical history, a more complicated treatment plan including bone augmentation and subsequent placement of standard length implants presents difficulties and potentially a greater risk of implant failure. However, some complications have been reported with short implants including an increased crown-to-implant ratio, occlusal overload, and failure in the posterior maxilla (**Table 1**).[6,9]

Short implants have high success rates in areas with less than ideal bone height. Although previous studies report higher failure and complication rates for short implants in the maxilla and mandible,[4,8,10-12] short-term[8,13,14] and long-term studies[15-17] have shown success rates approaching those for traditional length implants. Considering that short implants are used in mostly atrophic regions of the jaw, these positive results are impressive. A recent study directly compared 6-mm with greater than 10-mm implants with sinus augmentation, which demonstrated 95% to 100% implant survival without a significant difference between groups after 1 and 3 years. Mean implant stability was similar at placement and 1 year, but significantly higher in the grafted group after 3 years. Although patient satisfaction was high in both groups, treatment cost and overall treatment time was significantly lower in the short implant group.[7] One of the most important considerations when discussing the longevity of short implants is their ability to withstand consistent, long-term crestal bone loss. A longer implant provides more bone-to-implant contact, and therefore, may provide increased longevity if crestal bone loss continues over many years. In addition, finite element studies demonstrate increased stress distribution around the crestal bone with short implants and increased crown height.[18] However, the development of enhanced or roughened surface implants has increased survival and success of short implants in more complex patients and situations. Furthermore, newer implant designs that decrease the amount of force transferred to the crestal bone because of a decreased coronal implant diameter may also provide improvements to facilitate shorter implant placement.[4] A recent study demonstrated similar crestal or marginal bone loss between short and standard implants, or less bone loss around short implants,[7,19] and other comparisons showed more favorable patient morbidity, cost, and treatment time with short implants.[19-22] Even though more studies are available to demonstrate the high survival and success rates of short implants, the definition of short implants is inconsistent, minimal long-term studies exist, and few direct comparative studies are available.

A Cochrane systematic review by Esposito and colleagues[23] evaluated the need for augmentation versus placement of short implants. They reviewed articles evaluating prostheses failures, implant failures, and complications and concluded that there were more statistically significant implant failures and complications in the vertically augmented group versus short implant group.[17,24] Because vertical augmentation, especially in the posterior mandible, is less predictable than other bone grafting techniques, and is associated with complications, these issues may be avoided entirely with the use of short implants.[24-26] The

Table 1 Short implants	
Advantages	**Disadvantages**
• Avoidance of Bone Augmentation Procedures • Decreased healing time • Decreased treatment morbidity • Less invasive placement procedure • Less surgical skill required for implant success • Lower surgical and materials cost • Simplified Implant removal	• Increased crown to implant ratio • Decreased success rates in posterior maxilla • Less ability to withstand occlusal overload

success of short implants is intimately related to the type of bone the implant is placed into, with type IV bone having the least predictable long-term outcome for any size implant.[27,28] Therefore, the partially edentulous posterior maxilla with minimal alveolar bone between the maxillary sinus and the alveolar ridge may not be the ideal site for short implant placement. Moreover, the sinus augmentation procedure is the most predictable and well-studied technique in the short- and long-term to increase bone height for placement of dental implants.[29] For these reasons, it is paramount that short implant studies, specifically in the posterior maxilla, provide long follow-up periods, include a large number of patients, and consider medically compromised patients. It is true that sinus augmentation is a complex grafting procedure with many potential complications, and requires a skilled clinician and cooperative patient.[6,29] Even though sinus augmentation does have its challenges, vertical augmentation of the posterior mandible to allow for longer implant placement is significantly more complicated. Major bone resorption, often greater than 50%, is seen when vertical or onlay grafts are performed to increase height in the posterior mandible.[29] In addition, the inferior alveolar nerve is the limiting anatomic structure, which may cause great morbidity if encountered.[30] Therefore, short implants are extremely popular in this region, where the bone is dense and well corticated. The potential benefits of short implants over a bone graft and traditional length implant are related to increased efficiency and predictability of surgery, decreased cost, treatment time, and morbidity associated with simpler, less invasive procedures. However, the number of short implant studies with long-term follow-up, less than or equal to 6-mm implants, are not nearly as common as grafting with conventional implant length. This is particularly true for the posterior maxilla, where the sinus augmentation procedure is so well-documented.

IMPLANTS IN THE GROWING PATIENT

Complete or partial edentulism in children or adolescents can result from trauma, congenital anodontia, or congenital and acquired defects to the alveolar processes.[31] Currently, the most common solution to edentulism in the growing patient is a removable prosthesis that allows unaltered growth of the craniofacial complex. Removable partial dentures are extremely difficult to use in children because of psychosocial problems, loss or fracture of the prosthesis, lack of normal jaw function, increased decay and gingival problems, and alveolar resorption from continued pressure on the underlying bone and soft tissue. They also require significant compliance from the child, and need to be remade at regular intervals.[32] Fixed partial dentures are also not the best solution in children because of needing to prepare healthy teeth and difficulty with ideal alveolar and gingival contours.[31] For these reasons, dental implants are an attractive solution to missing teeth in a child. They combat all of the negative issues with removable partial dentures including increased confidence and patient acceptance, restoration of function, and preservation of alveolar bone.[33,34] Unfortunately, implants in growing patients behave in a similar manner to ankylosed primary teeth, inert to the dynamic osseous landscape surrounding them.[31,35,36] To date, the arbitrary age for placing dental implants in children is 15 in girls and 18 in boys.[37] Because of vertical alveolar growth in particular, implants can become infraocclusal in relation to the adjacent dentition, or become submerged in the bone to the point of being irretrievable or disrupting alveolar bone formation.[38,39] Although implant prostheses that have become infraoccluded can be replaced with a compensating restoration, change in implant position is unpredictable and may cause esthetic and functional problems (**Table 2**).

The maxilla develops in a downward and forward direction relative to the skull base with distinct growth phases. Passive growth of the maxilla occurs until roughly age 7 when anteroposterior, transverse, and vertical growth accelerate dramatically. Anteroposterior growth originating from the palatine/maxillary suture, and transverse growth originating from the mid-palatine suture, continues until the onset of puberty, and the eruption of the permanent second molar, respectively. Vertical growth continues with the resorption of bone on the nasal surface and deposition on the oral aspects of the maxilla. Implant success in growing patients is acutely

Table 2	
Implants in the growing patient	
Advantages	**Disadvantages**
• Avoidance of RPD or FDP • Increased confidence • Decreased alveolar resorption • Restoration of function • Increased treatment acceptance	• Few potential implant sites • Implant submersion • Potential for growth restriction • Implant ankylosis

dependent on these temporal landmarks.[40,41] Implants placed in growing bone behave as ankylosed structures as opposed to natural dentition. Thus, an osseointegrated implant in the developing anterior maxilla over time is submersed in the bone as apposition on the alveolar crest proceeds. Implants in the central anterior maxilla may become exposed in the nasal cavity because of resorption of the nasal floor during remodeling. This phenomenon may account for the decreased success rates for implants placed in the maxilla especially in regions presenting with little bone to begin with. There is evidence that success can be achieved with maxillary implants near the end of the pubertal growth spurt when maxillary development is near completion.[42] The mandible grows in a more uniform fashion throughout puberty, except the transverse dimension of the anterior mandible, which reaches full size early in development and remains stable throughout late childhood. The stability of the anterior mandible makes it the best location to use implants in the growing patient.[40–42] This should be avoided, however, during the mixed dentition stage during dental development because of adverse effects on the adjacent developing tooth structures.[41]

Although there is potential for the partial submersion of implants in regions of the growing arch that permit a "growing" into the implant, this idea has yet to be investigated in the literature. It has been shown that craniofacial development patterns are not negatively affected by the placement of endosseous implants in the growing patient if placed in the proper position at the correct stage of development.[43] The combination of these factors makes implant placement in the growing patient a feasible treatment modality when taking into account the anatomy of the edentulous area, progression through the growth phase, growth patterns of the specific region, and the presence of natural dentition. Ideally, an osseointegrated implant would provide an effective prosthesis that restores function, improves esthetics, and decreases the amount of bone loss in the edentulous growing arch. Studies demonstrate 80% to 96% implant survival over 5 to 7 years in children with cleft lip and palate and children without clefts ages 9 to 18.[34,44,45] In general, children have excellent healing potential and good blood supply, which makes them potential outstanding implant candidates.[45] However, craniofacial growth patterns differ temporally and between patients making it difficult to gauge bone migration for the purposes of a dental implant.

Ectodermal dysplasia (ED) is one of the most common indications for implant placement in children. ED is a group of more than 100 disorders characterized by hypoplasia or aplasia of at least one ectodermally derived structure (nails, hair, skin, teeth, sweat glands). Children with ED present with lack of facial support, underdeveloped alveolar ridges, anodontia or hypodontia, decreased vertical dimension of occlusion, and reduced salivary flow.[46–48] A significant problem in patients with ED is the reduced alveolar bone present because of the lack of natural dentition.[43] This decreased ridge height can present anywhere, in either arch presenting with hypodontia, and require creative solutions from the surgical and restorative team, including dental implants.[33,43] Several authors[31,49,50] have shown excellent implant survival and that implants may even stimulate alveolar growth in patients with ED. The major factor in the success of dental implants in patients with ED is the amount of residual alveolar bone, which is frequently compromised by hypodontia leading to aplasia of the alveolar ridge. The stimulation of ridge growth is an added benefit in the use of implants for the treatment of ED. Furthermore, the robust vascularity and bone healing observed in younger patients may facilitate early implant placement in these patients.[45]

Overall, the survival of implants in growing patients is high, but poses some problems based on anatomy and growth of the maxilla and mandible. Survival rates are generally higher in the mandible as compared with the maxilla.[31] In addition, continued transverse growth across the midpalatal suture makes cross-arch stabilization in the maxilla a potential problem during growth.[37,39] In contrast, mandibular implants placed during growth have been shown to have minimal effect in the anterior, especially because alveolar growth is minimal when teeth are missing.[51,52] However, the posterior mandible is where most anteroposterior growth occurs, and implants can end up positioned in infraocclusion.[51] The importance of individualized treatment planning by an astute provider well versed in craniofacial development patterns and growth phases provides the most appropriate care for growing patients. Although there are risks of continued growth and change in implant position, the benefits of implant therapy especially in patients with clefts or ED are physical, functional, and psychological because these patients are at an age of transition and development and the importance of a functioning smile cannot be overstated.

MINI IMPLANTS

Other than for orthodontic anchorage, mini implants (diameter <3.0 mm) are currently used for stabilization of removable partial prosthetics, definitive anchorage of denture teeth particularly in the edentulous mandible, and more recently, replacement of teeth in the atrophic arch.[53] Mini implants have several advantages including low cost, ease of use in narrow or atrophic alveolar ridges, simple surgical technique, and shortened treatment time if used for immediate loading.[54–57] Mini implants in the edentulous or partially edentulous arch are indicated when the facial-lingual width of the bone is insufficient for the placement of a traditional width implant.[58] Mini implants are also used in the anterior maxilla because of decreased palatolabial bone width and/or insufficient interdental space. Interdental space is also a common limiting factor in the region of the mandibular incisors. In the atrophic posterior mandible, insufficient buccolingual bone width is the common indication for mini implant placement.[59] This treatment option is limited by the bone height requirement for mini implants and by the inherent weakness of smaller diameter, single-piece implant body.[60] Although there are certain specific clinical scenarios where mini implants may be a viable treatment option, careful case selection and risk evaluation are essential. Mini implants have shown good results in the short-term but there is a marked lack of literature supporting their success as a long-term, definitive treatment (**Table 3**).[58,61] In fact, documented cases of 798 patients with 3095 implants from nine studies only show 5-year follow-up in two of the studies,[54,62,63] and most of the implants are from a single study.[55]

The decreased diameter of mini implants presents several challenges to their long-term success. To maximize strength, thread size is decreased resulting in less surface area available for osseointegration and decreased loading. The one-piece design limits the available abutment options further complicating their use in implant splinting. Mini implants naturally have a greater risk of fracture with 16-fold less bending fracture resistance compared with 4-mm implant designs. Mini implants are at risk for use fracture within even the first year of loading.[60] Narrower implants are more susceptible to stress at the implant-bone interface.[64] Mini implants also have other disadvantages, such as the need for multiple implants to splint for prosthesis, lack of resistance to occlusal loading, and that they must be more parallel because of their one-piece design.[54,65]

The use of mini implants temporarily has been successful in the literature for several promising applications. Anchorage of a removable overdenture during the healing period following the placement of standard implants allows patients to retain an aesthetic appearance and some function.[66,67] Mini implants have also been used to retain a temporary prosthesis to protect a vulnerable bone graft during the healing period. Because of the decreased extent of integration of mini implants, their utility as temporary fixtures is a highlight. The adoption of mini implants in the context of fixed single or multiunit restoration is best kept as a secondary option to traditional diameter, and even narrow diameter implants. Because of the combination of decreased fracture resistance, propensity for implant failure, limited abutment options, and need for immediate restoration, mini implants do not represent a reliable replacement for definitive treatment with bone augmentation and placement of a traditional diameter implant. Although they have been used since 1994 and are Food and

Table 3
Mini-implants for definitive prosthetic rehabilitation

Author (Published)	Follow up (mo)	Implants Placed (n)	Failed Implants (n)	Implant Success (%)
Elsyad et al,[56] 2011	36	112	4	96.4
Balaji et al,[57] 2010	24	11	1	90.1
Jofre et al,[84] 2010	36	90	5	94.4
Morneburg & Pröschell,[85] 2008	40–104	134	6	95.5
Cho et al,[86] 2007	13–36	34	2	94.1
Shatkin et al,[55] 2007	Up to 60	2514	145	94.2
Griffitts et al,[69] 2005	Unknown	116	3	97.4
Mazor et al,[59] 2004	Up to 60	32	1	96.9
Vigolo & Givani,[63] 2000	60	52	3	94.2

Drug Administration approved for interim and long-term prosthodontic treatment, few long-term studies on mini implant survival and success are available.[54,61,68] Even though the studies have minimal support for long-term survival and success, the interest in mini implants will continue to increase among clinicians and patients for several reasons: decreased cost, access to care for patients with limited finances, patients with challenging defects, medically compromised patients, and dentists with no or minimal surgical training.[53,54,57,69]

IMMEDIATE PLACEMENT OF IMPLANTS INTO INFECTED EXTRACTION SOCKETS

Extraction sites with a history of periapical, endodontic, or periodontal infection have traditionally been given a healing period of several months up to a year before being treated definitively with implant therapy. This allows for the resolution of infection and minimizes the likelihood of a premature failure caused by complications, such as retrograde peri-implantitis or the inability of the implant to osseointegrate concurrently with infection resolution.[70] Extraction sockets undergo significant remodeling during the healing period, which may result in unfavorable dimensional discrepancies between the healed site and the adjacent teeth. This is especially apparent in the anterior maxilla because of the palatolabial change in edentulous sites.[71] Immediate implant placement in the esthetic zone has been shown to reduce the amount of postextraction remodeling of the periodontal tissues resulting in a more satisfactory esthetic result. Postextraction, alveolar bone undergoes several changes that result in this discrepancy and make immediate implant placement advantageous. The vertical height of the alveolar ridge decreases, as does the buccolingual or palatolabial width of the ridge. The socket gradually fills in with bone resulting in a short, thin, and solid residual ridge. This multidimensional remodeling occurs for up to a year postextraction. The placement of an immediate implant can prevent much of this remodeling and maintain the natural position of the tooth and the height and contour of the alveolar bone. This has been shown to be a viable treatment modality when infection is not present in the extraction site. More recently, clinicians have begun to place implants in previously infected extraction sites after using a clinical sequence to clean and disinfect the site before placement.

Immediate placement into infected extraction sockets is often contraindicated because of how bacteria affect healing.[70,72–75] In fact, previous studies with machine surface implants had increased implant failure in extraction sites with periapical disease.[76] However, more recent studies showed better results with implants in infected sites. Crespi and colleagues[77] achieved a 100% success rate for 275 implants placed in sites with endodontic or periodontal pathology with a 4-year follow-up. The investigators used an infection control procedure including prophylactic amoxicillin, saline rinse, socket debridement, a 7-day postsurgical course of amoxicillin, and a 15-day course of chlorhexidine mouthrinse. Fugazotto[78] published a 98.8% success rate for 418 implants placed with a mean follow-up time of 67.3 months. All 418 implants were placed in sites that demonstrated a periapical lesion suggestive of active infection. The infected sockets were treated with curettage, soft tissue debridement, and autologous bone and membranes were placed when indicated. Patients were given a 10-day course of amoxicillin and a 5-day course of etodolac. They were not prescribed a chlorhexidine rinse.

For the immediate implant to be ultimately successful a careful debridement of the infected socket and tissues must be performed before implant placement. Several procedures have been cited in the literature and most include curettage, irrigation, and careful removal of all granulation tissue present in the socket. Other procedures cite the inclusion of a systemic antibiotic regimen, prophylactic antibiotics, antibiotic socket irrigation, chlorhexidine rinse, erbium laser debridement, platelet-rich plasma, bone grafting, or guided bone regeneration.[79,80] Success rates in recently published studies using these procedures are similar to the success rates of implants placed in noninfected sockets.[81–83] Because there is no standardized procedure in the literature, or experimentation focusing on the specific procedure, there seems to currently be little evidence for the use of antibiotics and chlorhexidine rinses or other adjunct therapy. Prophylactic antibiotics have been shown in the literature to decrease the incidence of implant failure when compared with control groups in nonaffected sites. The success rates of studies using these additional procedures are similar to those that do not, given that careful debridement, curettage, and removal of all granulation tissue is performed.[83] Studies questioning the benefits and drawbacks of these diverse procedures are needed to establish a more specific treatment guideline in the future.

The immediate placement of implants into sites presenting with periapical, endodontic, or periodontal pathology has been shown to have similar success rates to placement in uninfected sites given that the proper socket cleaning procedure is meticulously performed (**Table 4**). Preoperative

Table 4
Implants in infected sites

Author (Published)	Follow up (mo)	Implants Placed (n)	Failed Implants (n)	Implant Success (%)
Pecora et al,[87] 1996	16.3	7	1	85.7
Villa & Rangert,[88] 2005	15–44	97	0	100
Lindeboom et al,[89] 2006	12	25 (IP) 25 (DP)	2 (IP) 0 (DP)	92(IP) 100(DP)
Rabel & Kohler,[90] 2006	12	95	4	95.8
Casap et al,[79] 2007	12–72	30	1	96.7
Siegenthaler et al,[80] 2007	12	13(INF) 16[a]	0	100
Villa & Rangert,[91] 2007	12	76	2	97.4
Del Fabbro et al,[81] 2009	Mean 18.5	61	1	98.4
Crespi et al,[77] 2010	48	275 total 78 (NI) 197 (INF)	0 (NI) 2 (INF)	100 (NI) 98.9 (INF)
Crespi et al,[77] 2010	24	30 total 15 (INF) 15[a]	0	100
Bell et al,[92] 2011	Mean 19.75	922 total 285 (INF)	15 total 7 (INF)	98.4 total 97.5 (INF)
Truninger et al,[93] 2011	36	29 total 13 (INF) 16[a]	0	100
Fugazzotto,[78] 2012	Mean 67.3	418	5	98.8
Fugazzotto,[78] 2012	Mean 64	128 total 64 (INF) 64[a]	4 total 3 (INF) 1[a]	96.9 total 95.3 (INF) 98.4[a]
Jofre et al,[94] 2012	Mean 15	31	0	100
Jung et al,[2] 2012	60	27 total 12 (INF) 15[a]	0	100
Meltzer,[95] 2012	3–24	77	1	98.7
Marconcini et al,[96] 2013	12	20	0	100

Abbreviations: DP, Delayed Placement; INF, Infected; IP, Immediate Placement; NI, Noninfected.
[a] Control site.

antibiotics have been demonstrated to decrease failure rate with immediate implant placement and are thus advised. Although postoperative antibiotic procedures have not been thoroughly optimized, or their effectiveness proven for this specific clinical application, it is prudent to use an antibiotic course, including a chlorhexidine rinse at this point.

SUMMARY

Dental implants are a mainstream treatment protocol to replace missing teeth. Because they enjoy a high survival and success rate, patients and clinicians continue to increase the demand for more economical, less time consuming, and less complicated surgical procedures. In dentistry, providers are able to use clinical judgment to use materials and procedures to modify standard practices. These patient and clinician demands have led to shorter length and narrower diameter implants, immediately placed implants into infected sites, and the use of implants in children. With all new techniques and procedures, case reports and case series are the first publications to appear in the literature, and there are many favorable reports to justify their use. However, appropriate well designed, long-term studies are not always available to support clinical practice. This article reviews some of the controversial topics in implant dentistry, and presents the evidence that supports and challenges these newer techniques. Because long-term studies are often not available, especially for implants in infected sites, mini implants, and implants in the growing patient, the field continues to evolve. The reader and clinician must stay abreast of these topics and continue to modify his or her practice as more literature is published and more information becomes available.

REFERENCES

1. Pjetursson BE, Thoma D, Jung R, et al. A systematic review of the survival and complication rates of implant-supported fixed dental prostheses (FDPs) after a mean observation period of at least 5 years. Clin Oral Implants Res 2012; 23(Suppl 6):22–38.
2. Jung RE, Zembic A, Pjetursson BE, et al. Systematic review of the survival rate and the incidence of biological, technical, and aesthetic complications of single crowns on implants reported in longitudinal studies with a mean follow-up of 5 years. Clin Oral Implants Res 2012;23(Suppl 6):2–21.
3. Jimbo R, Albrektsson T. Long-term clinical success of minimally and moderately rough oral implants: a review of 71 studies with 5 years or more of follow-up. Implant Dent 2015;24:62–9.
4. Villarinho EA, Triches DF, Alonso FR, et al. Risk factors for single crowns supported by short (6-mm) implants in the posterior region: a prospective clinical and radiographic study. Clin Implant Dent Relat Res 2017;19(4):671–80.
5. Monje A, Suarez F, Galindo-Moreno P, et al. A systematic review on marginal bone loss around short dental implants (<10 mm) for implant-supported fixed prostheses. Clin Oral Implants Res 2014;25:1119–24.
6. Thoma DS, Cha JK, Jung UW. Treatment concepts for the posterior maxilla and mandible: short implants versus long implants in augmented bone. J Periodontal Implant Sci 2017;47:2–12.
7. Bechara S, Kubilius R, Veronesi G, et al. Short (6-mm) dental implants versus sinus floor elevation and placement of longer (≥10-mm) dental implants: a randomized controlled trial with a 3-year follow-up. Clin Oral Implants Res 2016. [Epub ahead of print].
8. Annibali S, Cristalli MP, Dell'Aquila D, et al. Short dental implants: a systematic review. J Dent Res 2012;91:25–32.
9. Telleman G, Raghoebar GM, Vissink A, et al. A systematic review of the prognosis of short (<10 mm) dental implants placed in the partially edentulous patient. J Clin Periodontol 2011;38:667–76.
10. Mezzomo LA, Miller R, Triches D, et al. Meta-analysis of single crowns supported by short (<10 mm) implants in the posterior region. J Clin Periodontol 2014;41:191–213.
11. Sun HL, Huang C, Wu YR, et al. Failure rates of short (≤ 10 mm) dental implants and factors influencing their failure: a systematic review. Int J Oral Maxillofac Implants 2011;26:816–25.
12. Srinivasan M, Vazquez L, Rieder P, et al. Survival rates of short (6 mm) micro-rough surface implants: a review of literature and meta-analysis. Clin Oral Implants Res 2014;25:539–45.
13. Renouard F, Nisand D. Short implants in the severely resorbed maxilla: a 2-year retrospective clinical study. Clin Implant Dent Relat Res 2005;7(Suppl 1):S104–10.
14. Ferrigno N, Laureti M, Fanali S, et al. A long-term follow-up study of non-submerged ITI implants in the treatment of totally edentulous jaws. Part I: ten-year life table analysis of a prospective multicenter study with 1286 implants. Clin Oral Implants Res 2002;13:260–73.
15. Nedir R, Nurdin N, Abi Najm S, et al. Short implants placed with or without grafting into atrophic sinuses: the 5-year results of a prospective randomized controlled study. Clin Oral Implants Res 2017; 28(7):877–86.
16. Malo P, de Araujo Nobre M, Rangert B. Short implants placed one-stage in maxillae and mandibles: a retrospective clinical study with 1 to 9 years of follow-up. Clin Implant Dent Relat Res 2007;9:15–21.
17. Lai HC, Si MS, Zhuang LF, et al. Long-term outcomes of short dental implants supporting single crowns in posterior region: a clinical retrospective study of 5-10 years. Clin Oral Implants Res 2013; 24:230–7.
18. Bulaqi HA, Mousavi Mashhadi M, Safari H, et al. Effect of increased crown height on stress distribution in short dental implant components and their surrounding bone: a finite element analysis. J prosthetic dentistry 2015;113:548–57.
19. Esposito M, Pistilli R, Barausse C, et al. Three-year results from a randomised controlled trial comparing prostheses supported by 5-mm long implants or by longer implants in augmented bone in posterior atrophic edentulous jaws. Eur J Oral Implantol 2014;7: 383–95.
20. Pistilli R, Felice P, Cannizzaro G, et al. Posterior atrophic jaws rehabilitated with prostheses supported by 6 mm long 4 mm wide implants or by longer implants in augmented bone. One-year post-loading results from a pilot randomised controlled trial. Eur J Oral Implantol 2013;6:359–72.
21. Gulje FL, Raghoebar GM, Vissink A, et al. Single crowns in the resorbed posterior maxilla supported by either 6-mm implants or by 11-mm implants combined with sinus floor elevation surgery: a 1-year

randomised controlled trial. Eur J Oral Implantol 2014;7:247–55.

22. Thoma DS, Haas R, Tutak M, et al. Randomized controlled multicentre study comparing short dental implants (6 mm) versus longer dental implants (11-15 mm) in combination with sinus floor elevation procedures. Part 1: demographics and patient-reported outcomes at 1 year of loading. J Clin Periodontol 2015;42:72–80.

23. Esposito M, Felice P, Worthington HV. Interventions for replacing missing teeth: augmentation procedures of the maxillary sinus. Cochrane Database Syst Rev 2014;(5):CD008397.

24. Felice P, Cannizzaro G, Checchi V, et al. Vertical bone augmentation versus 7-mm-long implants in posterior atrophic mandibles. Results of a randomised controlled clinical trial of up to 4 months after loading. Eur J Oral Implantol 2009;2:7–20.

25. Esposito M, Grusovin MG, Felice P, et al. The efficacy of horizontal and vertical bone augmentation procedures for dental implants: a Cochrane systematic review. Eur J Oral Implantol 2009;2:167–84.

26. Stellingsma K, Bouma J, Stegenga B, et al. Satisfaction and psychosocial aspects of patients with an extremely resorbed mandible treated with implant-retained overdentures. A prospective, comparative study. Clin Oral Implants Res 2003;14:166–72.

27. Jaffin RA, Berman CL. The excessive loss of Branemark fixtures in type IV bone: a 5-year analysis. J Periodontol 1991;62:2–4.

28. He J, Zhao B, Deng C, et al. Assessment of implant cumulative survival rates in sites with different bone density and related prognostic factors: an 8-year retrospective study of 2,684 implants. Int J Oral Maxillofac Implants 2015;30:360–71.

29. Aghaloo TL, Moy PK. Which hard tissue augmentation techniques are the most successful in furnishing bony support for implant placement? Int J Oral Maxillofac Implants 2007;22(Suppl):49–70.

30. Ucer C, Yilmaz Z, Scher E, et al. A survey of the opinion and experience of UK dentists part 3: an evidence-based protocol of surgical risk management strategies in the mandible. Implant Dent 2017;26(4):532–40.

31. Mankani N, Chowdhary R, Patil BA, et al. Osseointegrated dental implants in growing children: a literature review. J Oral Implantol 2014;40:627–31.

32. Agarwal N, Kumar D, Anand A, et al. Dental implants in children: a multidisciplinary perspective for long-term success. Natl J Maxillofac Surg 2016;7:122–6.

33. Wang Y, He J, Decker AM, et al. Clinical outcomes of implant therapy in ectodermal dysplasia patients: a systematic review. Int J Oral Maxillofac Surg 2016;45:1035–43.

34. Wermker K, Jung S, Joos U, et al. Dental implants in cleft lip, alveolus, and palate patients: a systematic review. Int J Oral Maxillofac Implants 2014;29:384–90.

35. Thilander B, Odman J, Grondahl K, et al. Aspects on osseointegrated implants inserted in growing jaws. A biometric and radiographic study in the young pig. Eur J Orthod 1992;14:99–109.

36. Odman J, Grondahl K, Lekholm U, et al. The effect of osseointegrated implants on the dento-alveolar development. A clinical and radiographic study in growing pigs. Eur J Orthod 1991;13:279–86.

37. Cronin RJ Jr, Oesterle LJ. Implant use in growing patients. Treatment planning concerns. Dent Clin North Am 1998;42:1–34.

38. Rossi E, Andreasen JO. Maxillary bone growth and implant positioning in a young patient: a case report. Int J Periodontics Restorative Dent 2003;23:113–9.

39. Oesterle LJ, Cronin RJ Jr, Ranly DM. Maxillary implants and the growing patient. Int J Oral Maxillofac Implants 1993;8:377–87.

40. Brahim JS. Dental implants in children. Oral Maxillofac Surg Clin North Am 2005;17:375–81.

41. Op Heij DG, Opdebeeck H, van Steenberghe D, et al. Age as compromising factor for implant insertion. Periodontol 2000 2003;33:172–84.

42. Mishra SK, Chowdhary N, Chowdhary R. Dental implants in growing children. J Indian Soc Pedod Prev Dent 2013;31:3–9.

43. Johnson EL, Roberts MW, Guckes AD, et al. Analysis of craniofacial development in children with hypohidrotic ectodermal dysplasia. Am J Med Genet 2002;112:327–34.

44. Carmichael RP, Sandor GK. Use of dental implants in the management of cleft lip and palate. Atlas Oral Maxillofac Surg Clin North Am 2008;16:61–82.

45. Ledermann PD, Hassell TM, Hefti AF. Osseointegrated dental implants as alternative therapy to bridge construction or orthodontics in young patients: seven years of clinical experience. Pediatr Dent 1993;15:327–33.

46. Stanford CM, Guckes A, Fete M, et al. Perceptions of outcomes of implant therapy in patients with ectodermal dysplasia syndromes. Int J Prosthodont 2008;21:195–200.

47. Pinheiro M, Freire-Maia N. Ectodermal dysplasias: a clinical classification and a causal review. Am J Med Genet 1994;53:153–62.

48. Lesman-Leegte I, Jaarsma T, Sanderman R, et al. Depressive symptoms are prominent among elderly hospitalised heart failure patients. Eur J Heart Fail 2006;8:634–40.

49. Escobar V, Epker BN. Alveolar bone growth in response to endosteal implants in two patients with ectodermal dysplasia. Int J Oral Maxillofac Surg 1998;27:445–7.

50. Guckes AD, Scurria MS, King TS, et al. Prospective clinical trial of dental implants in persons with ectodermal dysplasia. J Prosthet Dent 2002;88:21–5.

51. Oesterle LJ, Cronin RJ Jr. Adult growth, aging, and the single-tooth implant. Int J Oral Maxillofac Implants 2000;15:252–60.

52. Skieller V, Bjork A, Linde-Hansen T. Prediction of mandibular growth rotation evaluated from a longitudinal implant sample. Am J Orthod 1984;86:359–70.

53. Christensen GJ. The 'mini'-implant has arrived. J Am Dent Assoc 2006;137:387–90.

54. Bidra AS, Almas K. Mini implants for definitive prosthodontic treatment: a systematic review. J Prosthet Dent 2013;109:156–64.

55. Shatkin TE, Shatkin S, Oppenheimer BD, et al. Mini dental implants for long-term fixed and removable prosthetics: a retrospective analysis of 2514 implants placed over a five-year period. Compend Contin Educ Dent 2007;28:92–9 [quiz: 100–1].

56. Elsyad MA, Gebreel AA, Fouad MM, et al. The clinical and radiographic outcome of immediately loaded mini implants supporting a mandibular overdenture. A 3-year prospective study. J Oral Rehabil 2011;38:827–34.

57. Balaji A, Mohamed JB, Kathiresan R. A pilot study of mini implants as a treatment option for prosthetic rehabilitation of ridges with sub-optimal bone volume. J Maxillofac Oral Surg 2010;9:334–8.

58. Davarpanah M, Martinez H, Tecucianu JF, et al. Small-diameter implants: indications and contraindications. J Esthet Dent 2000;12:186–94.

59. Mazor Z, Steigmann M, Leshem R, et al. Mini-implants to reconstruct missing teeth in severe ridge deficiency and small interdental space: a 5-year case series. Implant Dent 2004;13:336–41.

60. Misch C. Dental implant prosthetics. 2nd edition. Atlanta(GA): Elsevier Health Sciences; 2014.

61. Klein MO, Schiegnitz E, Al-Nawas B. Systematic review on success of narrow-diameter dental implants. Int J Oral Maxillofac Implants 2014; 29(Suppl):43–54.

62. Zhao HY, Ooyama A, Yamamoto M, et al. Down regulation of c-Myc and induction of an angiogenesis inhibitor, thrombospondin-1, by 5-FU in human colon cancer KM12C cells. Cancer Lett 2008;270: 156–63.

63. Vigolo P, Givani A. Clinical evaluation of single-tooth mini-implant restorations: a five-year retrospective study. J Prosthet Dent 2000;84:50–4.

64. Baggi L, Cappelloni I, Di Girolamo M, et al. The influence of implant diameter and length on stress distribution of osseointegrated implants related to crestal bone geometry: a three-dimensional finite element analysis. J Prosthet Dent 2008;100:422–31.

65. Lee JH, Frias V, Lee KW, et al. Effect of implant size and shape on implant success rates: a literature review. J Prosthet Dent 2005;94:377–81.

66. Ahn MR, An KM, Choi JH, et al. Immediate loading with mini dental implants in the fully edentulous mandible. Implant Dent 2004;13:367–72.

67. el Attar MS, el Shazly D, Osman S, et al. Study of the effect of using mini-transitional Implants as temporary abutments in implant overdenture cases. Implant Dent 1999;8:152–8.

68. Barber HD, Seckinger RJ. The role of the small-diameter dental implant: a preliminary report on the Miniplant system. Compendium 1994;15:1390, 1392.

69. Griffitts TM, Collins CP, Collins PC. Mini dental implants: an adjunct for retention, stability, and comfort for the edentulous patient. Oral Surg Oral Med Oral Pathol Oral Radiol Endod 2005;100:e81–4.

70. Chrcanovic BR, Martins MD, Wennerberg A. Immediate placement of implants into infected sites: a systematic review. Clin Implant Dent Relat Res 2015;17(Suppl 1):e1–16.

71. Naves MM, Horbylon BZ, Gomes CF, et al. Immediate implants placed into infected sockets: a case report with 3-year follow-up. Braz Dent J 2009;20: 254–8.

72. Schwartz-Arad D, Chaushu G. The ways and wherefores of immediate placement of implants into fresh extraction sites: a literature review. J Periodontol 1997;68:915–23.

73. Quirynen M, Gijbels F, Jacobs R. An infected jawbone site compromising successful osseointegration. Periodontol 2000 2003;33:129–44.

74. Rosenquist B, Grenthe B. Immediate placement of implants into extraction sockets: implant survival. Int J Oral Maxillofac Implants 1996;11:205–9.

75. Becker W, Becker BE. Guided tissue regeneration for implants placed into extraction sockets and for implant dehiscences: surgical techniques and case report. Int J Periodontics Restorative Dent 1990;10:376–91.

76. Alsaadi G, Quirynen M, Komarek A, et al. Impact of local and systemic factors on the incidence of oral implant failures, up to abutment connection. J Clin Periodontol 2007;34:610–7.

77. Crespi R, Cappare P, Gherlone E. Immediate loading of dental implants placed in periodontally infected and non-infected sites: a 4-year follow-up clinical study. J Periodontol 2010;81:1140–6.

78. Fugazzotto P. A retrospective analysis of immediately placed implants in 418 sites exhibiting periapical pathology: results and clinical considerations. Int J Oral Maxillofac Implants 2012;27: 194–202.

79. Casap N, Zeltser C, Wexler A, et al. Immediate placement of dental implants into debrided infected dentoalveolar sockets. J Oral Maxillofac Surg 2007; 65:384–92.

80. Siegenthaler DW, Jung RE, Holderegger C, et al. Replacement of teeth exhibiting periapical pathology by immediate implants: a prospective, controlled clinical trial. Clin Oral Implants Res 2007;18:727–37.

81. Del Fabbro M, Boggian C, Taschieri S. Immediate implant placement into fresh extraction sites with chronic periapical pathologic features combined with plasma rich in growth factors: preliminary results of single-cohort study. J Oral Maxillofac Surg 2009;67:2476–84.

82. Waasdorp JA, Evian CI, Mandracchia M. Immediate placement of implants into infected sites: a systematic review of the literature. J Periodontol 2010;81: 801–8.

83. Chrcanovic BR, Albrektsson T, Wennerberg A. Dental implants inserted in fresh extraction sockets versus healed sites: a systematic review and meta-analysis. J Dent 2015;43:16–41.

84. Jofre J, Conrady Y, Carrasco C. Survival of splinted mini-implants after contamination with stainless steel. Int J Oral Maxillofac Impl 2010;25(2):351–6.

85. Morneburg TR, Proschel PA. Success rates of micro-implants in edentulous patients with residual ridge resorption. Int J Oral Maxillofac Implants 2008; 23(2):270–6.

86. Cho SC, Froum S, Tai CH, et al. Immediate loading of narrow diameter implants with overdentures in severely atrophic mandibles. Pract Proced Aesthet Dent 2007;19(3):167–74.

87. Pecora G, Andreana S, Covani U, et al. New directions in surgical endodontics; immediate implantation into an extraction site. J Endod 1996;22(3): 135–9.

88. Villa R, Rangert B. Early loading of interforaminal implants immediately installed after extraction of teeth presenting endodontic and periodontal lesions. Clin Implant Dent Relat Res 2005;7(Suppl 1):S28–35.

89. Lindeboom JA, Tjiook Y, Kroon FH. Immediate placement of implants in periapical infected sites: a prospective randomized study in 50 patients. Oral Surg Oral Med Oral Pathol Oral Radiol Endod 2006;101(6):705–10.

90. Rabel A, Kohler SG. Microbiological study on the prognosis of immediate implant and periodontal disease. Mund Kiefer Gesichtschir 2006;10(1): 7–13.

91. Villa R, Rangert B. Immediate and early function of implants placed in extraction sockets of maxillary infected teeth: a pilot study. J Prosthet Dent 2007;97(6 Suppl):S96–108.

92. Bell CL, Diehl D, Bell BM, et al. The immediate placement of dental implants into extraction sites with periapical lesions: a retrospective chart review. J Oral Maxillofac Surg 2011;69(6):1623–7.

93. Truninger TC, Philipp AO, Siegenthaler DW, et al. A prospective, controlled clinical trial evaluating the clinical and radiological outcome after 3 yeas of immediately placed implants in sockets exhibiting periapical pathology. Clin Oral Implants Res 2011; 22(1):20–7.

94. Jofre J, Valenzuela D, Quintana P, et al. Protocol for immediate implant replacement of infected teeth. Implant Dent 2012;21(4):287–94.

95. Meltzer AM. Immediate implant placement and restoration in infected sites. Int J Periodontics Restorative Dent 2012;32(5):e169–73.

96. Maroncini S, Barone A, Gelpi F, et al. Immediate implant placement in infected sites: a case series. J Periodontol 2013;84(2):196–202.

UNITED STATES POSTAL SERVICE ®

Statement of Ownership, Management, and Circulation
(All Periodicals Publications Except Requester Publications)

1. Publication Title	2. Publication Number	3. Filing Date
ORAL & MAXILLOFACIAL SURGERY CLINICS OF NORTH AMERICA	006 – 362	9/18/2017

4. Issue Frequency	5. Number of Issues Published Annually	6. Annual Subscription Price
FEB, MAY, AUG, NOV	4	$385.00

7. Complete Mailing Address of Known Office of Publication *(Not printer) (Street, city, county, state, and ZIP+4®)*

ELSEVIER INC.
230 Park Avenue, Suite 800
New York, NY 10169

Contact Person
STEPHEN R. BUSHING

Telephone *(Include area code)*
215-239-3688

8. Complete Mailing Address of Headquarters or General Business Office of Publisher *(Not printer)*

ELSEVIER INC.
230 Park Avenue, Suite 800
New York, NY 10169

9. Full Names and Complete Mailing Addresses of Publisher, Editor, and Managing Editor *(Do not leave blank)*

Publisher *(Name and complete mailing address)*

ADRIANNE BRIGIDO, ELSEVIER INC.
1600 JOHN F KENNEDY BLVD. SUITE 1800
PHILADELPHIA, PA 19103-2899

Editor *(Name and complete mailing address)*

JOHN VASSALLO, ELSEVIER INC.
1600 JOHN F KENNEDY BLVD. SUITE 1800
PHILADELPHIA, PA 19103-2899

Managing Editor *(Name and complete mailing address)*

PATRICK MANLEY, ELSEVIER INC.
1600 JOHN F KENNEDY BLVD. SUITE 1800
PHILADELPHIA, PA 19103-2899

10. Owner *(Do not leave blank. If the publication is owned by a corporation, give the name and address of the corporation immediately followed by the names and addresses of all stockholders owning or holding 1 percent or more of the total amount of stock. If not owned by a corporation, give the names and addresses of the individual owners. If owned by a partnership or other unincorporated firm, give its name and address as well as those of each individual owner. If the publication is published by a nonprofit organization, give its name and address.)*

Full Name	Complete Mailing Address
WHOLLY OWNED SUBSIDIARY OF REED/ELSEVIER, US HOLDINGS	1600 JOHN F KENNEDY BLVD. SUITE 1800 PHILADELPHIA, PA 19103-2899

11. Known Bondholders, Mortgagees, and Other Security Holders Owning or Holding 1 Percent or More of Total Amount of Bonds, Mortgages, or Other Securities. If none, check box ▶ ☐ None

Full Name	Complete Mailing Address
N/A	

12. Tax Status *(For completion by nonprofit organizations authorized to mail at nonprofit rates) (Check one)*
The purpose, function, and nonprofit status of this organization and the exempt status for federal income tax purposes:
☒ Has Not Changed During Preceding 12 Months
☐ Has Changed During Preceding 12 Months *(Publisher must submit explanation of change with this statement)*

13. Publication Title	14. Issue Date for Circulation Data Below
ORAL & MAXILLOFACIAL SURGERY CLINICS OF NORTH AMERICA	FEBRUARY 2017

15. Extent and Nature of Circulation			Average No. Copies Each Issue During Preceding 12 Months	No. Copies of Single Issue Published Nearest to Filing Date
a. Total Number of Copies *(Net press run)*			1138	1075
b. Paid Circulation (By Mail and Outside the Mail)	(1)	Mailed Outside-County Paid Subscriptions Stated on PS Form 3541 *(Include paid distribution above nominal rate, advertiser's proof copies, and exchange copies)*	767	744
	(2)	Mailed In-County Paid Subscriptions Stated on PS Form 3541 *(Include paid distribution above nominal rate, advertiser's proof copies, and exchange copies)*	0	0
	(3)	Paid Distribution Outside the Mails Including Sales Through Dealers and Carriers, Street Vendors, Counter Sales, and Other Paid Distribution Outside USPS®	152	96
	(4)	Paid Distribution by Other Classes of Mail Through the USPS *(e.g., First-Class Mail®)*	0	0
c. Total Paid Distribution *(Sum of 15b (1), (2), (3), and (4))*		▶	919	840
d. Free or Nominal Rate Distribution (By Mail and Outside the Mail)	(1)	Free or Nominal Rate Outside-County Copies included on PS Form 3541	70	70
	(2)	Free or Nominal Rate In-County Copies Included on PS Form 3541	0	0
	(3)	Free or Nominal Rate Copies Mailed at Other Classes Through the USPS *(e.g. First-Class Mail)*	0	0
	(4)	Free or Nominal Rate Distribution Outside the Mail *(Carriers or other means)*	0	0
e. Total Free or Nominal Rate Distribution *(Sum of 15d (1), (2), (3) and (4))*		▶	70	70
f. Total Distribution *(Sum of 15c and 15e)*		▶	989	910
g. Copies not Distributed *(See Instructions to Publishers #4 (page #3))*		▶	149	165
h. Total *(Sum of 15f and g)*		▶	1138	1075
i. Percent Paid *(15c divided by 15f times 100)*			92.92%	92.31%

* If you are claiming electronic copies, go to line 16 on page 3. If you are not claiming electronic copies, skip to line 17 on page 3.

16. Electronic Copy Circulation	Average No. Copies Each Issue During Preceding 12 Months	No. Copies of Single Issue Published Nearest to Filing Date
a. Paid Electronic Copies ▶	0	0
b. Total Paid Print Copies (Line 15c) + Paid Electronic Copies (Line 16a) ▶	919	840
c. Total Print Distribution (Line 15f) + Paid Electronic Copies (Line 16a) ▶	989	910
d. Percent Paid (Both Print & Electronic Copies) (16b divided by 16c × 100) ▶	92.92%	92.31%

☒ I certify that 50% of all my distributed copies (electronic and print) are paid above a nominal price.

17. Publication of Statement of Ownership
☒ If the publication is a general publication, publication of this statement is required. Will be printed
in the **NOVEMBER 2017** issue of this publication.
☐ Publication not required.

18. Signature and Title of Editor, Publisher, Business Manager, or Owner

Stephen R. Bushing — Date 9/18/2017

STEPHEN R. BUSHING - INVENTORY DISTRIBUTION CONTROL MANAGER

I certify that all information furnished on this form is true and complete. I understand that anyone who furnishes false or misleading information on this form or who omits material or information requested on the form may be subject to criminal sanctions (including fines and imprisonment) and/or civil sanctions (including civil penalties).

PS Form **3526**, July 2014 *(Page 1 of 4 (see instructions page 4))* PSN: 7530-01-000-9931 PRIVACY NOTICE: See our privacy policy on www.usps.com.

PS Form **3526**, July 2014 *(Page 3 of 4)* PRIVACY NOTICE: See our privacy policy on www.usps.com

Moving?

Make sure your subscription moves with you!

To notify us of your new address, find your **Clinics Account Number** (located on your mailing label above your name), and contact customer service at:

Email: journalscustomerservice-usa@elsevier.com

800-654-2452 (subscribers in the U.S. & Canada)
314-447-8871 (subscribers outside of the U.S. & Canada)

Fax number: 314-447-8029

Elsevier Health Sciences Division
Subscription Customer Service
3251 Riverport Lane
Maryland Heights, MO 63043

Printed and bound by CPI Group (UK) Ltd, Croydon, CR0 4YY

08/05/2025

01864703-0018